ADVANCES IN

Operative Orthopaedics

VOLUME 3

ADVANCES IN

Operative Orthopaedics

VOLUME 1

Instrumentation to Correct Spinal Deformities in Children and Adolescents--Analysis of Traditional and New Instrumentation Methods, *by Dennis R. Wenger, Jon R. Davids, and Choon-Sung Lee*

The Management of Childhood Spasticity, *by William L. Oppenheim, Loretta A. Staudt, and Warwick J. Peacock*

Neuromuscular Blockade in the Management of Cerebral Palsy, *by James F. Mooney, III, L. Andrew Koman, and Beth P. Smith*

Current Concepts in the Evaluation and Treatment of Osteosarcoma of Bone, *by Franklin H. Sim, Frank J. Frassica, James S. Miser, and K. Krishnan Unni*

The Treatment of Giant Cell Tumor of Bone, *by Michael Rock and Rodolfo Capanna*

Management of Ewing's Sarcoma, *by Douglas J. Pritchard*

VOLUME 2

Current Concepts in Shoulder Instability, *by Garth Bradford Wright, Mark David Miller, and Daniel Thomas Hinkin*

Revision Anterior Cruciate Ligament Surgery, *by Darren L. Johnson*

Meniscus Transplantation, *by Dieter Kohn*

Proprioception in Sports Medicine, *by Scott M. Lephart, Freddie H. Fu, and Paul A. Borsa*

Update on Lumbar Discectomy, *by Troy D. Lowell and Thomas J. Errico*

Update on Cervical Spine Trauma, *by Edward J. Dohring and Paul A. Anderson*

Differential Diagnosis and Surgical Treatment of Metastatic Spine Tumors, *by John P. Kostuik*

Peripheral Nerve Regeneration: Strategies to Augment Specificity, *by Thomas M. Brushart*

Treatment of Complex Distal Radius Fractures, *by Hill Hastings II*

Corrosion of Metallic Implants, *by Joshua J. Jacobs, Jeremy L. Gilbert, and Robert M. Urban*

Ultrasound in the Management of Developmental Dysplasia of the Hip, *by James R. Kasser*

Critical Evaluation of Percutaneous Epiphysiodesis, *by J. Richard Bowen and James T. Guille*

Myeloma of Bone, *by Frank J. Frassica, Deborah A. Frassica, and Franklin H. Sim*

Staging of Bone and Soft-Tissue Sarcomas Revisited, *by Thomas E. Nelson and William F. Enneking*

Endoscopic Carpal Tunnel Release, *by David J. Bozentka and A. Lee Osterman*

ADVANCES IN

Operative Orthopaedics

VOLUME 3

Editor-in-Chief
Richard N. Stauffer, M.D.
Professor and Chairperson, Department of Orthopaedic Surgery, The Johns Hopkins University School of Medicine, Baltimore, Maryland

Editors
Michael G. Erlich, M.D.
Professor and Chairman, Brown University School of Medicine, Providence, Rhode Island

Freddie H. Fu, M.D.
Blue Cross of Western Pennsylvania Professor of Orthopaedic Surgery, Vice Chairman and Chief, Division of Sports Medicine, Department of Orthopaedic Surgery, University of Pittsburgh School of Medicine; Head Team Physician, Athletic Department, University of Pittsburgh, Pennsylvania

John P. Kostuik, M.D.
Professor, Department of Orthopaedic Surgery and Neurosurgery, The Johns Hopkins University School of Medicine; Chief, Spine Division of Orthopaedics, The Johns Hopkins Hospital, Baltimore, Maryland

Paul R. Manske, M.D.
Chairman and Fred C. Reynolds Professor of Orthopaedic Surgery, Washington University Medical School, St. Louis, Missouri

Franklin H. Sim, M.D.
Professor of Orthopedic Surgery, Mayo Medical School, Consultant, Orthopedic Surgery, Mayo Clinic and Foundation, Rochester, Minnesota

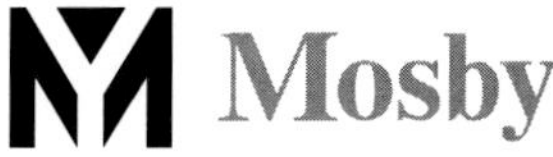

St. Louis Baltimore Boston Carlsbad Chicago Naples New York Philadelphia Portland
London Madrid Mexico City Singapore Sydney Tokyo Toronto Wiesbaden

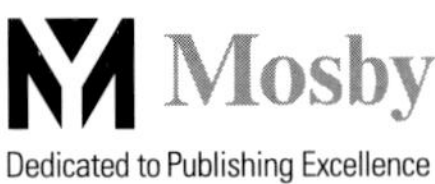

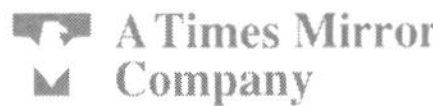

Vice President and Publisher, Continuity Publishing: Kenneth H. Killion
Director, Editorial Development: Gretchen C. Murphy
Acquisitions Editor: Linda Steiner
Developmental Editor: Catherine Flanagan
Manager, Continuity—EDP: Maria Nevinger
Project Specialist: Denise M. Dungey
Assistant Project Supervisor: Sandra Rogers
Freelance Staff Supervisor: Barbara M. Kelly
Vice President, Professional Sales and Marketing: George M. Parker
Senior Marketing Manager: Eileen M. Lynch
Marketing Specialist: Lynn D. Stevenson

Mosby–Year Book, Inc.
11830 Westline Industrial Drive
St. Louis, Missouri 63146

Editorial Office:
Mosby–Year Book, Inc.
200 North LaSalle Street
Chicago, Illinois 60601

International Standard Serial Number: 1069-7284
International Standard Book Number: 0-8151-7941-3

Contributors

Donald L. Bartel, Ph.D.
Professor, Cornell University, Ithaca, New York; Senior Scientist, Hospital for Special Surgery, New York, New York

Gregory Biddulph, M.D.
Department of Orthopedics, University of Utah Medical Center, Salt Lake City, Utah

Joel A. Block, M.D.
Assistant Professor, Departments of Internal Medicine and Biochemistry, Rush Medical College of Rush University, Chicago, Illinois

Robin Bruce, P.T.
Physical Therapist, Lexington Clinic Sports Medicine Center, Lexington, Kentucky

Don A. Coleman, M.D.
Department of Orthopedics, University of Utah Medical Center, Salt Lake City, Utah

Sherman S. Coleman, M.D.
Department of Orthopedics, University of Utah Medical Center, Salt Lake City, Utah

Scott F. Dye, M.D.
Assistant Clinical Professor, Department of Orthopaedic Surgery, University of California, San Francisco, School of Medicine, San Francisco, California

Jeffrey J. Eckardt, M.D.
Professor, Department of Orthopaedic Surgery, Chief of Section of Orthopaedic Oncology, University of California, Los Angeles, UCLA School of Medicine, Los Angeles, California

Frederick R. Eilber, M.D.
Professor of Surgery, Chief, Division of Surgical Oncology, University of California, Los Angeles, UCLA School of Medicine, Los Angeles, California

Frank J. Frassica, M.D.
Associate Professor, Orthopaedic Oncology, Chief, Division of Adult and Reconstructive Surgery, Johns Hopkins University School of Medicine, Baltimore, Maryland

Steven Gitelis, M.D.
Professor of Orthopaedic Surgery, Director, Section of Orthopaedic Oncology, Department of Orthopaedic Surgery, Rush Medical College of Rush University, Chicago, Illinois

Allan E. Gross, M.D.
A.J. Latner Professor and Chairman, Division of Orthopaedic Surgery, University of Toronto Faculty of Medicine, Mount Sinai Hospital, Toronto, Ontario, Canada

William L. Healy, M.D.
Department of Orthopaedic Surgery, Lahey Clinic, Burlington, Massachusetts

Michael H. Heggeness, M.D., Ph.D.
Associate Professor, Baylor College of Medicine, St. Luke's Episcopal Hospital Center for Orthopaedic Research and Education, Department of Orthopaedic Surgery, Houston, Texas

Michael J. Hejna, M.D., Ph.D.
Department of Orthopaedic Surgery, Rush Medical College of Rush University, Chicago, Illinois

Andreas B. Imhoff, M.D.
Shoulder Service Center for Sports Medicine, Department of Orthopaedic Surgery, University of Pittsburgh, Pittsburgh, Pennsylvania

Parviz Kambin, M.D.
Clinical Associate Professor, University of Pennsylvania School of Medicine; Chief, Division of Spinal Surgery, Department of Orthpaedic Surgery, Graduate Hospital; Director, Disk Treatment and Research Center, Graduate Hospital, Philadelphia, Pennsylvania

Cynthia Kelly, M.D.
Fellow of Orthopaedic Surgery, Section of Orthopaedic Oncology, University of California, Los Angeles, UCLA School of Medicine, Los Angeles, California

W. Ben Kibler, M.D.
Medical Director, Lexington Clinic Sports Medicine Center, Lexington, Kentucky

Steve Li, Ph.D.
Scientist, Department of Biomechanics, Hospital for Special Surgery, New York, New York

Beven Livingston, P.T., A.T.C.
Clinical Specialist, Lexington Clinic Sports Medicine Center, Lexington, Kentucky

Abid A. Qureshi, M.D.
Department of General Surgery, Rush-Presbyterian-St. Luke's Medical Center, Chicago, Illinois

Pietro Ruggieri, M.D.
Professor of Orthopedics, Department of Orthopedics, University of Bologna, Rizzoli Institute, Bologna, Italy

Kary R. Schulte, M.D.
Shoulder Service Center for Sports Medicine, Department of Orthpaedic Surgery, University of Pittsburgh, Pittsburgh, Pennsylvania

Franklin H. Sim, M.D.
Professor of Orthopedic Surgery, Mayo Medical School, Consultant, Department of Orthpedic Oncology, Mayo Clinic, Rochester, Minnesota

William G. Ward, M.D.
Assistant Professor, Department of Orthopaedic Surgery, Bowman Gray Medical Center, Winston-Salem, North Carolina

Jon J.P. Warner, M.D.
Director, Shoulder Service Center for Sports Medicine, Department of Orthopaedic Surgery, University of Pittsburgh, Pittsburgh, Pennsylvania

Rong-Sen Yang, M.D., Ph.D.
Visiting International Fellow of Orthopaedic Surgery, Section of Orthopaedic Oncology, University of California, Los Angeles, UCLA School of Medicine, Los Angeles, California

Preface

In this third volume of the Mosby–Year Book series, we have again endeavored to include manuscripts dealing with subjects of current popularity and interest to orthopaedists. The hallmark of subjects included, however, remains those topics which are contemporary and yet well-supported by a scientific base.

The first "cluster" of three chapters, dealing with total joint replacement, is introduced by a subject of special timeliness. In this new era of cost consciousness engendered by managed medical care, Dr. Healy is a pioneer of sorts. He was one of the first to raise the practice of cost containment to a near science--or at least to quantify and document the dollar savings that can be realized by a hospital through a change to more fiscally responsible practices. Following his lead, we personally have saved our hospital about $5,000,000 over a 5-year period. We challenge the reader to get involved also.

Donald Bartel, Ph.D., a well-recognized orthopaedic bioengineer, describes the growing concerns regarding wear and the use of polyethylene as a bearing surface for total joint replacement. The third chapter is authored by Alan Gross—one of the foremost experts on the use of allografts to replace bony defects—and should prove to be of assistance to those of us who encounter the all too frequent patient who needs very difficult total joint revision.

Dr. Jeff Eckardt "bridges" the transition from the total joint replacement chapters to orthopaedic oncology and the chapters on chondrosarcoma by Steve Gitelis with his work, "Endoprosthesis in Tumor Reconstruction." The chapter on fibrous dysplasia by Dr. Ruggieri is appropriately followed by Dr. Sherman Coleman's chapter on congenital pseudoarthrosis of the tibia, as the latter condition may well represent some sort of regional, localized mesenchymal dysplasia related to fibrous dysplasia of bone.

Dr. Kambin describes the role of minimally invasive surgery in the treatment of spine problems—techniques that are rapidly gaining in popularity. Dr. Michael Heggeness discusses fractures of the osteoporotic spine, and offers some new thoughts about how to deal with this problem that occurs with ever-increasing frequency in our aging population.

As ever, we, the editors and publishers of this series, hope that you will find much of substance that will be thought-provoking and helpful in your care of patients.

Richard N. Stauffer, M.D.

Contents

Mosby Document Express

Copies of the full text of journal articles referenced in this book are available by calling Mosby Document Express, toll-free, at 1-800-55-MOSBY.

With Mosby Document Express, you have convenient 24-hour-a-day access to literally every journal reference within this book. In fact, through Mosby Document Express, virtually any medical or scientific article can be located and delivered by FAX, overnight delivery services, international airmail, electronic transmission of bitmapped images (via Internet), or regular mail. The average cost of a complete delivered copy of an article, including copyright clearance charges and first-class mail delivery, is $12.

For inquiries and pricing information, please call the toll-free number shown above.

Cost Containment in Total Joint Arthroplasty

William L. Healy, M.D.
Department of Orthopaedic Surgery, Lahey Clinic, Burlington, Massachusetts

Total joint arthroplasty is one of the most successful medical innovations of the last half century. Total hip replacement and total knee replacement can predictably relieve pain and improve function in 90% of the patients for 10 years or more. These procedures have been evaluated by disease-specific, procedure-specific, patient outcome, health status, and economic instruments, all of which suggest that joint replacement is a cost-effective and clinically successful operation.[1–7]

Despite its widespread success, total joint arthroplasty has been targeted for cost control because of its high cost per procedure and its increasing prevalence in an aging population. Since 1980, the volume of total hip and total knee surgery has increased each year.[8] In 1993, hip, knee, and shoulder replacement operations in the United States increased 9.7% to 454,654 procedures; hip replacements increased 7.4%, whereas knee replacements increased 12.6%. Two hundred twenty-two thousand five hundred sixty-two primary hip replacements were performed, as well as 26,730 hip replacement revisions. One hundred eighty-nine thousand primary knee replacements were performed along with 16,354 knee replacement revisions.

During the past few years, Americans have expressed a desire to spend less on health care, and total joint arthroplasty has been targeted for cost control. This may be a problem for patients who need total joint arthroplasty and for health professionals who make a living providing total joint arthroplasty. These operations are being performed more frequently in an economy in which fewer dollars are available to pay for the operation. Therefore, it is timely and appropriate to consider cost containment in total joint arthroplasty.

PRIMARY TOTAL JOINT ARTHROPLASTY

In an effort to define and understand the economics of total joint arthroplasty, the hospital cost of total hip and total knee replacement operations during the 1980s was analyzed at the Lahey Clinic. Hospital bills were evaluated, and charges were assigned to hospital service centers. Charges were converted to cost by government-mandated hospital-specific cost-to-charge ratios. These cost-to-charge ratios provide a reasonably accurate estimate of cost. Economic comparisons were made with actual dollars and inflation-adjusted dollars.[9, 10]

Advances in Operative Orthopaedics, vol. 3

The findings in both the hip and knee studies were similar. The hospital cost to deliver hip and knee replacement at the Lahey Clinic during the 1980s was controlled at the rate of inflation. The hospital cost of hip replacement increased 2% in inflation-adjusted dollars from 1981 to 1990, whereas the hospital cost for knee replacement decreased 15% in inflation dollars from 1983 to 1991.

The most significant decrease in hospital cost associated with joint replacement was room cost (Figs 1 and 2). Room cost decreased as the length of stay decreased. Nationally, the average hospital length of stay decreased from 14 days in 1985 to 8 days in 1993 for hip replacements and from 13 days in 1985 to 7.7 days in 1993 for knee replacements.[8]

The most significant increase in hospital cost associated with joint replacement was implant cost (see Figs 1 and 2). In total hip arthroplasty, hip implant costs increased 212% in actual dollars, whereas the consumer price index increased 43.8% during this interval. In total knee arthroplasty, knee implant costs increased 118% in actual dollars, whereas the consumer price index increased 37% during this same interval.

The hospital cost for primary total joint arthroplasty at the Lahey Clinic during the 1980s was controlled at the rate of inflation by utilization review. Joint replacement was successfully delivered with shorter length of stay, less operating room time, fewer radiographs, fewer transfusions, fewer physical/occupational therapy sessions, and fewer tests

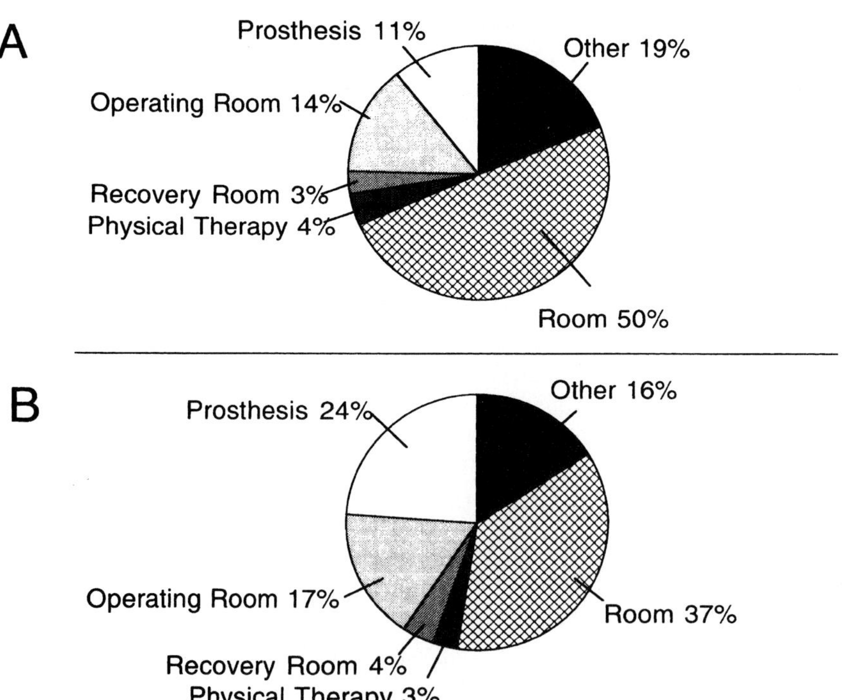

FIGURE 1.

A, allocation of costs for total hip arthroplasty in 1981 at the Lahey Clinic. **B,** allocation of costs for total hip arthroplasty in 1990 at the Lahey Clinic. (From Barber TC, Healy WL: *J Bone Joint Surg Am* 75:323, 1993. Used by permission.)

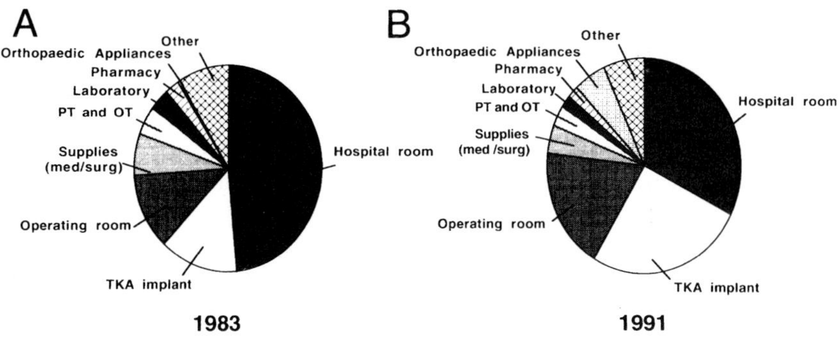

FIGURE 2.
A, allocation of costs for total knee arthroplasty *(TKA)* in 1983 at the Lahey Clinic. **B,** allocation of costs for TKA in 1991 at the Lahey Clinic. *PT* = physical therapy; *OT* = occupational therapy. (From Healy WL, Finn D: *J Bone Joint Surg Am* 76:803, 1994. Used by permission.)

and medications. The question that must be asked is, "If volumes of service decreased, why did the total hospital cost for joint replacement not decrease?" The answer is that unit costs for services and supplies associated with joint replacement increased universally. The most significant increase in the hospital cost of total joint arthroplasty was implant costs, and implant costs cannot be controlled by utilization review because one patient requires at least one prosthesis.

IMPLANT COST AND HOSPITAL PAYMENT

Implant prices for total joint arthroplasty increased an average of 8% per year during the 1980s. During the early 1990s, this rate of increase has been smaller as implant vendors have become more sensitive to pricing in the marketplace. All orthopaedic implant vendors shared in the annual price increases, and little discrepancy was noted between vendors for similar implants. Average selling prices of hip and knee implants generally showed increases of 4% to 5% from 1992 to 1993.

In sharp contradistinction to the rise in implant prices, Medicare payments to hospitals for total joint arthroplasty under diagnosis-related group (DRG) 209 increased only 2% during the 1980s. This increase in Medicare DRG 209 hospital payment has been less than 2% during the early 1990s, and some managed care contracts pay hospitals less than Medicare for joint replacement operations. Prices for total joint implants have increased faster than hospital payment for total joint arthroplasty. These disparate rates of increase create a problem for hospitals because the joint replacement implant is consuming more of the hospital payment for the operation each year.

In 1995, many hospitals are having trouble breaking even or making a profit on primary total joint replacement.[11–13] Surgeons at the Hospital for Special Surgery in New York City reviewed 1,020 primary total hip replacements performed in 1992. Overall, the hospital lost $238 per case, or 1.5% of hospital cost, while delivering those operations. When the patients were stratified by age, they noted that the hospital made $2,622, or

18%, profit on patients less than 65 years of age. In sharp contrast, the hospital lost $1,899, or 12%, on patients between 65 and 80 years of age, and they lost $5,677, or 29%, on patients 80 years of age and older.[13] As patients became older and potentially sicker, the hospital lost money delivering total joint arthroplasty. As the Medicare budget is cut, this trend at the Hospital for Special Surgery is problematic because about two thirds of joint replacement operations are performed on Medicare patients.

Total joint arthroplasty can be profitable for a hospital when the patients are covered by commercial or indemnity insurance. However, when hospital payment for total joint arthroplasty is provided by Medicare or health maintenance organization contracts, many hospitals lose money on joint replacement. This is a growing problem in states where the payer mix is shifting from commercial insurance to Medicare/managed care at the same time as commercial insurance companies are negotiating payment schedules for total joint replacement closer to Medicare payment schedules.

In an attempt to contain the hospital cost of total joint arthroplasty, it is appropriate to focus on implant cost. Implant cost is a fixed cost in total joint arthroplasty, and it is the single largest expense in a joint replacement operation. The American Academy of Orthopaedic Surgeons encouraged orthopaedic surgeons to work toward cost containment of orthopaedic implants in May 1992 in the position statement "Containing the Cost of Orthopaedic Implants." The Academy emphasized that implant selection should be by surgeons; however, they strongly advised surgeons to collaborate with hospitals to contain implant cost.[14] The *Journal of Bone and Joint Surgery* has also encouraged surgeons to control implant costs.[15] Surgeons are the prime consumers of orthopaedic implants, and it is surgeons who ultimately have the ability to control implant costs.

If surgeons need an incentive to work to control the cost of total joint arthroplasty, they should consider their own surgeon payment and a comparison of surgeon payment and implant cost. Medicare payments to surgeons for primary hip replacement (CPT 27130) and primary knee replacement (CPT 27447) will decrease 19% and 20%, respectively, from 1991 to 1996. Furthermore, when implant cost was compared with surgeon payment at the Lahey Clinic in October 1990, the price the hospital paid for the implant ($2,947) was greater than the payment the surgeon received for performing the operation ($2,468). Parts cost more than labor. The same problem was identified in knee replacement; in November 1991, implants cost the hospital $3,100, and the surgeon was paid $2,600.

REVISION TOTAL JOINT ARTHROPLASTY

The economic conditions identified in primary total joint arthroplasty are magnified for revision total joint arthroplasty. First of all, the prevalence of revision arthroplasty may be increasing faster than primary arthroplasty. In 1992, primary total hip arthroplasty increased 9%, whereas revision total hip arthroplasty increased 18%.[11] This trend was corrected somewhat in 1993 when primary hip and knee replacements increased 7.8% and 12.8% whereas revision hip and knee replacements increased 5.1% and 9.8%.[3] In either case, volumes of revision operations are increasing each year.

Work and time associated with primary and revision total hip arthroplasty have been compared, and revision arthroplasty requires significantly more work. Revision hip replacement at the Lahey Clinic is associated with more complex, more detailed preoperative evaluation and 78% longer operating room time than primary hip replacement.[16] Ritter et al.[17] in Indiana documented a similar work increase for revision hip replacement vs. primary hip replacement. They noted that revision hip replacement operating room time was 78% greater than primary hip replacement operating room time. Medicare statistics in 1992 demonstrated that patients undergoing revision hip replacement have a 15% longer hospital stay than patients having primary hip replacement and patients having revision hip replacement generate 20% higher hospital charges than patients having primary hip replacement.[18]

Lavernia et al.[19] at the Good Samaritan Hospital (Johns Hopkins) compared primary and revision total hip replacement. They found that revision surgery was associated with 109% increased operating room time and a 92% increased length of stay compared with primary hip replacement. Hospital charges for patients having revision were 59% higher than for patients having primary replacement, and implant charges for patients having revision were 25% higher than for patients having primary replacement.

Despite increasing work and risk associated with revision total joint arthroplasty, surgeon payment and hospital payment are not increased for revision operations. Barrack et al.[20] at Tulane University documented significant increases in operating room time, blood loss, bone grafting, complications, and length of stay in revision surgery vs. primary total hip replacement. However, they also noted that surgeon reimbursement was not significantly greater for revision surgery as opposed to primary surgery. Ritter et al.[17] also looked at surgeon reimbursement and noted that although surgeons spent 78% more time in the operating room for revision hip replacement, they received only 31% more reimbursement for revision hip replacement compared with primary hip replacement.

One of the biggest problems in revision hip replacement is that the operation, which has more work and more supplies associated with it, receives a fixed hospital payment that is similar to that for primary hip replacement. Hospitals spend more money on services and supplies to deliver revision hip replacement; however, hospitals do not receive a significantly larger payment for revision total hip arthroplasty. In fact, hospital payment may be less for revision total hip arthroplasty than for primary total hip arthroplasty. This has led to a situation in which few hospitals in this country specialize in and encourage revision total hip replacement. In 1992, 2,468 hospitals reported surgeons performing 1 revision or more, 1,234 hospitals reported 5 or fewer revisions, and only 3 hospitals reported 200 revision hip operations or more.[18] The ultimate result of such a trend could be disastrous.

COST CONTAINMENT

Cost control is a relatively new problem in total joint arthroplasty. During most of the last two decades, indemnity health insurance companies paid all bills submitted for total joint arthroplasty. The procedure was universally hailed as successful. Patients were happy with the procedure, and payers paid for the procedure. Hospitals were happy because their beds were filled with paying patients. However, with the introduction of DRG 209 hospital payments and the evolution of case pricing by managed care organizations and insurance companies, hospitals are receiving fixed payments for total joint arthroplasty operations. Under these fixed payment systems, hospital costs for total joint arthroplasty are frequently greater than hospital payment for the operation.

Cost control strategies for total joint arthroplasty begin with utilization review. Utilization of services and supplies creates hospital charges and costs. By reducing the volume of services and supplies used to deliver joint replacement operations, a hospital can save significant dollars. Critical pathways have been used to reduce variability in practice patterns and increase the efficiency and cost-effectiveness of delivering total joint operations.

Cost shifting has been a popular method for acute care hospitals to control costs and increase profit from total joint replacement. After joint replacement, patients can be transferred from the acute care hospital to a rehabilitation hospital or a skilled nursing facility soon after surgery.[21] Transfer might occur on postoperative day 2 or 3, and in some facilities, the rehabilitation hospital or skilled nursing facility may be on the same campus, hospital, or floor as the acute care hospital. This practice permits the acute care hospital to receive the entire case price payment for the procedure while at the same time reducing utilization and hospital cost for the operation. This method of cost shifting does not reduce the overall cost to society for total joint arthroplasty; the rehabilitation unit is also reimbursed. However, the individual acute care hospital delivering the service profits. Cost shifting may, in fact, raise the total cost for joint replacement because the rehabilitation facility is paid from another source.

During the 1980s, hospitals and surgeons effectively reduced the quantity of services and supplies used to deliver joint replacement.[22] Sommers et al.[22] at Stanford demonstrated that utilization control lowered the cost of primary hip replacement by $2,045 from 1984 to 1986. Utilization control measures were largely instituted by payers, but hospitals and surgeons adjusted so that patient outcome was not compromised. The most significant saving effected by these utilization review measures was a reduction in the length of hospital stay for total joint replacement.

In 1991, Schwartz and Mendelson[23] reported their study on the effect of utilization review on general hospital populations. They documented that utilization review initiatives could effect significant reductions in length of stay. However, they noted that by the end of the decade, the decreases in length of stay were becoming smaller, and they warned that the maximum cost saving benefits may have already been realized from utilization review. Furthermore, they suggested that utilization review may not be associated with cost reductions in the future.

During the next decade, cost containment in total joint arthroplasty will require control of the unit costs associated with total joint arthroplasty. Levine et al.[24, 25] from the Hospital for Special Surgery in New York City suggested that this goal can be achieved by instituting programs in cost awareness, cost containment, and cost reduction. When the entire team of hospital personnel associated with joint replacement was educated regarding supply costs for joint replacement, cost savings were achieved. Unused joint implants that were suitable for reuse were recycled. Less expensive surgical gloves were ordered. Length of stay for joint replacement was reduced. Cost awareness is the first step in cost containment.

Froimson[26] contained the cost of total joint arthroplasty at Mt. Sinai Hospital in Cleveland by a policy of rational use of resources. Education of all members of his team led to cost containment for total joint arthroplasty. In 1989, joint replacement at Mr. Sinai lost $2,500 per case for more than 200 cases. Total joint arthroplasty was responsible for a half-million-dollar loss in one hospital. Their program for the rational use of resources evaluated preoperative assessment, admission procedures, implant cost, operating room efficiency, and postoperative care. Their efforts reduced length of stay from 10.1 to 7.8 days and implant cost from $3,900 to $2,900 per case, and the hospital stopped losing money on total joint arthroplasty operations.

The cost most directly under the control of the orthopaedic surgeon is implant cost. Surgeons choose the implants for their patients. Cost has not been a priority for surgeons during the last decade, but implant design has evolved to the point where most hip and knee implants have similar features, depending on the method of fixation. It can be argued that joint implants are essentially generic commodities designed to relieve pain and improve function in place of a diseased joint. Although implant prices have increased steadily during the past decade, there is no evidence that the joint replacement operation provides greater relief of pain, improved function, or more durability with more expensive implants.

One method for reducing implant costs for total joint replacement is to purchase implants by competitive bid. Zuckerman et al.[27] at the Hospital for Joint Diseases in New York City reported a 23% reduction in money spent on joint implants as a direct result of a competitive bid process. For a competitive bid process to be successful, surgeons must be willing to unite and standardize their use of specific implants, and they must be willing to change to cost-effective implants. Surgeons who are trained with one system of implants may find it difficult to change because of concerns for the patient's welfare. However, patient outcome is generally related to surgical skill and rehabilitation rather than to a specific implant. With appropriate training, orthopaedic surgeons can adapt to new joint implant systems.

Implant standardization can also reduce the unit cost of total joint implants. Implant standardization is a method of implant selection whereby an objective recommendation of implant choice is based on a patient's projected demand category. The Lahey Clinic implant standardization program has been developed by using age, weight, expected activity, health, and bone stock as patient criteria related to demand from a joint implant. Surgeons assign patients and implants to demand categories to standardize implant selection.[28–30]

The Lahey Clinic implant standardization program was able to save 25% of the cost of hip implants and 9% of the cost of knee implants during a retrospective review. The advantages of an implant standardization program are that costs can be controlled without any reduction in the quality of joint replacement. Furthermore, a surgeon is not placed in the position of having to choose between a more or less expensive implant for a patient.

CONCLUSION

Total joint arthroplasty is a clinically successful procedure. The perceived health care cost crisis in the United States has led to a need to control the cost of total joint arthroplasty. Utilization review initiatives during the past decade have controlled the hospital cost for total joint arthroplasty at the rate of inflation. Further control of the cost of total joint arthroplasty will involve control of unit costs. The most significant unit cost that can be controlled is the implant cost for total joint replacement. Orthopaedic surgeons control the choice of joint implants, so they can also help control the cost of total joint implants. The challenge for orthopaedic surgeons who perform total joint arthroplasty is to implant the right joint in the right patient at the right cost.

REFERENCES

1. Schulte KR, Callaghan JJ, Kelley SS, et al: The outcome of Charnley total hip arthroplasty with cement after a minimum twenty-year follow-up: The results of one surgeon. *J Bone Joint Surg Am* 75:961–975, 1993.
2. Wiklund I, Romanus B: A comparison of quality of life before and after arthroplasty in patients who had arthrosis of the hip joint. *J Bone Joint Surg Am* 73:765–769, 1991.
3. Rorabeck CH, Bourne RB, Laupacis A, et al: A double-blind study of 250 cases comparing cemented with cementless total hip arthroplasty: Cost-effectiveness and its impact on health-related quality of life. *Clin Orthop* 298:156–164, 1994.
4. Laupacis A, Bourne RB, Rorabeck C, et al: The effect of elective total hip replacement on health-related quality of life. *J Bone Joint Surg Am* 75:1619–1626, 1993.
5. Rand JA, Ilstrup DM: Survivorship analysis of total knee arthroplasty: Cumulative rates of survival of 9200 total knee arthroplasties. *J Bone Joint Surg Am* 73:397–409, 1991.
6. Scuderi GR, Insall JN, Windsor RE, et al: Survivorship of cemented knee replacements. *J Bone Joint Surg Br* 71:798–803, 1989.
7. Wright J, Ewald FC, Walker PS, et al: Total knee arthroplasty with the kinematic prosthesis. Results after five to nine years: A follow-up note. *J Bone Joint Surg Am* 72:1003–1009, 1990.

8. Mendenhall S: 1993 hip and knee implant review. *Orthop Network News* 5:1–6, 1994.
9. Barber TC, Healy WL: The hospital cost of total hip arthroplasty: Comparison between 1981 and 1990. *J Bone Joint Surg Am* 75:321–325, 1993.
10. Healy WL, Finn D: The hospital cost and the cost of the implant for total knee arthroplasty: Comparison between 1983 and 1991 for one hospital. *J Bone Joint Surg Am* 76:801–806, 1994.
11. Gutterson WA: *Financial Analysis of Primary Total Hip Arthroplasty*. Boston, Mass Simmons College Graduate School for Health Studies, Health Care Administration, April 1994.
12. Meyers SJ, Reuben JD, Moye LA, et al: The actual inpatient cost of primary and revision total joint replacements. Presented at a meeting of the American Academy of Orthopaedic Surgeons, New Orleans, Feb 1994.
13. Evans BJ, Bear BJ, Salvati EA, et al: Relationship of age to hospital cost and reimbursement for primary total hip arthroplasty. Presented at a meeting of the American Academy of Orthopaedic Surgeons, New Orleans, Feb 1994.
14. American Academy of Orthopaedic Surgeons: *Containing the Cost of Orthopaedic Implants*. Rosemont, Ill, American Academy of Orthopaedic Surgeons, May 1992.
15. Clark CR: Cost containment: Total joint implants (editorial). *J Bone Joint Surg Am* 76:799–800, 1994.
16. Healy WL: The cost of primary and revision total hip arthroplasty, in Galante JO, Rosenberg AG, Callaghan JJ (eds): *Total Hip Revision Surgery*. New York, Raven Press, 1995, pp 231–237.
17. Ritter MA, Carr KD, Keating EM, et al: Revision total joint arthroplasty: Does Medicare reimbursement justify time spent? Presented at a meeting of the American Association of Hip and Knee Surgeons, Dallas, Nov 14, 1993, p 93.
18. Mendenhall S: A closer look at revisions. *Orthop Network News* 4:6, 1993.
19. Lavernia CJ, Tsao A, Drakeford M, et al: Revision and primary hip and knee arthroplasty: The cost analysis. Presented at the 60th Annual Meeting of the American Academy of Orthopaedic Surgeons, San Francisco, Feb 18–23, 1993, p 326.
20. Barrack RL, Hoffman DJ, Tejeiro WV, et al: Surgeon work input and risk in primary versus revision total joint arthroplasty. *J Arthroplasty*, in press.
21. Lombardi AV Jr, Mallory TH, Vaughn BK, et al: Clinical benefit, patient acceptance and satisfaction, and cost effectiveness of early discharge and transfer to a skilled nursing facility following primary and revision total hip and total knee arthroplasty. *Orthop Trans* 16:709, 1992.
22. Sommers LS, Schurman DJ, Jamison JQ, et al: Clinician-directed hospital cost management for total hip arthroplasty patients. *Clin Orthop* 258:168–175, 1990.
23. Schwartz WB, Mendelson DN: Hospital cost containment in the 1980s: Hard lessons learned and prospects for the 1990s. *N Engl J Med* 324:1037–1042, 1991.
24. Levine DB, Cole BJ, Rodeo S: Cost awareness and cost containment at the Hospital for Special Surgery: Strategies in total hip replacement cost centers. *Clin Orthop*, 1995, in press.
25. Levine DB, Killen AR, Keenan M, et al: Cost awareness and containment for the 1990s: Recycling orthopaedic implants. *Contemp Orthop* 25:376–381, 1992.
26. Froimson AI: The rational use of resources in total joint arthroplasty. Presented at a meeting of the American Academy of Orthopaedic Surgeons, New Orleans, Feb 1994.
27. Zuckerman JD, Kummer FJ, Frankel VH: The effectiveness of a hospital-based

strategy to reduce the cost of total joint implants. *J Bone Joint Surg Am* 76:807–811, 1994.
28. Healy WL, Kirven FM, Iorio R, et al: Implant standardization for total hip arthroplasty: A cost reduction program. *J Arthroplasty* 10:177–183, 1995.
29. Healy WL, Kirven FM, Iorio R, et al: Knee implant standardization: A cost reduction program. Presented at a meeting of the American Academy of Orthopaedic Surgeons, Orlando, Fla, Feb 1995.
30. Healy WL: Economic considerations in total hip arthroplasty and implant standardization. *Clin Orthop* 311:102–108, 1995.

Use of Polyethylene for Joint Replacement Prostheses

Donald L. Bartel, Ph.D.
Professor, Cornell University, Ithaca, New York; Senior Scientist, Hospital for Special Surgery, New York, New York

Steve Li, Ph.D.
Scientist, Department of Biomechanics, Hospital for Special Surgery, New York, New York

---

Polyethylene continues to be used for one of the articulating surfaces in most total joint replacements. This has been true since it was first used for the acetabular component in total hip replacements by Charnley in the 1960s. Other polymeric materials have been tried, but only polyethylene has withstood the test of time. Furthermore, it is likely that polyethylene will continue to be the material of choice for the foreseeable future. First, it has performed well in good designs. Second, it would be prohibitively expensive to introduce a new material to replace it because of regulatory requirements and the extensive testing that would be required to establish its biocompatibility, physical properties, wear characteristics, and biological response to debris.

Debris, both polymeric and metallic, limits the lifetime of current joint replacements. Particles are produced when damage is caused by relative motion at interfaces of bone-implant systems. Bits of debris can migrate to the surrounding biological tissues, where their effect is to increase the risk of late infection and late loosening of the joint replacement. Particles may be produced at articulating surfaces, at interfaces between modular components, and at fixation interfaces.

Interfaces for fixation and at modular connections should be designed to eliminate or minimize the amount of relative motion at these locations. Consequently, in well-designed joint replacements, the amount of debris generated at these sites is small.

On the other hand, the articulating surface of polyethylene components is particularly vulnerable to damage because the contact stresses are high and the relative motion between the components is large. Contact between articulating surfaces causes some damage to both components. In the absence of three-body wear, the greatest amount of debris by far is generated from damage to the polyethylene component. Consequently, most of the attention in recent years had been focused on minimizing the in vivo damage done to these elements of total joint replacements.

In this chapter we address four major aspects of the use of polyeth-

Advances in Operative Orthopaedics, vol. 3

ylene for joint replacement prostheses. First, we provide a brief history of the use of polyethylene to tell why this material is being emphasized. Second, we describe the properties of polyethylene in its current forms. We then discuss the stress environment caused by contact and how design and material properties interact to affect these stresses. Finally, we offer some comments on how to assess polyethylene component designs and provide an evaluation of current design concepts.

HISTORY OF BEARING MATERIALS

Since the advent of total hip replacements, relatively few polymeric materials have been used clinically. These include polytetrafluoroethylene (PTFE), polyacetal, high-density polyethylene (HDPE), ultrahigh-molecular-weight polyethylene (UHMWPE), and carbon fiber–reinforced UHMWPE.

Charnley chose PTFE as a bearing material because of its general chemical inertness and low coefficient of friction. The PTFE material he used was Fluon, a product of Imperial Chemical Industries (private correspondence from J. Charnley to C. Homsy, 1966). The more familiar name for these types of materials, Teflon (Dupont), has been used widely and incorrectly to describe this material. Clinical failures with Fluon acetabular cups generally occurred within 1 to 2 years. The failures were generally attributed to the low resistance to deformation of PTFE and its poor abrasive wear characteristics.

After the poor clinical experience with PTFE, Charnley and his group looked to other polymers. Credit for introducing polyethylene for orthopedic applications is given to Harry Craven, who tested a material called high-molecular-weight polyethylene that was given to him by a salesman of plastic gears. This material family remains the primary choice for the polymeric bearing surfaces in total joint replacements today. The terms ultrahigh molecular weight and high density are often used interchangeably in the orthopedic literature. This is incorrect; the properties of the two materials are significantly different (Table 1). In particular, note that the impact strength of UHMWPE is higher than that for HDPE and that the density of UHMWPE is much lower than that of HDPE. A density difference of 0.02 g/cc is very significant for polyethylene materials.

In the 1970s and 1980s there were efforts to find a material with better wear properties than UHMWPE. The two most notable attempts involved the use of polyacetal (Delrin) in the Christiansen hip, and Poly II, a carbon fiber–reinforced UHMWPE used in tibial inserts and patellar components.

Polyacetal (sometimes referred to as polyoxymethylene) was introduced because it had the potential advantages of higher yield strength, higher crystallinity, and ease of manufacturing as compared with UHMWPE. Polyacetal can be formed into parts via injection molding processes, which are more rapid and much less expensive than machining the comparable part. The early results have been summarized and reviewed by Dumbleton.[2] In 1970 Delrin was used in the Christiansen endoprostheses and in Christiansen total hip replacements. The Christiansen total hip sys-

TABLE 1.
Physical Property Ranges for Polyethylene

Property	HDPE*†	UHMWPE	Units
Melting point	130 – 137‡	125 – 135	°C
Density	0.952 – 0.965	0.930 – 0.945	g/cc
Tensile yield	26.2 – 33.1	19.3 – 21	MPa
Elongation at break	10 – 1200	200 – 350	%
Tensile modulus	0.9 – 1.6	0.8 – 1.0	GPA
IZOD impact	0.4 – 4.0	>20, no break	ft-lb/in
Shore D hardness	66 – 73	60 – 65	

*HDPE = high-density polyethylene; UHMWPE = ultrahigh-molecular-weight polyethylene.
†Data for HDPE obtained from *Encyclopedia of Plastics,* New York, Modern Plastics, 1990.
‡The ranges of properties are dependent on the supplier and grade of the material. For instance, HDPE is made by Allied, Amoco, Chevron, Bamberger, Dow, Schulman, Schuman, Phillips, USI, and Union Carbide. Each of these companies also makes several grades of HDPE. The main suppliers of UHMWPE resins are Hoechst/Celanese and Himont.

tem actually had two bearing surfaces made of Delrin. The metal femoral ball was connected to a Delrin sleeve that was free to rotate and fit over the metal trunion of the femoral stem. Additionally, the acetabular cup was also made of a Delrin resin. Christiansen total hips were first made with Delrin 550, then with Delrin 150, and in the later stages when the device was made by injection molding, with Delrin 100. By 1976 approximately 3,500 patients had received the endoprosthesis, and 2,400 patients had received the total hip system. Based on the successful early results of these surgeries, the Food and Drug Administration (FDA) recommended that Christiansen devices using Delrin be downgraded to class II devices.[2]*

However, by the mid 1980s, several groups reported a high rate of revision of these devices. In 1983, Sudman, in a study comparing 113 Charnley total hip replacements using UHMWPE as the bearing surface with 90 Christiansen total hip replacements using Delrin, reported that the revision rate for the Delrin devices was almost eight times higher than for the polyethylene devices at the 5- to 7-year time period.[3] Alho and coworkers also reported significantly better results when the Charnley device was used instead of the Christiansen device, but they warned that it was difficult to separate design factors from materials.[4] In still another study, Mathiesen and coworkers examined 12 retrieved Delrin cups and 11 UHMWPE cups at comparable implantation times and found that the Delrin cups had higher wear rates and higher coefficients of friction at

*The FDA classifies medical devices. A class II device is more readily available to the public than devices that are still restricted to clinical trials.

the time of removal than the UHMWPE cups.[5] Although Delrin continues to be used occasionally in some clinical trials,[6] it is no longer used for total joint replacements.

It is estimated that over 20,000 devices containing Delrin were implanted between 1970 and 1986. It should be pointed out that the relative contribution of design and material properties to the clinical failure of these devices has never been determined. Furthermore, this experience also points out that short-term clinical results (less than 5 years) can be misleading.

Carbon fiber–reinforced polyethylene (Poly II) was introduced to reduce the creep (cold flow) of UHMWPE. The composite consisted of short, randomly oriented carbon fibers in UHMWPE and was made into tibial inserts and patellar components. Although Poly II did have significantly higher creep resistance, it required extraordinary quality control processes and had lower fatigue resistance than unreinforced UHMWPE. Its use was discontinued shortly after introduction into the marketplace.[7,8]

Ultrahigh-molecular-weight polyethylene remains the material of choice. Its combination of abrasion resistance, strength, resistance to deformation, and fatigue strength makes it well suited for total joint replacements. Three general grades of UHMWPE are currently used in orthopedic implants, 1900 from Himont and 412 and 415 GUR from Hoechst/Celanese. Details of these resins will be discussed in a later section. Components can be molded directly from UHMWPE powder or machined from ram-extended bar stock or molded sheets.

In 1990, a more highly crystalline form of UHMWPE called Hylamer orthopaedic bearing polymer (DePuy-Dupont) was introduced, and in 1993 Hyalmer M orthopedic bearing polymer (DePuy-Dupont) and ArCom polyethylene were introduced to the marketplace. The Hylamer family of materials consists of conventional UHMWPE materials that have been processed to produce higher crystallinity[9] and generate higher strength, creep resistance, and resistance to oxidation. ArCom polyethylene is made by molding 1900 resin into a cylindrical shape. The resin specifications and molding conditions are unreported at this time. Tibial inserts and acetabular cups are then machined from the cylinders. Neither ArCom's physical properties nor any characterization has yet been reported.[10,11]

POLYETHYLENE

PLAIN POLYETHYLENE

Polyethylene is produced in powder form by using Ziegler-type catalysis. The most common forms of UHMWPE are 1900 from Himont and 4120 and 4150 GUR from Hoechst/Celanese. The 4120 and 4150 grades were formerly called 412 and 415 GUR, respectively. In the middle of 1994, Hoechst/Celanese added a zero to all their resin grades. For medical uses, the "HP" designation is added to the name; the current resins are 4120HP and 4150HP. The HP resins are sold as higher-purity materials, but few data are available at this time. Over 90 million lb of UHMWPE was produced in 1993. Orthopaedic applications account for a very small frac-tion of this amount. If it is estimated that 400,000 total joint replacements were done in 1993[12] and that each joint used 0.25 lb of polymer, then approximately 100,000 lb was implanted, only 0.1% of the annual production. Because the medical uses of UHMWPE consume such a small portion of the total amount produced, no specially formulated medical grade of polyethylene is currently available. Until recently[13–15] little attention has been paid to the nature of the material used in implants, the methods of manufacturing, and the quality of the material. Furthermore, it is only within the last few years that efforts have been made to control, alter, or improve the material for specific use as an orthopedic implant.

The 412 GUR and 1900 resins have approximate molecular weights of 2 million; the molecular weight of 415 GUR is approximately 5 million. All of these resins can be made to conform to guidelines for "medical-grade" UHMWPE as described in American Standard Test Methods (ASTM) F648.[16] However, given the number of resins available and the processing variables introduced by the fabricators, it is not surprising that wide variations have been found in the properties of polyethylene used for orthopedic implants. In one study, 16 lots of 415 GUR, 6 lots of 412 GUR, and 2 lots of Himont 1900 UHMWPE were evaluated for tensile properties. The bars were all ram-extruded by the same company.[13] Table 2 shows the wide range of material properties found in this study.

From the values shown, it is clear that yield strengths can vary by as much as 26%, modulus by 33%, elongation to break by 126%, and creep by as much as 475% depending on which lot of material is used. Note that the highest and lowest values of modulus came from two different lots of the same resin, 415 GUR. Table 3 shows that large variations in molecular weight have also been observed in retrieved components of the same design from the same manufacturer.[17] The large variation in the molecular weights strongly suggests that different resins were used in these devices.

Ultrahigh-molecular-weight polyethylene components can fail by frank fracture of the component or by damage to the articulating surfaces. As will be discussed later, surface damage is a critical problem because of the polyethylene debris that is produced. Hood et al.[18] characterized the damage of UHMWPE components into distinct types, including abrasion, burnishing, pitting, delamination, and fracture. Eyerer and others[15, 19, 20] suggested that oxidation of the UHMWPE may also contribute to damage to the material. Based on these observations, potential benefits

TABLE 2.
Variations in Properties of Ultrahigh-Molecular-Weight Polyethylene Used for Implants

Property	Lowest Value	Resin	Highest Value	Resin
Yield strength	19.6 MPa	412	24.7 MPa	415
Modulus	1.2 GPa	415	1.6 GPa	415
Elongation	190%	1900	430%	412
Creep at 27 MPa	0.4%	1900	2.3%	412

TABLE 3.
Molecular Weight Variations of Ultrahigh-Molecular-Weight Polyethylene From Retrieved Knee Prostheses

Prosthesis	Manufacturer	Years (Implanted)	Molecular Weight (Millions)
Kinematic	Howmedica	0	3.4
		6	1.3
		2	0.8
		0.8	0.8
Duocondylar	Johnson & Johnson	9	3.7
		8	3.7
		9.5	0.9
Marmor	Richards	9	4.6
		8	4.7
		6	4.4

could be gained if the currently used UHMWPE could be made stronger, tougher, more abrasion resistant, and more resistant to chemical attack.

MODIFIED POLYETHYLENE

Fiber-Reinforced Polyethylene

There are two historic examples where manufacturers have tried to improve polyethylene wear performance by changing material properties or manufacturing processes. One of the first attempts to alter polyethylene properties was a material called Poly II.[21] Poly II, a carbon fiber–reinforced UHMWPE, was used for tibial inserts and patellar components. The purpose of the randomly oriented fibers was to provide improved resistance to creep, increased strength, and improved wear characteristics.[21, 22] As described and summarized by Wright et al.,[8] Poly II did indeed have better creep resistance and higher modulus than nonreinforced UHMWPE. However, Poly II did not exhibit improved wear properties.[23] Further, the higher modulus of Poly II led to higher contact stresses, and finally, the fatigue resistance of Poly II was less than that of conventional UHMWPE.[24] The use of Poly II was discontinued in the late 1980s.

Heat-Pressed Polyethylene

A second approach was introduced by Howmedica in an attempt to provide a smooth bearing surface and achieve final contour geometries. A heat treatment process was developed in which a hot, polished metal surface was brought into contact with a "rough-cut" tibial insert. This process melted the surface of the polyethylene and provided a very smooth surface. The contact time of the process was such that only the top 2 to 3 mm of the polyethylene device was altered. This caused a line of demarcation within the polyethylene component that can clearly be seen in a cross-sectional micrograph of a new, unused component (Fig 1). This line of demarcation served as a focal point for delamination in vivo (Fig 2). As will be seen later, the maximum shear stresses from contact between

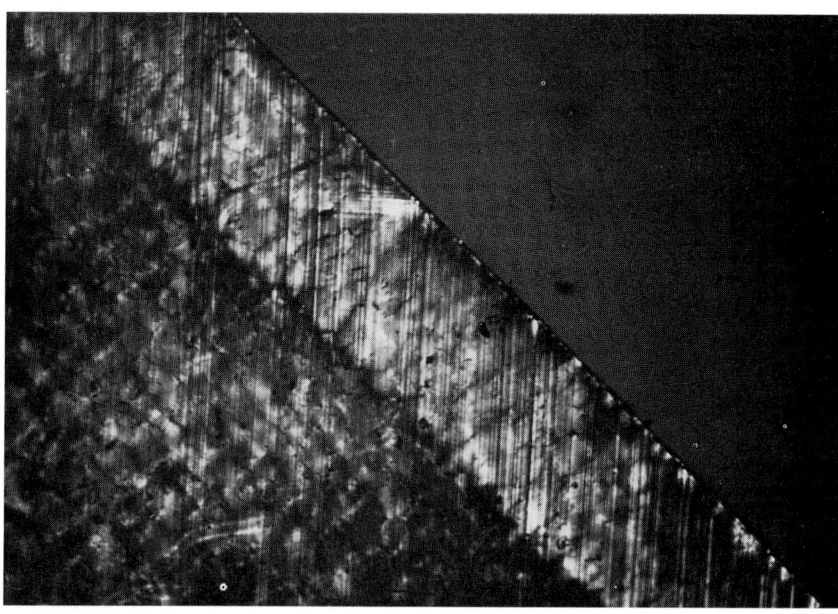

FIGURE 1.
Cross section of a heat-pressed component before implantation.

the articulating surfaces reach their maximum in this region. Bloebaum et al. discuss this device and its performance at length.[25]

Enhanced Polyethylene

As has been shown by a number of investigators, the crystallinity of HDPE and UHMWPE can be modified by processing the material with tempera-

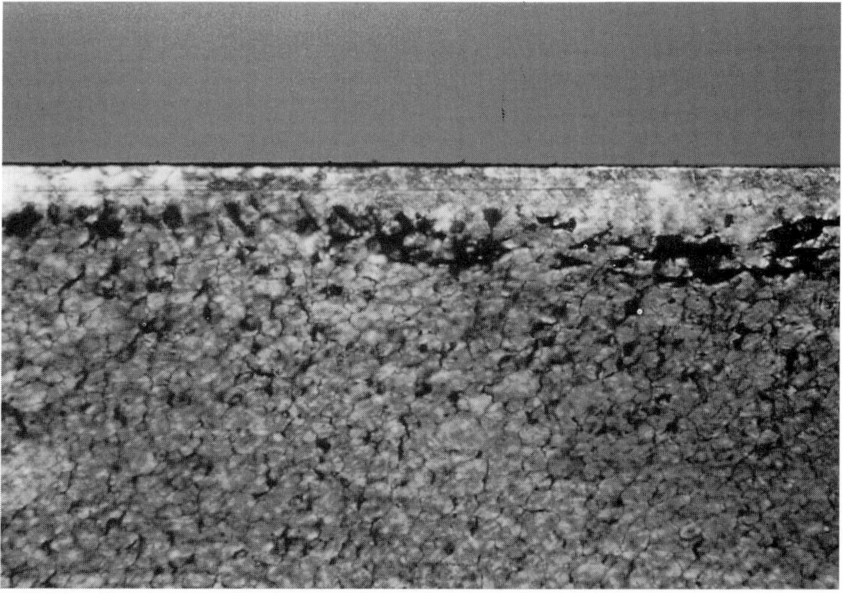

FIGURE 2.
Cross section of a retrieved component that was heat-pressed. Note that delamination occurred at the junction of the melted and unmelted zones.

ture and pressure.[26–30] However, early attempts were preoccupied with the resulting morphology of the material, and as a result, few of the reports provided physical property data along with morphologic information; no one had targeted a set of properties that would be advantageous in total joint arthroplasty. Furthermore, the processing procedures were generally done with rheometers or small vessels and, consequently, were not commercially viable.

Early work by Lupton and Regester[31] suggested that some of the properties of UHMWPE could be changed by subjecting UHMWPE to a heat, pressure, and cooling cycle. Lupton and Regester reported making a modified UHMWPE that had higher density, a higher melting point, and higher crystallinity than the precursor. The material was described as having an absence of chain fold spacing of 50 to 2,000 A (the typical range for UHMWPE) and the presence of chain fold spacing of about 10,000 A as determined by low-angle x-ray diffraction. The modulus of the materials was reported to be in the range of 340,000 to 500,000 psi (2.3 to 3.4 GPa). The process was conducted on a small scale, and samples were not homogeneous; the center of the sample had properties significantly different from those of the outside edges.

The process was recently extended to produce materials that can be used in orthopaedic devices. This procedure allows the conversion of currently available UHMWPE stock materials to a higher crystalline form. Typically, the crystallinity of 415 GUR bar stock material is around 50% as determined by differential scanning calorimetry. The high-pressure, high-temperature process can provide materials with higher crystallinity. This increase in crystallinity causes a change in the chemical and physical properties of the materials as shown in Table 4.[32]

DEBRIS IN TOTAL JOINT REPLACEMENTS

One of the greatest concerns in joint replacements today is the effect of particulate debris on the useful lifetime of the device. Willert and Semlitsch were among the first to mention the connection between generated debris and revision.[33] They reported the results of tissue examinations from 123 patients who had total joint replacement revisions. This study

TABLE 4.
Effect of Crystallinity on the Physical Properties of Ultrahigh-Molecular-Weight Polyethylene

Property	415 GUR	Hylamer M	Hylamer
Crystallinity (%)	40	57	86
Density (g/cc)	0.934	0.946	0.955
Melting point (°C)	135	147	149
Yield strength (MPa)	23.3	26.5	28.6
Ultimate tensile strength (MPa)	33.8	37.9	40.7
Modulus (GPa)	1.39	2.01	2.52
Creep at 7 MPa (%)	2.3	1.2	0.9
Elongation (%)	339	369	334

includes various types of implants and materials. Most of the metal components were made from CoCr alloy; the plastic components were made from UHMWPE, polyester, and polymethyl methacrylate. There were both metal-on-metal and metal-on-plastic devices. Indications for revision were malposition of the implant, loosening, fracture of the implant, periarticular calcification, or pain. They proposed that

> In small amounts, the foreign body particles are eliminated via the perivascular lymph spaces. Where this transport system is insufficient to handle the volume, however, the foreign body response may extend to the whole environment surrounding the joint. In such cases, there may be loosening of the cemented prosthetic parts because of deterioration of contiguous bone anchors by the tissue membrane lining the bone cement.

They also found that tissue response was most sensitive to polyethylene debris.

In succeeding years several investigators called attention to the problems of polyethylene wear, but its overall significance was not generally recognized.[34–37] The clearest evidence for the association of polyethylene debris and loosening was provided in 1988 by Howie et al.,[35] who conducted an experiment with New Zealand white rabbits that showed that the interface between bone and a cement plug in the distal end of the femur could be directly affected by the injection of polyethylene particles into the knee space. This was the first direct evidence that polyethylene could cause histologic and osteolytic responses that could lead to implant loosening.

Since that time, the study of the effects of particulate debris and osteolysis has greatly expanded. It is now known that polyethylene particles can cause the production of factors such as prostaglandin E_2, interleukin-1 (IL-1), and IL-2, which are known to stimulate bone lysis. Polyethylene debris particles can also cause the release of these factors in in vitro experiments. However, there is much work to be done before extension of these experiments can be made to the in vivo situation.[38, 39, 63, 64]

Osteolysis has mostly been associated with total hip replacements on both the acetabular and the femoral sides. However, it has recently been reported in total knee replacements as well.[40] It is interesting to note that although total knee replacements do not generally have the longevity of total hip replacements, the incidence of osteolysis is substantially smaller for knee replacements. The reasons for this are not known. At the time of this writing there are several critical questions for which there are no answers. There is no dose-response relationship known for polyethylene debris and osteolysis. That is, we do not know how sensitive osteolysis is to the size of the particles or the rate at which they are introduced to a particular site. There is a general belief that the small particles (less than 1 μm in diameter) are the most damaging, but Howie and colleagues were able to interrupt the bone-cement interface with much larger particles.

There are other debris particles in the system from the metal and bone cement (when used). However, the relative activity of these materials vs. that of polyethylene is not precisely known because of the inability to match debris particle sizes between materials. This is related to the problem of not knowing the dose-response behavior of these materials.

A good article that provides an overview of the interactions between implant materials and the surrounding biological environment can be found in a review by Galante et al.[41]

BIOCOMPATIBILITY

In addition to the physical property requirements a material must have to be a successful bearing surface, it must also be biocompatible. Biocompatibility is a necessary requirement for all materials that are used in implants, but it is not well defined. Perhaps the simplest definition is one that was proposed from the proceedings of a Consensus Conference of the European Society of Biomaterials.[42] Biocompatible means "the ability of a material to perform with an appropriate host response in a specific application." This definition indicates that every material must be evaluated in each application or device in which it is used. The methods for these evaluations have been discussed in detail in several references[42–46] that propose a series of tests to evaluate the biological activity of the material of interest and provide a method to assess risk (Table 5).

There are no FDA regulations that dictate a set of required tests. However, ASTM F748 provides a guide for tests that might be appropriate. These guides are based on general information concerning the material, including the type of device it is used in, the length of implantation, and the implant site. In the specific case of orthopaedic devices, protocols are provided to evaluate the interaction between the material in question and bone for long time periods and the interaction between the material and soft tissue.

The first three tests from ASTM F748 are in vitro tests for screening materials. Cytotoxicity is a comparative test in which the material or substance extracted from the material is placed in contact with cells from a standard line. The number of cells killed by the material or the extract is compared with that for positive and negative control materials. The carcinogenicity and mutagenicity tests also compare the response of cultured cells to the material with the response of the cells to positive and negative control materials. After exposure of the cells to the material, the cells are evaluated for chromosomal aberrations, DNA damage, and gene mutations. It should be emphasized that these tests are not foolproof and are

TABLE 5.
Suggested Tests for Biocompatibility

Test	Environment
Cytotoxicity	Cell culture
Carcinogenicity	
Mutagenicity	
Systemic injection—acute toxicity	Animal intramuscular implantation
Pyrogenicity	Intracutaneous injection
Long-term implantation	Animal

not sensitive to all carcinogenic materials. Other factors such as surface morphology, dose, location, etc., are not addressed in these tests. However, if the cytotoxicity, carcinogenicity, and mutagenicity responses for the materials are higher than for the negative controls, the material is probably not suitable for implantation.

The next phase of testing consists of short-term animal tests, which are also screening tests involving a comparison of the material's response to the response of positive and negative controls. These tests are generally shorter than 30 days.

The final stage of testing consists of long-term animal implantation. These tests can range from 3 months to several years depending on the material, the implantation site, and the type of device.

It should be noted that using these tests to predict actual risk to human patients is complicated by many factors. The first is the dose, or the amount of material used in the test, and the second is the rate at which the materials are introduced into the system. The amount of material used and the rate at which they are introduced into the in vitro or in vivo system are generally much higher than encountered in the actual implant. For example, pure metallic Ni and Co are carcinogenic when injected in solution into rat muscles, but epidemiologic study of implants containing these metals suggests that the risk of tumors is extremely small.

Bulk UHMWPE passes all of the aforementioned tests in that it generally behaves as the negative control, which means that there is little or no response of cells or tissues greater than that of control (presumably safe) materials. However, the biological response to very small debris particles of UHMWPE is great and can ultimately lead to loosening of the implant.

DESIGN

STRESSES CAUSED BY CONTACT

When contact occurs between metal and polyethylene components, both surfaces deform, but the metal component deforms such a small amount that it behaves like a rigid body when compared with polyethylene. Thus when an artificial joint is loaded, the polyethylene is squeezed between the rigid metal component and the supporting material—bone, cement, or metal backing. Furthermore, in the region of contact, the articulating surface of the polyethylene is forced to generally conform to the shape of the metal surface. The resulting deformation causes compressive, tensile, and shear stresses in the polyethylene.

The stresses associated with damage to the articulating surfaces occur both at the surface and within the polyethylene component. Two types of stresses can be applied to the surface—compressive stresses (contact stresses), which act perpendicular to the surface, and shear stresses from friction, which act on the surface in a tangential direction. Metal and polyethylene were originally chosen for bearing surface materials to produce low-friction total joint replacements.[47] When prostheses are properly manufactured (and undamaged), the friction between the metal and polyethylene components is quite small and may be ignored.

The only stress acting *on* the surface in this case is contact stress. However, if either one of the surfaces is damaged, the friction may be too large to ignore when stresses in the polyethylene are determined.

The stresses acting on the surface produce normal and shear stresses within the polyethylene. At the surface, the largest compressive stresses are the contact stresses that act perpendicular to the surface (σ_r, Fig 3). They decrease nonlinearly with depth through the thickness of the polyethylene. Joint contact also produces compressive and tensile stresses within the polyethylene component that act at a tangent to the articulating surface. Tangential compressive stresses occur because the polyethylene under the center of the contact area expands radially as the component is compressed. This expansion is resisted by the surrounding material. Tangential compressive stresses are produced to resist this expansion (σ_t, see Fig 3).

Tangential tensile stresses near the articulating surface occur because the surface must stretch as the polyethylene conforms to the shape of the metal component when the joint is loaded. The stretching occurs near the edge of the contact area (see Fig 3). The resulting tensile stresses are largest at the surface of the component.

Surface damage is most likely due to combinations of stress components. The combined stresses associated with surface damage are the maximum principal stress, the minimum principal stress, and the maximum shear stress. The maximum and minimum principal stresses are the *algebraically* largest and smallest normal stresses. For frictionless contact, the maximum and minimum principal stresses are easily identified. The tangential stresses acting at the surface are the maximum principal stresses, and as just described, they are compressive near the center of

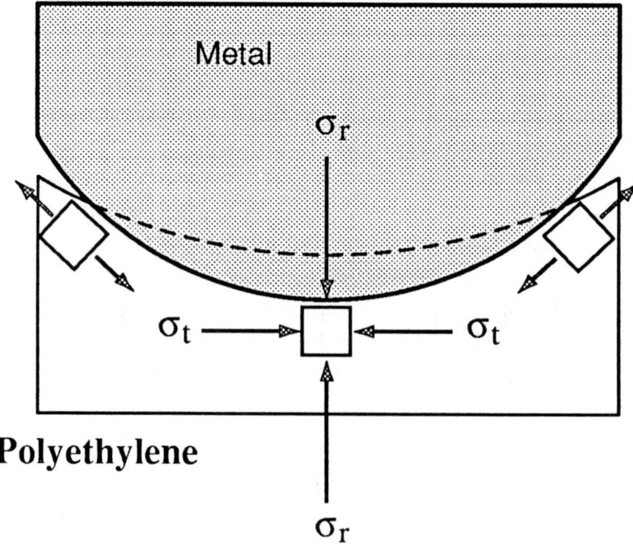

FIGURE 3.
Stresses on the surface of a polyethylene component.

contact and tensile near the edge of contact. The minimum principal stresses (the largest-magnitude compressive stress) are the contact stresses at the surface. When the principal stresses are unequal (the usual case), distortion, or shearing, occurs. The maximum shear stress occurs just below the surface (about 1 mm) for nonconforming joints such as knee joints and at the surface for conforming joints like hip joints. The maximum shear stress may be computed from Equation 1.

$$\tau_{max} = \frac{\sigma_{max} - \sigma_{min}}{2} \qquad \text{(Equation 1)}$$

The magnitude of the stress depends on the magnitude of the joint load. The joint loads transmitted across the articulating surfaces of lower extremity joints are typically several times body weight. For example, at the hip joint, loads of about three times body weight have been measured in instrumented prostheses.[48, 49] More conservative estimates of load (3000 newtons) have been used to design these joints.[50] The stresses from these large loads, in combination with the relative motion of the articulating surfaces, result in surface damage that increases with time of implantation (number of cycles of loading) and patient weight (magnitude of the loading).[51] This provides strong circumstantial evidence that surface damage in total joint replacements is the result of fatigue processes.

The size of the debris particles generated by these processes differs with the conformity of the joint. Conforming joints such as hip replacements produce small particles; nonconforming total knee replacements produce larger particles. Fatigue probably plays a role in both circumstances. In knee joints, where pitting is one of the most frequently observed damage modes, the surfaces of the pits show the same characteristics observed on the fracture surfaces of crack propagation specimens tested in the laboratory.[52] Although the wear of acetabular components is usually attributed to abrasive wear processes, fatigue processes similar to those that occur in knees may also be involved, but on a much smaller scale.[53, 54]

In total knee replacements, pits may be formed when cracks propagate from the surface into the polyethylene or when subsurface cracks propagate toward the surface. In the first case, the important stresses are the maximum principal stresses; in the latter, the important stress is the maximum shear stress. In a knee joint the contact area between the femoral and tibial components moves as the knee flexes and extends. Consequently, a point on the surface of the component will be subjected to varying stresses during the activities of daily living. The range (algebraic difference) of the stresses that act tangentially to the articulating surface (maximum principal stresses) varies between tension, when the point on the surface is at the edge of contact, and compression, when the point is at the center of contact.

As mentioned previously, the maximum shear stress in nonconforming knee joints occurs about 1 mm beneath the articulating surface. This is about the same depth at which pitting and delamination occurs and provides circumstantial evidence that subsurface cracking is associated with these two failure mechanisms. *Pits* can occur when subsurface cracks turn and propagate toward the surface. *Delamination* occurs when the crack continues to propagate parallel to the surface, eventually resulting in the formation of a sheet of material.

The risk of surface damage may be decreased by minimizing the stresses associated with the types of damage that can occur. Abrasive wear can be minimized by reducing contact stress. The range of the maximum principal stress and the magnitude of the maximum shear stress should be minimized to decrease the risk of damage from fatigue processes involving crack propagation. It has been shown that the range of maximum principal stress and the maximum shear stress decrease when contact stress is decreased. Therefore, the overall design goal is to choose a geometry of the articulating surface and material properties of the polyethylene that minimize contact stress.[52]

The articulating surface is not the only place where damage can occur. Debris can also be generated at the polyethylene-metal interface in metal-backed components. The existence of gaps or other features necessary for interchangeable modular components can lead to relative motion between the polyethylene and the metal when the joint is loaded. Screws and screw holes may also cause problems. For example, if the polyethylene contacts a screw head, relative motion between the screw and the polyethylene may generate debris. Screw holes can cause additional problems. In most designs employing screws for initial fixation, surgical flexibility is provided by having more holes than necessary. If the polyethylene rubs against the edge of a screw hole, debris may be generated. Furthermore, the unused screw holes provide channels for debris to migrate to the underlying bone.

The design of the polyethylene-metal interface in metal-backed components can also affect the contact stresses on the articulating surface. The stresses will be quite different if the polyethylene liner in an acetabular cup is in intimate contact with the backing than if it is not. Both the distribution and the magnitude of the contact stress will be affected.[55] Initial conformity between the liner and the metal backing does not necessarily eliminate the possibility of wear at this interface. Wear can eventually occur in components that are initially perfectly conforming as a result of in vivo changes in geometry and material properties.

Frank fracture of the polyethylene component must also be avoided. This has occurred in cemented acetabular cups when grooves that provide interlock with the cement compromised the structural integrity of all-polyethylene acetabular cups[56] and in uncemented cups when the polyethylene liner was supported only at the rim of the cup.[57] The latter case is an example of how failure of the rim and subsequent disassociation of the polyethylene component from the metal backing can occur if the cup or the rim is too thin to support the load. Cracking and fracture have also been observed in tibial components for total knee replacements.[58]

Wear at the liner-backing interface and frank fracture of polyethylene components are important design problems but are beyond the scope of this chapter. Here, we restrict further discussion to the stresses associated with damage to the articulating surface of fixed bearing designs where relative motion and large contact stresses are difficult to avoid if the joint is to provide normal anatomic function.

CONTACT STRESS: GENERAL CONSIDERATIONS

Contact stresses in acetabular components for total hip replacements and tibial components for total knee replacements are affected by changes in loading, conformity of the articulating surfaces, thickness of the polyethylene, and stiffness of the material. Contact stresses increase with increasing load. If the same prosthesis (same conformity, thickness, and material) is used in patients with different weights, the stresses will be higher in the heavier patients. The stresses are not directly proportional to the load (Fig 4). As the load between the contacting surfaces increases, the contact area also gets larger. Because of this inherently nonlinear interaction between the load and the contact area, one must examine the effects of changes in conformity, thickness, and material for a particular joint load. The load should be representative of the largest loads expected for joint function. As mentioned earlier, a load of 3,000 newtons has been used for design purposes.

The contact stresses, of course, are not uniform over the contact area. The metal component of a total joint replacement is a rigid indenter. The contact stress will be greatest where the surface displacement of the polyethylene is greatest. Consequently, the displacement of the polyethylene surface in a direction normal to the surface will be determined by the shapes of the two contacting surfaces. For example, if the indenter and the polyethylene are both spherical, as they are in an ideal total hip replacement, then the maximum displacement of the polyethylene will occur at the center of contact (Fig 5). Therefore, the maximum contact stress will occur at the center of the contact area, and the minimum contact stress (zero) will occur at the edge of contact. Furthermore, the shape of the contact area in this ideal case will be circular.

If the surfaces are not spherical because of either design or manufacturing variations, then the maximum contact stress may not be at the center of the contact area. For example, in Figure 6 the indenter is spherical

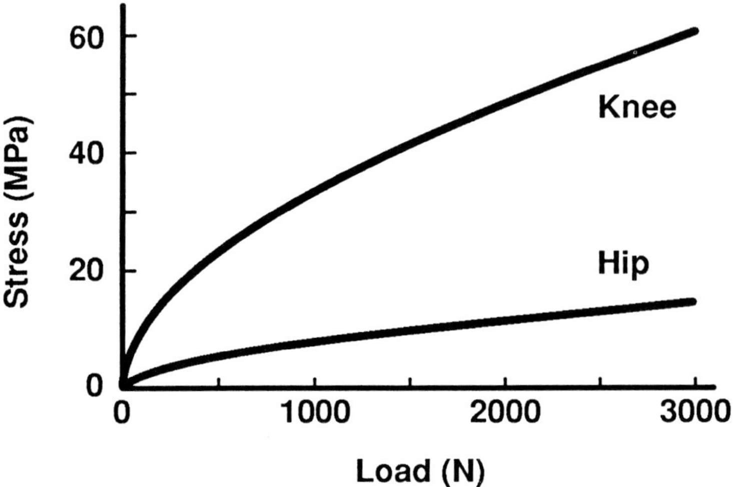

FIGURE 4.
Contact stress as a function of load and conformity.

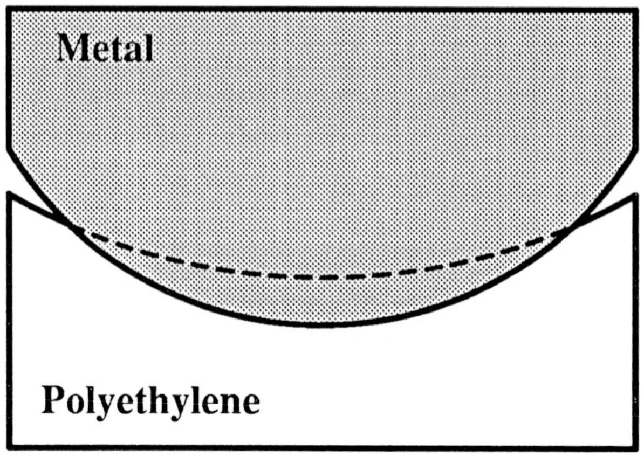

FIGURE 5.
Contact stresses are greatest where the displacement of the surface is greatest and depend on the geometry of the contacting surfaces. The *dashed line* indicates the surface of the undeformed polyethylene. The greatest deformation and highest contact stress will occur at the center because the displacement is greatest here.

but the acetabular surface has ripples in it. As a result, when the femoral head is pressed into the polyethylene, the largest displacement normal to the surface of the polyethylene component will be at locations like points A and C. Therefore, the greatest contact stresses will also occur at points A and C. The stress at point B in the contact area will be small because the deformation (difference between the dashed and solid lines) will be small at this location. Surface waviness can be caused by normal variations in manufacturing processes. So it is not surprising that experi-

Metal

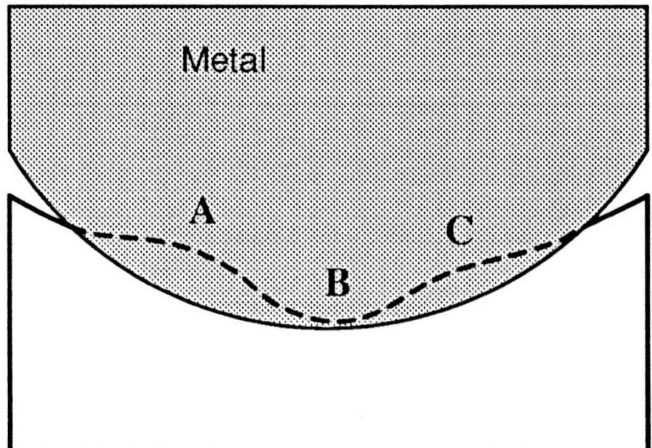

Polyethylene

FIGURE 6.
Surface irregularities cause variations in contact stress. The *dashed line* indicates the surface of the undeformed, initially wave polyethylene component. The greatest deformation and greatest contact stress will occur at points *A* and *C* because the compression of the polyethylene will be greatest there.

mental measurements show variations from ideal contact shapes and ideal contact stress distributions.

Similar observations can be made for nonspherical contact geometries. For example, the articulating surfaces of the femoral and tibial components of some total condylar knee geometries are toroidal. For ideal geometry, the contact area for these designs would be approximately elliptical, but slight variations in surface geometry can produce substantial variations in the contact stresses and the shape of the contact area. Other knee designs have intentional undulations in the articulating surface of the polyethylene component. These prostheses will have more pronounced variations in contact area geometry and contact stress than those with less complex surface shapes.

Even though such variations in surface geometry can occur, the fundamental behavior of polyethylene components can be described in terms of the size of the contact area based on the ideal shapes of the articulating surfaces. Changes in conformity, thickness, and material properties cause changes in the contact area. In general, changes that decrease the contact area will increase the stresses because the same load must be distributed over a smaller region. The contact area decreases when the conformity between the articulating surfaces decreases, when the thickness of the material decreases, and when the stiffness of the material increases.

When the articulating surfaces are nonconforming, the contact area over which the stresses are distributed will be smaller and the displacement of the surface at the center of contact will be greater than when a more conforming geometry is used. Therefore, the maximum contact stress will be greater than for a more conforming geometry.

The effects of changes in thickness on contact stresses may be understood as follows. Conceptually, the polyethylene may be considered to be supporting the metal indenter by a collection of parallel rods that are aligned along the direction of loading.* Each rod supports a portion, δP, of the total load P. The stiffness of a rod under axial load is given by

$$k_{rod} = \delta P/\Delta = EA/L \qquad \text{(Equation 2)}$$

where Δ is the displacement of the rod, E is the elastic modulus of the rod material, A is the cross-sectional area of the rod, and L is the length of the rod. As can be seen from Equation 2, the structural stiffness of the rod increases as the length of the rod decreases. In a similar way, the structural stiffness of polyethylene components increases with decreasing thickness. When the stiffness of the component increases, the indenter does not displace as much, the contact area decreases, and the contact stresses increase.

The rod analogy further shows that structural stiffness also increases when the elastic modulus of the rod material increases. Similarly, the structural stiffness of a polyethylene component increases when the elastic modulus increases. As a result, the contact area decreases and the stress increases.

*The rod analogy is, of course, limited because shear stress cannot be transferred from one rod to another.

STRESSES IN ACETABULAR COMPONENTS

For acetabular components, the maximum shear stress occurs very close to the articulating surface. This is consistent with the observation that retrieved acetabular components have many fewer pits than tibial components for total knee prostheses and delamination is rarely if ever seen in acetabular components. The fact that the maximum shear stress occurs at the surface in acetabular components has not yet been directly linked to the wear seen in these components. As noted previously, overall damage scores for acetabular components provide circumstantial evidence that the wear process is due to fatigue. It is possible that the large shear stresses at the surface may contribute to this process on a microscale. An interesting question, yet to be resolved, is whether or not the maximum shear stresses are independent of thickness and material properties when the contacting surfaces are perfectly conforming.

STRESSES IN TIBIAL COMPONENTS

The articulating surfaces for total knee replacements are much less conforming than for total hip replacements. As a result, all of the stresses associated with surface damage are greater in tibial components than in acetabular components because the contact areas are smaller for these less conforming devices. The stresses increase with decreasing thickness and increasing stiffness of the polyethylene in the same way they do for acetabular components.

Most knee replacements use femoral condyles that approximate the anteroposterior geometry of the natural condyles of the knee. As a result, the anteroposterior geometry of the condyle is more or less fixed. This in turn defines the minimum anteroposterior radius of the tibial component—it can be no smaller than the largest radius of the femoral component. In practice, the anteroposterior radius of the tibial component is greater than the minimum allowable value to provide some joint laxity in full extension. Good function of total knee replacements that spare the posterior cruciate ligament may require even larger anteroposterior radii on the tibial components because when the surfaces are too conforming, the posterior ligament may not function properly. In some cruciate-sparing designs, the posterior portion of the tibial plateau is flat or nearly flat. Consequently, anteroposterior conformity between the articulating surfaces may be further decreased.

These functional requirements limit what the designer can do to change the geometry in the anteroposterior direction. Consequently, changes in the lateral-medial geometry provide the greatest opportunities for increasing the conformity of the contacting surfaces. Conformity is maximized and contact stresses are minimized when the condyle and the plateau are flat in the lateral-medial direction, but this brings its own set of problems. It is well known that there is a tendency for the lateral condyle to lift off because of medially directed loads on the foot during normal gait.[59] When tilting occurs in a total knee replacement with articulating surfaces that are flat in the lateral-medial direction, two things happen. First, conformity between the femoral and tibial components is greatly decreased when the smaller radius on the outside of the prosthesis comes in contact with the polyethylene. As a result, the contact stresses and other stresses associated with surface damage may be dramatically increased. Second, with flat or nearly flat surfaces, tilting causes the contact area to move toward the edge of the polyethylene component. This can result in further increases in contact stress. In addition, the stresses associated with frank fracture of the component may also be increased.[58] Edge loading is also a disadvantage because it is associated with increased stresses on the cancellous bone.[60]

It is clear that articulating surfaces that are curved in the lateral-medial direction have distinct advantages because the contact area of the polyethylene does not shift to the edge when the femoral component tilts (Fig 7). When curved surfaces are used, maximum conformity will occur when the femoral and tibial radii in the lateral-medial direction are the same. However, this decreases the rotational laxity of the knee joint, which is necessary for the soft tissue structures around the joint to share load. If the soft tissues structures do not carry a portion of the load, then it will be transferred totally through the prosthetic components, and the risk of failure at the implant-bone interface will be increased. Therefore, the articulating surfaces in the lateral-medial direction must not be perfectly conforming. Radii must be chosen to minimize contact stress while providing an appropriate level of joint laxity.

EFFECTS OF MATERIAL ON CONTACT STRESSES

As the elastic modulus of the polyethylene is increased, the stresses on and within the polyethylene component as a result of contact are also increased. Therefore, modifications to polyethylene that increase the elastic modulus are only beneficial if the fatigue strength of the material is increased. When carbon fibers were introduced into the polyethylene, this was not the case.[24, 50] More recently, processes for enhancing polyethylene by using high temperature and high pressure have been introduced. These processes also increase the modulus of the polyethylene, but there is a concomitant increase in the strength of the material (see Table 4). Therefore there seems to be no disadvantage to using these materials, at least for acetabular components, even though higher stresses are produced. There may be other advantages with this material, such as resistance to in vivo oxidative degradation, that justify its use even if the stress-strength ratio is not substantially improved.

The stiffness of polyethylene also increases with time of implantation.[61] The overall density of polyethylene increases with time because

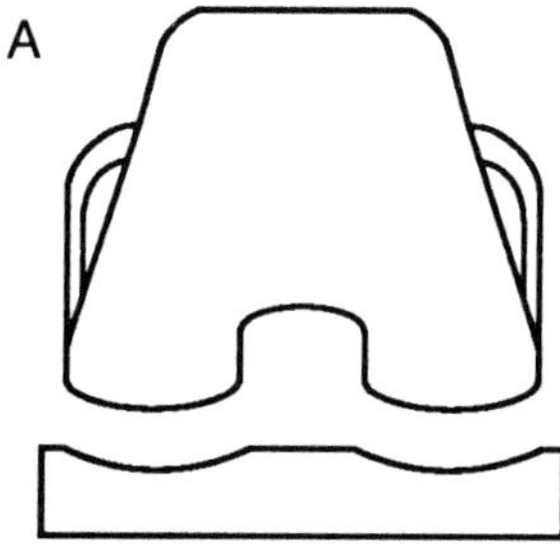

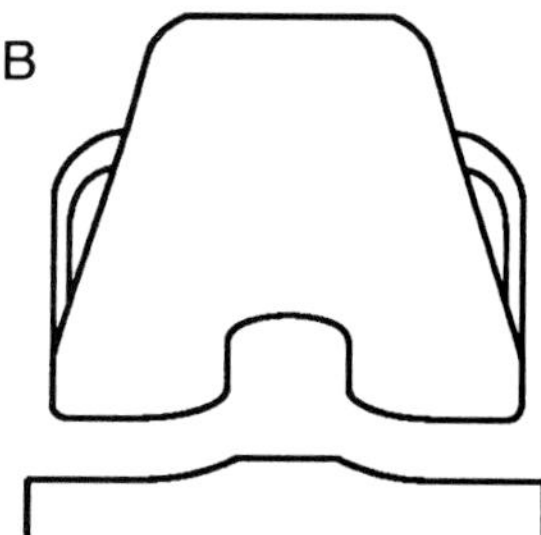

FIGURE 7.

Curved condyles and tibial plateaus **(A)** eliminate the edge loading that can occur with articulating surfaces that are flat **(B)** in the lateral-medial direction.

of postradiation aging, the oxidative environment of the body, and possibly loading. The increase in density is nonuniform through the thickness of the component and is greatest near the superior and inferior surfaces. As the density of polyethylene increases, the elastic modulus also increases.[62] Therefore, the stresses associated with surface damage also increase with time after irradiation and with time after implantation. Control of these degradative processes is one of the greatest challenges for improvement of polyethylene bearing surfaces and is an important topic for current research.

It should also be noted that heat-pressing the polyethylene surface increases the density of the material near the surface. More importantly, if the pressing results in temperatures near melting, a weakened zone of polyethylene is created at a depth where the maximum shear stresses are high.[25] The early delamination of some components that have been heat-pressed has been attributed to the use of this process.

Finally, it should be noted that the stress-strain relationship for polyethylene is nonlinear with decreasing stiffness at higher strains. Thus the effect of material properties on stresses in tibial components is much more complex, particularly for the most nonconforming geometries. In these cases, contact areas are so small that high strains are produced. If linearly elastic behavior is assumed and used to approximate stresses for these components to determine the effects of geometry and material properties on the stresses, the stresses predicted will be overestimated. However, the general effects of geometry and material properties on stresses can be easily demonstrated by linear analyses.

CURRENT STATE OF THE ART

Based on published long-term follow-up studies, successful total hip and knee replacements are available that have lives in excess of 10 years. These successful joints should provide revision-free service for patients 65 years and older. If such joints are placed in younger, more active individuals, the incidence of revision would probably increase, but the longer-term performance of joints that have been successful in the 10- to 15-year range is for the most part still unknown. In either case, the most successful design concepts are well known.

Successful existing designs provide a basis for evolutionary design changes. The objectives of design changes should be clearly stated and tested in much the same way that hypotheses in scientific experiments are tested. For example, a design goal for a knee joint could be to reduce the contact stress in a design while maintaining the torsional laxity in the baseline design. The desired improvement could be tested by using experimental or theoretical methods to demonstrate that the design goals were satisfied. Consequently, experimental and theoretical analyses of stresses on and within polyethylene components are absolutely essential for evaluating the expected performance of design modifications.

It is possible that some of the designs that have been successful in the 10- to 15-year period may be better than others in the longer term. Therefore, long-term survival analyses such as those currently underway in Scandinavia should be encouraged. Such studies provide the surgeon with a rational basis for choosing implants for particular classes of patients and provide a refined database of successful designs that can be further evolved.

The goals for design modifications require detailed information concerning in vivo performance. This information is determined from analyses of explanted components. To date, much of the information from retrieval analyses has been qualitative. Increasingly detailed, quantitative studies will be required to better define the reasons for damage or failure and to associate them with patient factors. Improved retrieval analyses are essential for the definition of relevant design goals.

If the lifetime of joint replacements could be extended by 10 years, they could be placed in patients 55 years and older with the expectation of revision-free service during the lifetime of the patient. Because the lifetimes of current successful designs are primarily limited by the amount of debris generated from the articulating surfaces and other implant interfaces, current research is directed toward choosing materials, processing methods, and component geometries that will minimize surface damage at these sites.

Even though much remains to be learned about polyethylene components, we already have information available that provides the basis for making reasonable choices between design concepts and for choosing specific designs within these general categories. The long-term successful designs are known. We also know the general effects of design variables such as thickness, conformity, and material properties on the stresses associated with surface damage. We know that it is always better to choose a thicker component than a thinner one when the use of a thicker component is consistent with the other goals of surgery. The effects of certain material modifications on performance are also well understood. Most of these fundamentals have been known in principle for some time. The key is to apply them rigorously.

REFERENCES

1. Waugh W: *John Charnley: The Man and the Hip*. New York, Springer-Verlag, 1990.
2. Dumbleton JH: Corrosion and degradation of implant materials: Delrin as material for joint prostheses—A review. *ASTM Special Publication* 684:41–60, 1979.
3. Sudmann E, Havelin LI, Lunde OD, et al: The Charnley vs. the Christiansen total hip arthroplasty: A comparative clinical study. *Acta Orthop Scand* 54:545–552, 1983.
4. Alho A, Soreide O, Bjersand A: Mechanical factors in loosening of Christiansen and Charnley arthroplasties. *Acta Orthop Scand* 55:261–266, 1984.
5. Mathiesen EB, Lindgren U, Reinholt FP: Wear of the acetabular socket. *Acta Orthop Scand* 57:193–196, 1986.
6. Bradley GW, Freeman MAR, Tuke MA: All polymer total knee replacement. *Am J Knee Surg* 5:3–8, 1992.
7. Wright TM, Rimnac CM, Faris PM, et al: Analysis of surface damage in retrieved carbon fiber–reinforced and plain polyethylene tibial components from posterior stabilized total knee replacements. *J Bone Joint Surg Am* 70:1312–1319, 1988.

8. Wright TM, Fukubayshi T, Burstein AH: The effect of carbon reinforcement on contact area, contact pressure, and time-dependent deformation in polyethylene tibial components. *J Biomed Mater Res* 15:719–730, 1981.
9. Li S, Howard EG: Process for manufacturing ultra high molecular weight polyethylene shaped articles. US Patent No. 5,037,928, issued August 6, 1991.
10. Biomet Inc: *ArCom Processed Polyethylene—A Technical Report*, Report No Y-BMT-279/033193. Warsaw, Ind, Biomet, 1993.
11. Biomet Inc: *Test Results ArCom Processed Polyethylene—Uniform Compression Molded Polyethylene*, Report No Y-BMT-325/093093. Biomet, 1993.
12. Zimmerman J: *Orthopaedics Review and 1992 Outlook*. New York, Shearson Lehman Brothers, March 17, 1992.
13. Li S, Howard EG: Characterization and description of enhanced UHMWPE for orthopaedic bearing surfaces. Presented at the 16th Annual Meeting of the Society for Biomaterials. Charleston, SC, May 20–23, 1990.
14. Li S: Special workshop on wear in joint replacement. Presented at the 36th Annual Meeting of the Orthopaedic Research Society, New Orleans, 1990.
15. Nagy EV, Li S: A fourier transform infrared technique for the evaluation of polyethylene orthopaedic bearing materials. Presented at the 16th Annual Meeting of the Society for Biomaterials, Charleston, SC, May 20–23, 1990.
16. Medical devices; Emergency medical services, in *ASTM 1991 Annual Book of ASTM Standards*, F648–84, 13.01. Philadelphia, ASTM, 1991, pp 201–203.
17. Landy M, Walker PS: Wear of UHMWPE components in 90 retrieved knee prostheses. *J Arthroplasty Suppl* S73–S85, 1988.
18. Hood RW, Wright TM, Burstein AH: Retrieval analysis of total knee prostheses: A method and its application to 48 total condylar prostheses. *J Biomed Mater Res* 17:829, 1983.
19. Eyerer P, Ke YC: Property changes of UHMW polyethylene hip cup endoprostheses during implantation. *J Biomed Mater Res* 18:1137, 1984.
20. Li S, Nagy EV: Chemical degradation of polyethylene in hip and knee replacements. Presented at the 38th Annual Meeting of the Orthopaedic Research Society, New Orleans, 1992.
21. Zimmer Inc: *Poly Two Carbon Polyethylene Composite*, Zimmer technical Report. Warsaw, Ind, Zimmer, 1977.
22. Ainsworth R, Farling G, Bardos D: An improved bearing material for joint replacement prostheses: Carbon fiber reinforced UHMWPE. Presented at the 23rd Annual Meeting of the Orthopaedic Research Society, 2:120, 1977.
23. McKellop H, Clarke I, Markolf K, et al: Friction and wear properties of polymer, metal, and ceramic prosthetic joint materials evaluated on a multichannel screening device. *J Biomed Mater Res* 15:619–653, 1981.
24. Connelly GM, Rimnac CM, Wright TM, et al: Fatigue crack propagation behavior of ultra-high molecular weight polyethylene. *J Orthop Res* 2:119–125, 1984.
25. Bloebaum RD, Nelson K, Dorr L, et al: Investigation of the early surface damage observed in retrieved heat pressed tibial inserts. *Clin Orthop* 269:120–127, 1991.
26. Bassett DC, Carder DR: Lamellar thickening and chain extended growth of polyethylene. *Polymer* 14:387–389, 1973.
27. Bassett DC, Turner B: On chain extended and chain folded crystallization of polyethylene. *Philosoph Mag* 29:285–307, 1974.
28. Bassett DC, Turner B: On the phenomenology of chain extended crystallization of polyethylene. *Philosoph Mag* 29:925–955, 1974.
29. Bassett DC, Turner B: Pressure quenching and chain extended crystallization of polyethylene. *J Polym Sci Polym Phys Educ* 13:1501–1509, 1975.

30. Rees DV, Bassett DC: Crystallization of polyethylene at elevated pressures. *J Polym Sci* 2:385–406, 1971.
31. Lupton J, Regester J: Physical properties of extended chain high density polyethylene. *J Appl Polym Sci* 18:2407, 1974.
32. Champion AR, Li S, Saum K, et al: The effect of crystallinity on the physical properties of UHMWPE. Presented at the 40th Annual Meeting of the Orthopaedic Research Society, New Orleans, 1994.
33. Willert HG, Semlitsch M: Reactions of the articular capsule to wear products of artificial joint prostheses. *J Biomed Mater Res* 11:157–164, 1977.
34. Dannenmaier WC, Haynes DW, Nelson CL: Granulomatous reaction and cystic bony destruction associated with high wear rate in a total knee prosthesis. *Clin Orthop* 198:224–230, 1985.
35. Howie DW, Vernon-Roberts B, Oakeshott R, et al: A rat model of resorption of bone at the cement-bone interface in the presence of polyethylene wear particles. *J Bone Joint Surg Am* 70:257, 1988.
36. Maguire JK, Coscia MF, Lynch MH: Foreign body reaction to polymer debris following total hip arthroplasty. *Clin Orthop* 216:213–223, 1987.
37. Nusbaum HJ, Rose RM, Paul IL, et al: Wear mechanisms for ultra high molecular weight polyethylene in the total hip prosthesis. *J Appl Polym Sci* 23:777–789, 1979.
38. Howie DW: Tissue response in relation to type of wear particles around failed hip arthroplasties. *J Arthroplasty* 5:337–348, 1990.
39. Jacobs JJ, Urban RM, Schajowicz F, et al: Particulate-associated endosteal osteolysis in Ti-based alloy cementless total hip replacement. *ASTM STP* 1144:52–60, 1992.
40. Peters PC, Engh GA, Dwyer KA, et al: Osteolysis after total knee arthroplasty without cement. *J Bone Joint Surg Am* 74:864–876, 1992.
41. Galante JO, Lemons J, Spector M, et al: The biological effects of implant materials. *J Orthop Res* 9:760, 1991.
42. Williams DF: *Definitions in Biomaterials*. New York, Elsevier, 1987.
43. Black J: *Orthopaedic Biomaterials*. New York, Churchill Livingstone, 1988, pp 303–319.
44. Leininger RI: *CRC Critical Reviews in Bioengineering*. Boca Raton, Fla, CRC Press, 1972, pp 333–380.
45. Park JB, Lakes RS: *Biomaterials*. New York, Plenum, 1992, pp 223–244.
46. Williams DF (ed): *Biocompatibility of Orthopaedic Implants*, vols 1 and 2. Boca Raton, Fla, CRC Press, 1982.
47. Charnley J: *Low Friction Arthroplasty of the Hip: Theory and Practice*. New York, Springer-Verlag, 1979.
48. Davy DT, Kotzar GM, Brown RH, et al: Telemetric force measurements across the hip after total arthroplasty. *J Bone Joint Surg Am* 70:45–50, 1988.
49. Kotzar GM, Davy DT, Goldberg VM, et al: Telemeterized in vivo hip joint force data: A report on two patients after total hip surgery. *J Orthop Res* 9:621–633, 1991.
50. Bartel DL, Bicknell VL, Wright TM: The effect of conformity, thickness, and material on stresses in ultra-high molecular weight components for total joint replacement. *J Bone Joint Surg Am* 68:1041–1051, 1986.
51. Wright TM, Burstein AH, Bartel DL: Retrieval analysis of total joint replacement components: A six-year experience, in Fraker A, Griffin C (eds): *Corrosion and Degradation of Implant Materials: Second Symposium*, ASTM STP 859. Philadelphia, American Society for Testing and Materials, 1985, pp 415–428.
52. Bartel DL, Rimnac CM, Wright TM: Evaluation and design of the articular surface, in Goldberg VM (ed): *Controversies of Total Knee Arthroplasty*. New York, Raven Press, 1991, pp 61–73.

53. Cooper JR, Dowson D, Fisher J: Birefringent studies of polyethylene wear specimens and acetabular cups. *Wear* 151:391–402, 1991.
54. Cooper JR, Dowson D, Fisher J: Macroscopic and microscopic wear mechanisms in ultra-high molecular weight polyethylene. *Wear* 153:378–384, 1993.
55. Kurtz SM, Bartel DL, Edidin, AA: The effect of gaps on contact stress and relative motion in a metal-backed acetabular component for total hip replacement. Presented at the 40th Annual Meeting of the Orthopaedic Research Society. New Orleans, 1994, p 243.
56. Salvati EA, Wright TM, Burstein AH, et al: Fracture of polyethylene acetabular cups: Report of two cases. *J Bone Joint Surg Am* 61:1239–1242, 1979.
57. Bono JV, Sanford L, Toussaint JT: Severe polyethylene wear in total hip arthroplasty. Observations from retrieved AML PLUS hip implants with an ACS polyethylene liner. *J Arthroplasty* 9:119–125, 1994.
58. Gunsallus KL, Bartel DL: Stresses and surface damage in PCA and total condylar polyethylene components. Presented at the 38th Annual Meeting of the Orthopaedic Research Society, New Orleans, 1992, p 329.
59. Burstein AH: Biomechanics of the knee, in Insall JN (ed): *Surgery of the Knee*. New York, Churchill Livingstone, 1984, pp 21–39.
60. Bartel DL, Burstein AH, Santavicca EA, et al: Performance of the tibial component in total knee replacement. *J Bone Joint Surg Am* 64:1026–1033, 1982.
61. Bostrom MP, Bennett AP, Rimnac CM, et al: The natural history of ultra high molecular weight polyethylene. *Clin Orthop* 309:20–28, 1994.
62. Kurtz SM, Rimnac CM, Bartel DL: A bilinear material model for UHMWPE in total joint replacements. Presented at the 40th Annual Meeting of the Orthopaedic Research Society, New Orleans, 1994, p 289.
63. Goldring MB, Goldring SR: Skeletal tissue response to cytokines. *Clin Orthop* 258:245–278, 1990.
64. Maloney WJ, Jasty M, Burke DW, et al: Biomechanic and histologic investigation of cemented total hip arthroplasty. *Clin Orthop* 249:120–140, 1989.

Revision Arthroplasty of the Hip With Restoration of Bone Stock

Allan E. Gross, M.D.
A.J. Latner Professor and Chairman, Division of Orthopaedic Surgery, University of Toronto, Faculty of Medicine, Mount Sinai Hospital, Toronto, Ontario, Canada

Revision surgery for loose hip and knee implants is now a major part of any orthopedic surgical program, and its volume is going to increase. Loose cemented hip and knee prostheses, particularly in a multiply revised implant, are associated with loss of bone stock because of wear particles and the loose cement acting as an abrasive.[1–9] Wear particles may cause bone lysis even in the presence of stable cemented or uncemented components.[10, 11] Also, each time a revision is carried out, the surgery itself leads to some loss of bone stock. Symptomatic loose knees or hip prostheses with associated loss of bone stock are going to continue to be a standard orthopedic problem occupying a significant portion of the surgical resources of any orthopedic division that performs implant surgery. The problem must therefore be dealt with if orthopedic surgeons are going to continue to replace arthritic joints.

There are surgical alternatives to this problem. Excision arthroplasty may be acceptable, but not when the bone loss is extensive.[12, 13] Arthrodesis is difficult to achieve and results in excessive shortening if bone loss is extensive.[14] The use of tumor or custom implants in which bone is replaced by metal may be acceptable in low-demand patients, but there are certain disadvantages. The large tumor implants may require the use of cement in the host bone, which can no longer provide the rough lattice necessary for good cement techniques. A stress riser is created at the junction of host bone and implant with both cemented and uncemented implants.[15–21] The prosthesis does not provide a biological anchorage for host bone and muscle.

Restoration of bone stock in association with a relatively conventional implant offers a more normal gradation of forces from the prosthesis to host bone. Reattachment of bone and muscle is possible. The implant may be of a more conventional design and may be less expensive. Restoration of bone stock also allows the surgeon to use uncemented or cemented implants, and most importantly, it may allow further revisions if necessary in the future.

Bone stock may be replenished by the patient's own bone or allograft bone. Using the patient's own bone is only applicable when a minimal

Advances in Operative Orthopaedics, vol. 3

amount of bone is required. Allograft bone offers quality and quantity and is applicable in certain situations in which there are major defects, i.e., proximal femoral or major pelvic column loss. There are also the obvious advantages to leaving the patient's iliac crest intact.

There are, of course, certain disadvantages to using allograft bone. The problems of disease transmission are well documented but can be minimized by adhering to the guidelines of the American Association of Tissue Banks.[22, 23] Banked bone is not always readily available but is becoming increasingly more so. Allograft bone has certain biological problems. It is not as osteoinductive as autograft bone, and nonunions may result.[24] This can be alleviated by autografting host-allograft junctions and obtaining rigid fixation. Resorption of allograft bone, particularly solid-fragment grafts, may lead to failure.[25, 26] This, of course, may also occur with autograft bone, but the process probably is slower. There may be problems like fracture or fragmentation of solid-fragment grafts if the biomechanics of the reconstruction are not correct or the level of demand is too high. This problem applies to both autografts and allografts. Whatever the problems are, however, there is no question that we are facing a large population of patients who are going to need restoration of bone stock before further revision surgery can be performed.

CLASSIFICATION OF BONE DEFECTS

It is important to have a functional and relatively simple classification of bone deficits associated with loose hip implants. There are more complicated classifications in the literature,[27, 28] but we have found that all of our grafts can fit into the following classification:

I. Pelvic side defects
   A. *Protrusio:* A contained cavitary defect with the acetabular walls and columns intact. Morsellized bone is usually used for this type of defect.
   B. *Minor column (shelf):* Loss of part of the rim plus the corresponding acetabular wall but less than 50% of the acetabulum. A structural graft is used, but less than half of the acetabulum is replaced. This is called a minor column or shelf graft.
   C. *Major column:* Loss of one or both columns with its corresponding acetabular wall and involving over 50% of the acetabulum. A major column structural graft involving over 50% of the acetabulum is used.

II. Femoral side defects
   A. *Intraluminal:* The canal is widened but the cortex is still intact and thought to be strong enough to support an implant.
   B. *Cortical*
      1. Cortical noncircumferential: Cortical defects that require only strut grafts.
      2. Circumferential
         a. Calcar: <3 cm in length.
         b. Proximal femur (large fragment): >3 cm in length.

These bone defects can be classified, in most cases, by plain radiographs (routine views, Judet views)[29]; computed axial tomography (CAT) may be helpful, particularly when first starting to do these types of reconstructions, but it is not usually necessary.

SYSTEMIC APPROACH

The goal of revision arthroplasty of the hip is to achieve a stable implant with restoration of anatomy. This may be achieved relatively easily or with great difficulty, depending on the available bone stock.

The primary goal is to implant new components against the host bone with restoration of anatomy and leg length. This can be done with or without the use of cement, depending on the characteristics of the patient and the preference of the surgeon.[30–45]

If the primary goal cannot be achieved, the secondary goal would be to achieve stable components and restore anatomy and leg length but with help from bone grafts or prosthetic design. If a bone graft is used, it is either morsellized or noncircumferential (cortical strut) so that the implant is supported primarily by host bone. Some implants are designed to compensate for minimal-to-moderate loss of bone stock. Oblong asymmetrical cups and femoral components with calcar replacing stems and several neck lengths are examples of this.[45, 46]

When the bone loss is more severe and the implants cannot be stabilized primarily against host bone, then a decision has to be made whether to sacrifice or to restore anatomy and leg length.

If the components can be stabilized primarily against host bone with acceptable sacrifice of anatomy, then the tertiary goal is achieved. A high hip center is an example of this.[45]

If the loss of bone stock is very severe and the components cannot be stabilized primarily against host bone, then structural grafts or custom implants must be used to restore anatomy and leg length. This is the quartenary goal.[47, 48]

We have used this approach to produce the following classification of revisions:

Type I: Uncemented or cemented components placed in host bone with restoration of anatomy and leg length.

Type II: Uncemented or cemented components supported primarily by host bone but with some minor support by bone graft (i.e., morsellized bone, cortical strut) or by prosthetic design (i.e., calcar replacing prosthesis, oblong cup), with restoration of anatomy and leg lengths (see Figs 3, 4, and 11).

Type III: Uncemented or cemented components supported primarily by host bone with acceptable loss of anatomy and leg length (high hip center) (see Fig 5).

Type IV: Uncemented or cemented components supported by structural grafts or custom prostheses with restoration of anatomy and leg length (see Figs 6, 7, and 10).

Several factors must be considered before deciding on the type of revision and what type of components to use.

PATIENT FACTORS

The level of demand of the patient is determined by age, height, weight, occupation, and lifestyle. For example, in a high-demand patient, restoration of bone stock and the use of uncemented components would seem more advisable.

In a low-demand patient who is unlikely to require another revision, the use of a long-stemmed cemented component is more acceptable than in a higher-demand patient who might require another revision.[38]

Loss of bone stock anatomy and leg length discrepancy are crucial factors in decision making. This must be determined accurately before surgery. In addition to plain radiographs, Judet views of the pelvis[29] and a CAT scan may be helpful for assessing bone stock.

Infection must be ruled out if suspected. A bone scan, gallium scan, indium scan, and hip aspiration may be helpful.[49–51] Even if these tests are negative, if at the time of surgery the findings on gross examination or on Gram stain or frozen section are suggestive of infection, then in the opinion of the author the reconstruction should be done in two stages if structural grafts are necessary.

SURGEON FACTORS

Surgeon factors play an important role in decision making about the type of revision and the components to be used. Some surgeons prefer to do all their revisions cementless,[30, 35, 36, 38, 52] whereas others use cement.[31, 40, 41] Some surgeons will not use bone grafts of any type, whereas others will use morsellized but not structural grafts.[53, 54] Surgeons who will not use structural grafts either use custom prostheses[55] or are willing to sacrifice some anatomy and leg length to place their components against host bone.[45] In some centers, excision arthroplasty[12, 13] or fusion[14] is more accepted by surgeons and patients than in others.

PRINCIPLES OF RESTORATION OF BONE STOCK IN REVISION SURGERY OF THE HIP

Bone grafts are classified into heterografts (bone from another species), allografts (bone from the same species), and autografts (bone taken from one part of the same individual). In revision situations, because of the quantity and quality of bone required, an allograft is more practical than an autograft. There are, however, certain advantages and disadvantages to each.

Autografts have the advantages of not being immunogenic, and even more importantly, they are best for inducing new bone formation in the host. Disadvantages are the quantity available, the strength, shape, and form of which cannot completely fill the deficit.

Allografts, on the other hand, are available in quantity and can be strong and completely fill the deficit. They are, however, immunogenic[56–58] and are not as effective as autografts for inducing new bone formation.[59]

Allografts bone can be further classified according to how it is used: (1) morsellized and (2) structural, either simulated or anatomic.

In a simulated structural graft, bone from another region is shaped to simulate the deficit. For example, the distal end of the femur can be sculpted to duplicate an acetabulum.

In an anatomic structural graft, the graft is the actual anatomic part being duplicated. For example, an acetabular allograft is used in whole or in part to replace an acetabular defect.

The advantages of a structural graft are restoration of anatomy and provision of structural support for the implant. The disadvantage of a structural graft is that revascularization and remodeling can lead to resorption and/or collapse, and the graft therefore weakens with time.

Structural grafts are indicated for uncontained defects in which it is necessary to restore anatomy and leg length and provide bone support for the implant. Acceptable compromises to the anatomy and leg lengths are preferable to structural grafts if adequate bone stock is available, i.e., a high hip center.[45, 60]

Morsellized bone is indicated for contained defects, where it serves as a filler scaffold. It can undergo revascularization and remodeling and strengthens with time. It cannot be used for early structural support.

All reconstructions will eventually fail whether they are synthetic or biological. As surgeons, our role is to prolong the time to failure and to make sure that when failure occurs, further reconstruction is possible. Bone grafts restore bone for future surgery.

GUIDELINES

1. Host bone should not be devascularized.
2. Autograft is best for bone induction and should be used to promote union, i.e., as a flying buttress for shelves, and at all allograft-host junctions.
3. Rigid fixation that goes from live bone to live bone and bridges the graft should be used.
4. Cement can be used in bone grafts because it strengthens them and delays vascularization and membrane formation.
5. Strong bone should be used for structural grafts.
6. A trochanteric osteotomy is used for complex reconstructions.
7. Structural grafts should not be used unless definitely necessary to provide support for an implant or restore anatomy and leg length.

Acceptable compromises to anatomy and leg length are preferable to structural grafts if adequate bone stock is available, i.e., a high hip center.

SURGICAL APPROACH

In our hospital, all revisions requiring the use of allograft bone are done in a laminar-flow operating room with body exhaust systems. If there is preoperative evidence of infection or any suggestion at the time of surgery (even with a negative Gram stain), the surgery is staged for any revision requiring the use of allograft bone.

All allograft bone is brought into the operating room at the beginning of the procedure, unwrapped, cultured, and immersed in warm povidone-iodine (Betadine). The bone is obtained from our own bone bank, where it has been deep-frozen at −70° C after being irradiated with 2.5 megarads.

The surgical approach is either transgluteal[61] or transtrochanteric. The transtrochanteric approach is used most commonly because of the need for extensive exposure and also because in many cases there is a pre-existing trochanteric nonunion.

Large-fragment proximal femoral grafts should be done via the transtrochanteric approach, and the trochanteric fragment should be kept as long as possible so that it will unite and also reinforce the allograft. The proximal portion of the femur is exposed by reflecting the vastus lateralis off the septum anteriorly while being careful to not strip any residual bone off of its soft tissue completely.

A Steinmann pin is inserted into the iliac crest as a reference point to adjust the leg length. The distance from the pin to the rough line (insertion of the vastus lateralis) is recorded before dislocation.

RECONSTRUCTION OF THE ACETABULUM IN REVISION ARTHROPLASTY OF THE HIP

Restoration of bone stock on the pelvic side in arthroplasty of the hip is a difficult and controversial procedure. The spectrum of surgical opinion goes from avoiding the use of bone graft if at all possible,[45, 60] to the use of morsellized bone only,[53, 54] to the use of complex structural grafts.[25, 47]

There is no question that structural grafts on the pelvic side have a guarded prognosis and should be avoided if possible.[47, 60] At the same time there are situations in which bulk allografts have to be used; if used properly it can yield acceptable results and restore bone stock for future surgery.[47]

SURGICAL TECHNIQUE

The acetabulum is prepared after the hip has been dislocated. After the acetabular prosthesis and the cement are removed, the membrane is excised carefully because of possible complete bony defects. The defect is then defined by visualization, by palpation, and by using a trial cup. At this point the defect must be defined so that the allograft can be prepared. If the defect is a contained cavity (protrusio), then morsellized bone can be used. If the defect is a minor or major column defect, then a bulk allograft is indicated. If a bulk allograft can be avoided by raising the acetabulum 1 or 2 cm to get into better bone stock, then this alternative should be used because better contact with host bone is obtained. Bulk allografts on the pelvic side should be avoided if possible, and in the majority of cases the acetabulum can be seated in host bone and supplemented with morsellized allograft (protrusio graft). If a major or minor column defect does exist and cannot be compensated for by raising or centralizing the acetabular bed, then a bulk allograft should be used. For bulk allografts we prefer to fashion true acetabular allografts, but male femoral heads or even distal femur can be used. If morsellized bone is needed, then female femoral heads should be used rather than sacrificing strong structural bone. We prefer to not use a bone mill because the bone becomes too mushy. The bone can be easily morsellized by hand with

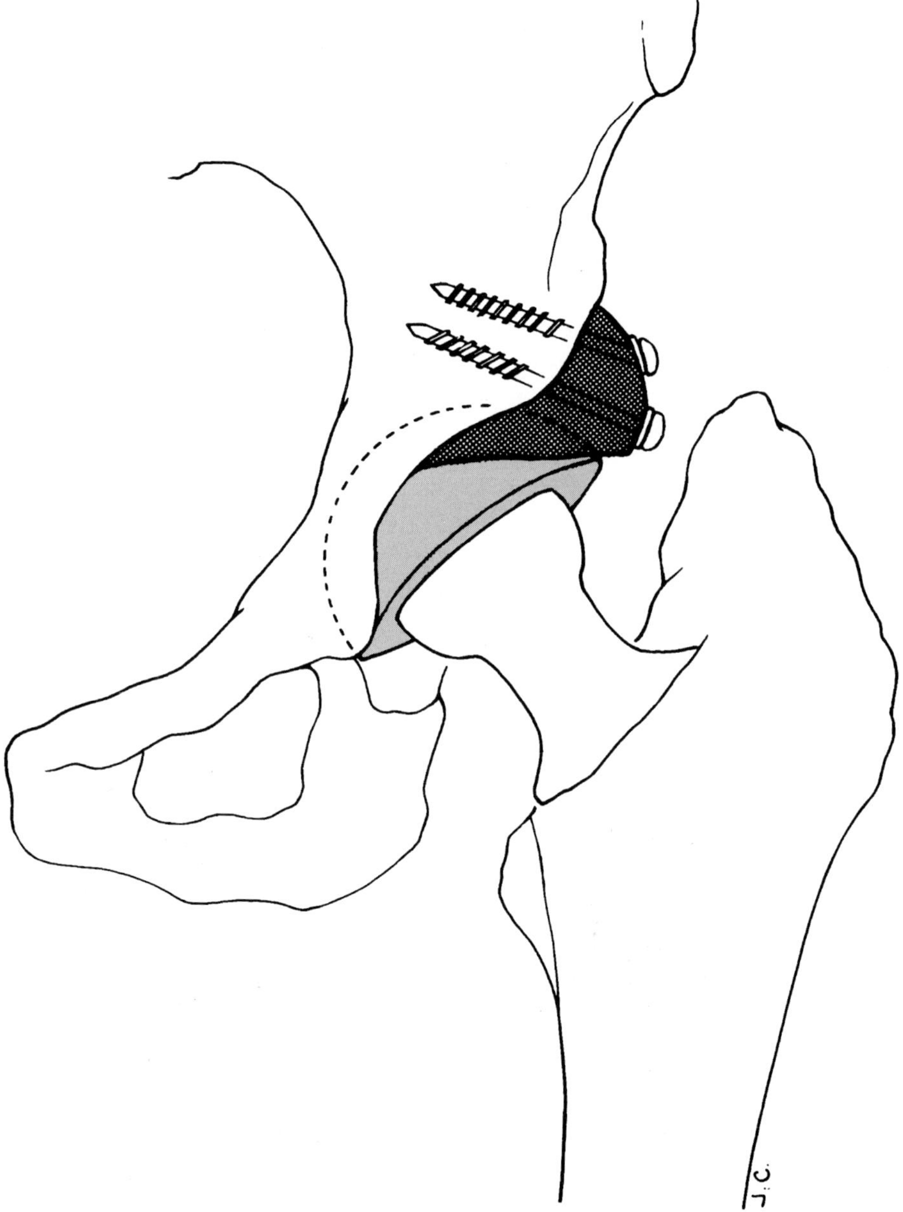

FIGURE 1.
Minor column (shelf) allograft. Note that half of the cup is seated in host bone. The graft is held by 2 × 4.5-mm cancellous screws.

curets and rongeurs and is fine enough to pack into cavities but still has some structural integrity. Morsellized bone can be packed into cavities by using acetabular reamers in reverse.

Minor column grafts can be fixed by two vertical to obliquely oriented cancellous screws (4.5 mm) (Fig 1). Reinforcement rings or reconstruction pelvic plates are used for the major column grafts (Fig 2). If possible, it is our preference to bridge these major column grafts from host bone to host bone with a plate or a reinforcement ring. It is best to not ream these grafts, but if it is necessary, the cartilage is reamed off and the subchondral bone left intact. It is done very lightly with the grafts fixed in position. If possible, the cancellous surfaces of the allografts should not be exposed to anything but host bone.

There are several options for acetabular prostheses. In the protrusio situation, morsellized bone, a reinforcement ring, and a cemented cup make a good reconstruction for moderate- to low-demand elderly patients. The best reconstruction for a protrusio defect in a higher-demand patient is morsellized bone with an uncemented, fixed large-diameter, metal-backed, porous-coated cup with direct contact with at least 50% host bone. In most cases screws are necessary to fix the cup. Bipolar or biarticulating cups are only used if nothing else is technically or biologically possible or if a more extensive procedure is not indicated because of the patient's health.

A shelf or minor column defect will allow contact with at least 50% host bone, and here we prefer to use an uncemented porous-coated cup, press-fit or fixed by screws. A cemented cup may, however, be used.

A major column graft involves more than 50% of the acetabulum,

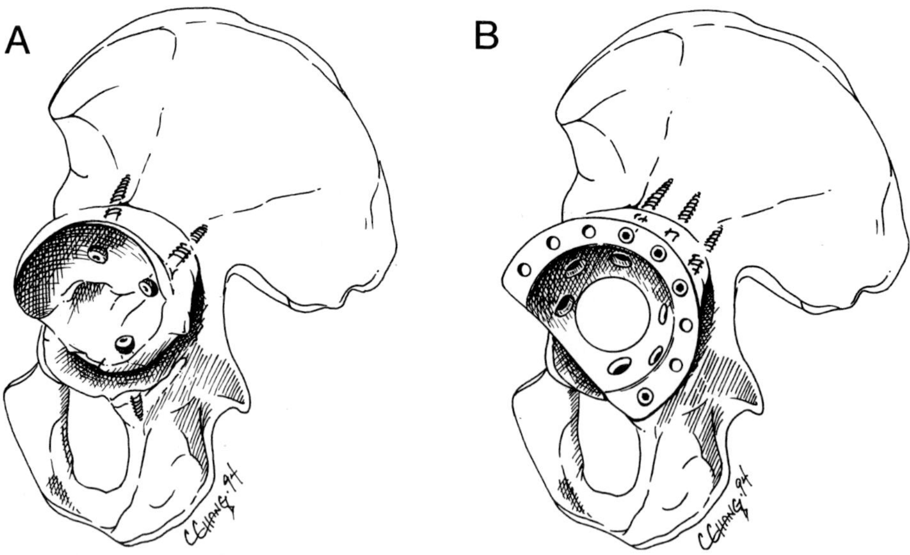

FIGURE 2.

Major column allograft. **A,** an acetabular allograft involving more than 50% of the acetabulum has been fixed to the host pelvis with three 4.5-mm cancellous screws. **B,** the graft is protected by a reinforcement ring that bridges the graft from host bone to host bone.

which means that the cup is mainly in contact with dead allograft bone. Under the circumstances, the cup should be cemented.

We attempt to obtain fixation of the porous-coated cups by press-fit antirotation lugs if possible. If not, we use screws to fix the metal backing in place. We have had no experience with screw-in cups.

POSTOPERATIVE CARE

Prophylactic intravenous antibiotics are used for 5 days, followed by 10 more days of oral antibiotics. We prefer a cephalosporin. If the patient is catheterized intraoperatively, we use gentamicin during the surgery and for the first 24 hours but then switch to sulfamethoxazole-trimethoprim (Septra) until the catheter is removed. Because of the extent of the surgery, we usually keep patients on bed rest and in abduction for 5 days. The patients are not allowed any weight bearing until union is obtained between the allograft and host, usually at 3 to 6 months.

PRINCIPLES OF SURGERY FOR ACETABULAR GRAFTING

1. Preoperatively decide on the type of bone (morsellized or bulk), type of fixation, and implant (Table 1).
2. Use an exposure that allows access to the anterior and posterior columns. Trochanteric osteotomy is advantageous in most cases.
3. Use internal fixation that goes from host bone to host bone if a structural graft involving over 50% of the acetabulum is used. Small grafts are fixed by cancellous screws oriented in an oblique-to-vertical direction.
4. If a structural graft is necessary, use strong bone, i.e., an acetabular allograft, distal femur, or a male femoral head.
5. If a structural graft involving over 50% of the acetabulum is used, cement the cup.
6. Do not expose the cancellous surface of the graft to the soft tissue of the host if possible.
7. Do not use structural grafts unless it is necessary to provide support for an implant or restore anatomy and leg length. Acceptable compromises to anatomy and leg length are preferable to structural acetabular grafts if adequate bone stock is available, i.e., high hip center.
8. Autograft should be used in the junction of the allograft and the host pelvis.

RESULTS

As of July 1, 1993, there have been acetabular revisions using morsellized allograft bone in 179 hips with an average follow-up of 4.57 years (range, 1 to 11), 56 shelf grafts (minor column) with an average follow-up of 5.12 years (range, 1 to 10), and 67 acetabular grafts (major column) with an average follow-up of 5.23 years (range, 1 to 10).

A follow-up study of 58 reconstructions of contained cavitary defects with morsellized bone was carried out.[47, 62] The follow-up average was 46.4 months (range, 26 to 87). Morsellized allograft bone was used with

TABLE 1.
Summary of Bone Deficits and Pelvic Reconstruction

Small defect
  Autograft
  Modified implant
Large defect (allograft)
  Contained cavitary defect (protrusio)
    Low-demand patient
      Morsellized bone, protrusio ring, and cemented cup
    High-demand patient
      Morsellized bone and large-diameter uncemented metal-backed cup (porous coated press-fit or held with screws)
  Structural defect (major or minor column defect)
    Minor column
      Uncemented or cemented cup (shelf)
    Major column
      Cemented cup

an uncemented porous-coated metal-backed cup in 32 hips, with a Mueller ring and a cemented cup in 15 hips, and with a biarticulating device (bipolar) in 11 hips.

A modified Harris hip scoring system was used[63] (Table 2). Failure was defined as a postoperative increase in score of less than 20 points or the need for further surgery as a result of problems with the allograft.

A successful outcome was seen in 100% of the reconstructions with the Mueller ring and a cemented cup and in 94% of the reconstructions using an uncemented cup. Only 64% of the reconstructions using the biarticulating device were successful.

Radiographic review demonstrated probable loosening (circumferential lucent lines of more than 2 mm) in 57% and definite loosening (migration or a change in orientation) in 14% of the reconstructions using reinforcement rings (average follow-up, 63 months). Possible loosening was seen in 5% of the uncemented cups at an average follow-up of 39 months. Of the bicentric reconstructions, 57% showed significant migration and less satisfactory pain reduction. Overall, the average medial migration of the bicentric devices was 3.2 mm (range, 0 to 10 mm), and superior migration averaged 17.0 mm (range, 0 to 60 mm). The superior lateral corner of the obturator foramen served as a landmark, and horizontal and vertical lines from the center of the femoral head were used to determine superior and medial migration. In contrast, cemented implants with reinforcement rings averaged 0.1 mm of medial migration (range, −1 to +1 mm) and 1.7 mm of superior migration (range, −6 to +12 mm). The fixed noncemented implants averaged 0.9 mm of medial migration (range, −3 to +4 mm) and 1.1 mm of superior migration (range, −9 to +9 mm).

Remodeling and resorption of the morsellized graft were observed. The final width of the bone graft was noted to be diminished in comparison with the immediate postoperative width. The percentage of resorp-

TABLE 2.
Modified Harris Hip Rating System

Pain
- 44 = None
- 40 = Slight
- 30 = Moderate, occasional
- 20 = Moderate
- 10 = Marked
- 0 = Disabled

Function
- Limp
  - 11 = None
  - 8 = Slight
  - 5 = Moderate
  - 0 = Severe
- Support
  - 11 = None
  - 7 = Cane, long walks
  - 3 = 1 Crutch
  - 2 = 2 Canes
  - 0 = 2 Crutches
- Distance walked
  - 11 = Unlimited
  - 8 = 6 Blocks
  - 5 = 3 Blocks
  - 2 = Indoors
  - 0 = Bed and chair

Activities
- Stairs
  - 4 = Normally
  - 2 = Without railing
  - 1 = Any manner
  - 0 = Unable
- Shoes and socks
  - 4 = With ease
  - 2 = With difficulty
  - 0 = Unable
- Sitting
  - 4 = Any chair, 1 hr
  - 2 = High chair
  - 0 = Unable to sit comfortably
- Public transportation
  - 1 = Able to use
  - 0 = Unable to use

Deformity
- Fixed adduction
  - 1 = <10
  - 0 = >10
- Fixed internal rotation
  - 1 = <10
  - 0 = >10
- Flexion contracture
  - 1 = <15
  - 0 = >15
- Leg length discrepancy
  - 1 = <3 cm
  - 0 = >3 cm

Range of motion
- Flexion
  - 1 = >90
  - 0 = <90
- Abduction
  - 1 = >15
  - 0 = <15
- Adduction
  - 1 = >15
  - 0 = <15
- External rotation
  - 1 = >30
  - 0 = <30
- Internal rotation
  - 1 = >15
  - 0 = <15
- Trendelenburg
  - 1 = Negative
  - 0 = Positive

tion was 5.7% (range, 0% to 27%) in the cemented cups, 50.6% (range, 17% to 100%) in the bicentric devices, and 26.4% (range, 0% to 83%) in the noncemented cups (Figs 3 and 4).

A follow-up study of bulk (major and minor column) acetabular allografts was performed.[47, 64] A modified Harris scoring system was used[63] (see Table 2). In this study there were 19 patients with 22 shelf (minor column) reconstructions with a mean follow-up of 40.8 months (range, 29 to 68). The mean preoperative score was 31, and postoperatively it was 72. Two grafts had complete graft resorption. Eight grafts showed a stress shielding type of resorption or remodeling in which the unloaded portion of the graft was resorbed. This affected the most lateral part of the graft and usually involved 3 to 7 mm. Acetabular implant migration occurred in 3 cases, 2 of which were bipolar prostheses. Of the 22 shelf (minor column) grafts, there were 3 failures, 2 for deep sepsis requiring further surgery and 1 for a dislocated cup. The overall success rate was 86% (Figs 5 and 6).

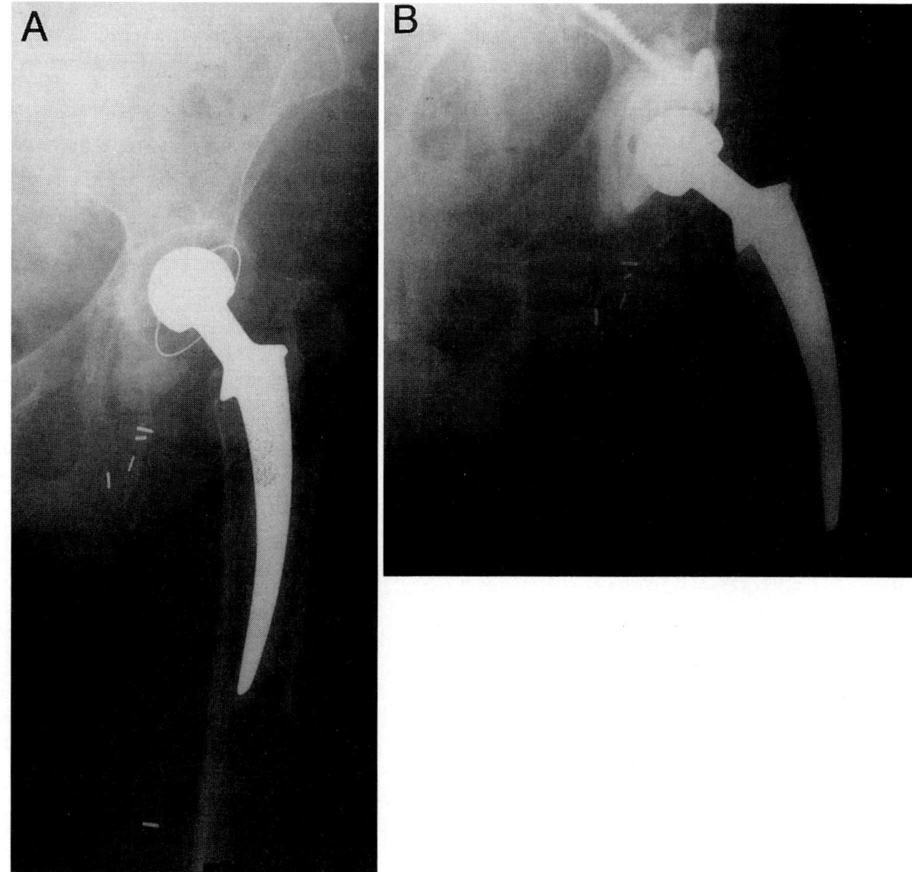

FIGURE 3.

Morsellized graft for a contained defect. **A,** preoperative radiograph of a 65-year-old female with a loose cemented acetabular component and superomedical protrusio. The pelvis bone defect is contained. **B,** the pelvis has been reconstructed with morsellized allograft bone, a roof reinforcement ring, and a cemented cup.

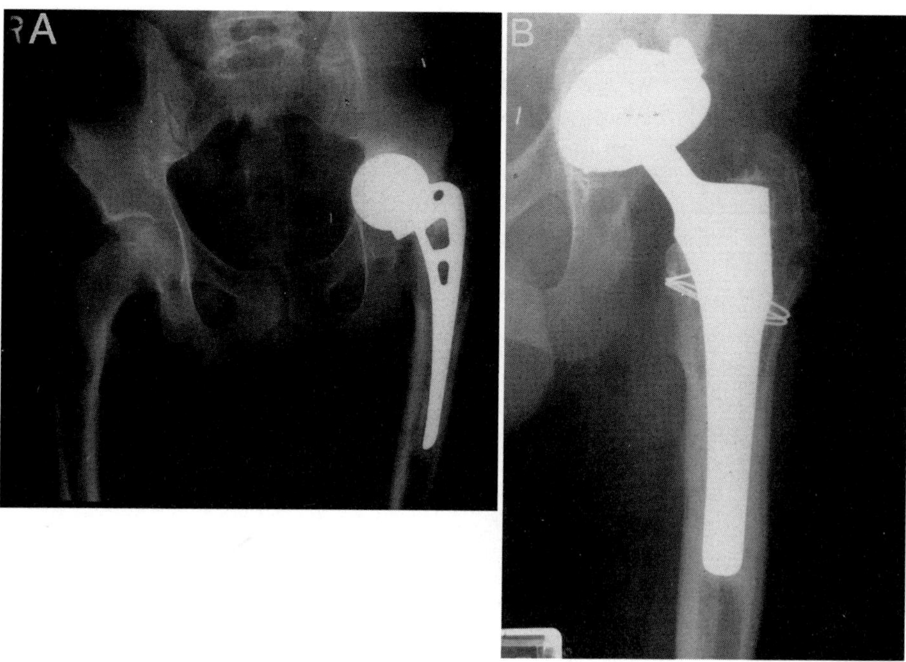

FIGURE 4.
Morsellized graft for a contained defect. **A,** severe superomedical protrusio in a 30-year old male 6 years after a Moore prosthesis was inserted for osteonecrosis. **B,** the revision has been performed with morsellized allograft bone and an uncemented cup.

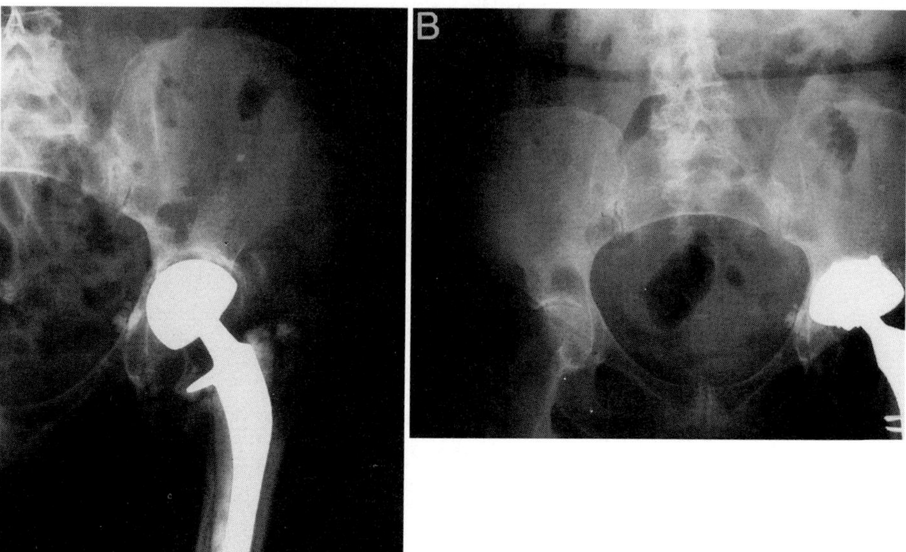

FIGURE 5.
High hip center. **A,** preoperative radiograph of a 75-year-old female with superomedical protrusis and a bipolar prosthesis. **B,** the patient has undergone revision to an uncemented cup placed in a high position against host bone rather than using a structural acetabular graft.

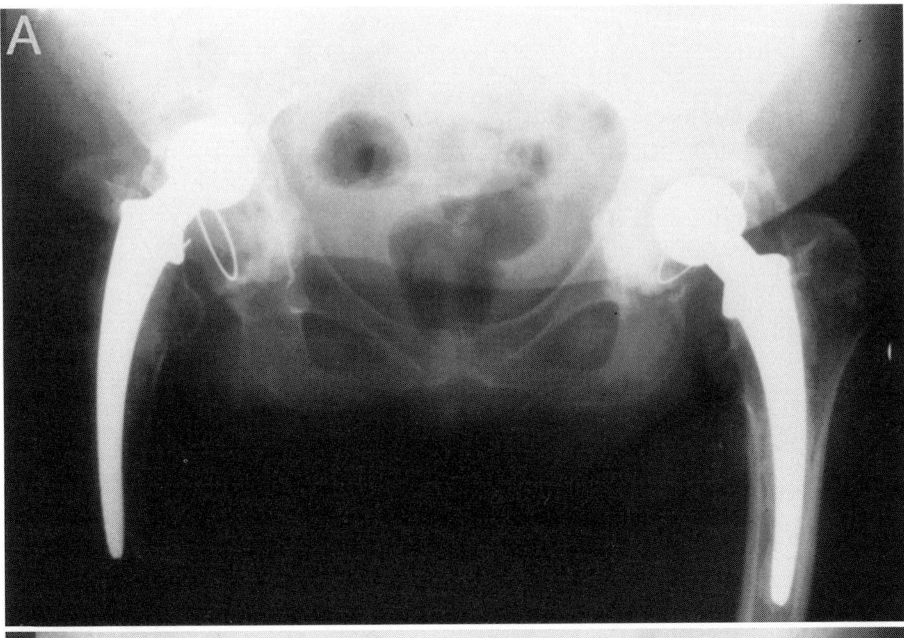

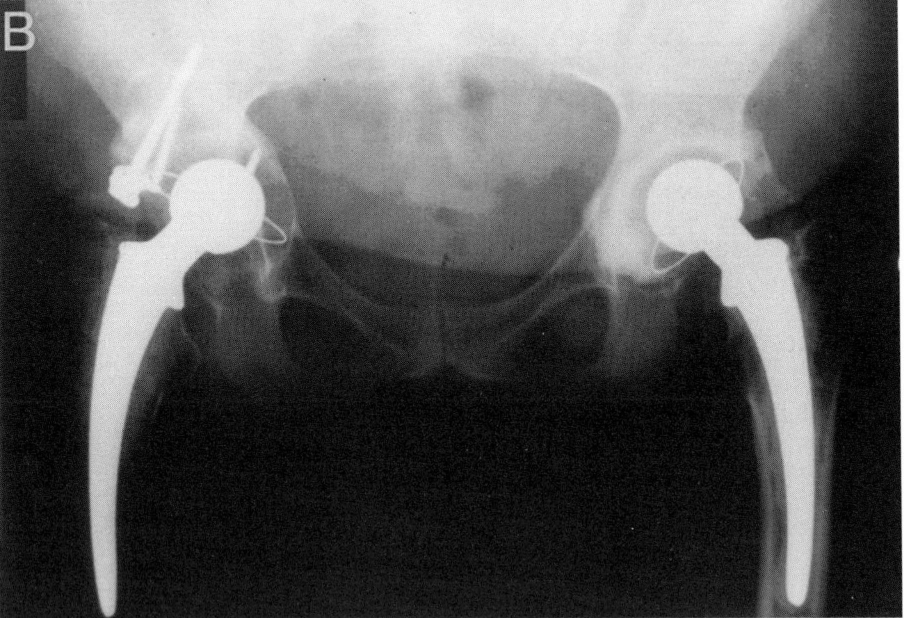

FIGURE 6.

Structural pelvic allograft (minor column). **A**, preoperative radiograph of a 45-year-old female with chronic dislocation of the hip and loss of pelvic bone stock. The bone defect is uncontained. **B**, 8 years after reconstruction with a structural pelvic allograft and uncemented cup. The graft involves less than 50% of the acetabulum and is therefore classified as a minor column graft.

In the major column group there were 28 reconstructions in 26 patients with a mean follow-up of 36 months (range, 24 to 71). The mean preoperative score was 29, and the mean postoperative score was 75.

There was one case of deep sepsis requiring excision in a reconstruction using femoral heads. A patient with flaccid paralysis (myelomenigocele) whose defect was reconstructed with an acetabular allograft required further surgery for recurrent dislocation.

Six of the remaining 14 patients with true acetabular allografts (i.e., reconstruction with acetabular allograft bone) required further surgery because of fracture or fragmentation of the graft. The subsequent reconstruction was greatly facilitated by the restored bone stock. Five of these six patients with reoperated acetabular allografts have a successful clinical score 2 years after reoperation. The last patient with a bipolar reconstruction remains a failure because of minimal increase in her clinical score after reoperation. Six allografts were associated with implant migration, and 5 of these cases involved a bipolar prosthesis that had eroded the allograft in varying amounts, 5 to 15 mm, in a proximal-medial direction. Only 1 of the 6 bipolar reconstructions was not associated with migration. The overall success rate for major column allografts was 71% (20 of 28 cases; Fig 7).

A more recent review of our cases revealed the following data as of July 1, 1993. Of 179 acetabular reconstructions using morsellized allograft bone, 9 have required revision (5%) at an average follow-up of 4.57 years. The reasons for revision were cup loosening in 4 and dislocation in 5. All revisions were successful.

Of 56 minor column (shelf) allografts, 4 revisions were necessary (7%) at an average follow-up of 5.12 years. Two were revised for loose cups, 1 for infection, and 1 for resorption. All were revised successfully.

Of 67 major column grafts, 25 revisions were necessary (37%) at an

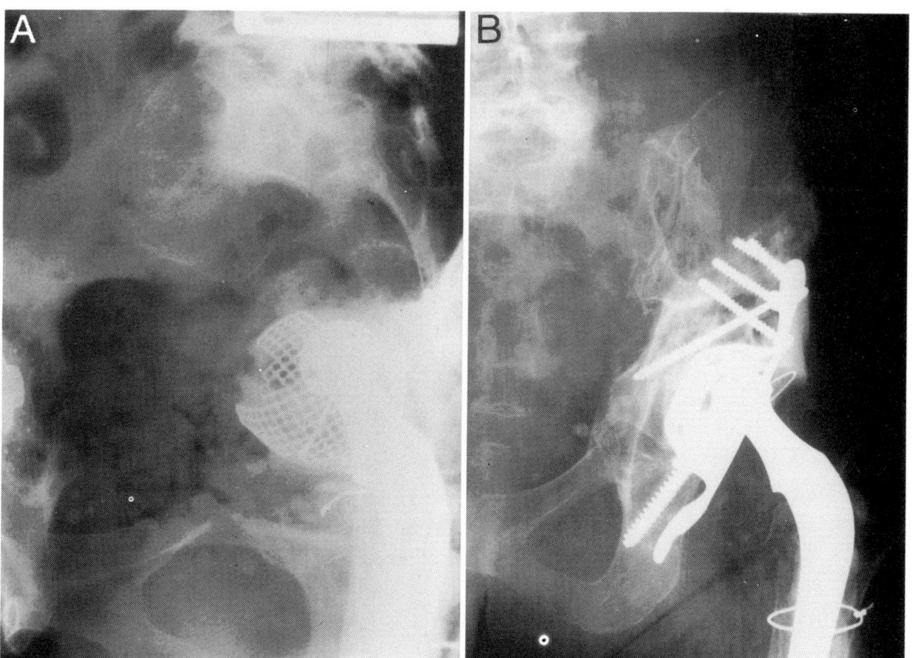

FIGURE 7.

Structural pelvic allograft (major column). **A,** preoperative radiograph of a 55-year-old female illustrating loss of all of the anterior column with a loose migrated cup. **B,** 10½ years after the major column acetabular allograft was fixed by screws and protected by a roof reinforcement ring. The cup is cemented.

average follow-up of 5.23 years. Ten were revised successfully and 6 underwent excision arthroplasty. The reasons for revision or excision were as follows: dislocation, 4 hips; loose cup, 10 hips; nonunion, 5 hips; fracture, 3 hips; infection, 2 hips; and nerve injury, 1 hip.

The 37% incidence of revisions of major column grafts is inflated because of the fact that 16 hips had 25 complications. The incidence of patients requiring further surgery was therefore 27% (16 of 60).

RECONSTRUCTION OF THE FEMUR IN REVISION ARTHROPLASTY OF THE HIP

SURGICAL TECHNIQUE

The acetabulum is reconstructed first so that the length of the femoral allograft can be determined. We use long-stemmed femoral components and therefore do not hesitate to cut a window for controlled cement removal and reaming. If a proximal femoral allograft is to be performed (Fig 8), then the residual proximal portion of the femur is split distally to good bone. As much soft tissue as possible is left attached to the residual bone for later use as a vascularized bone graft. The cement is then removed.

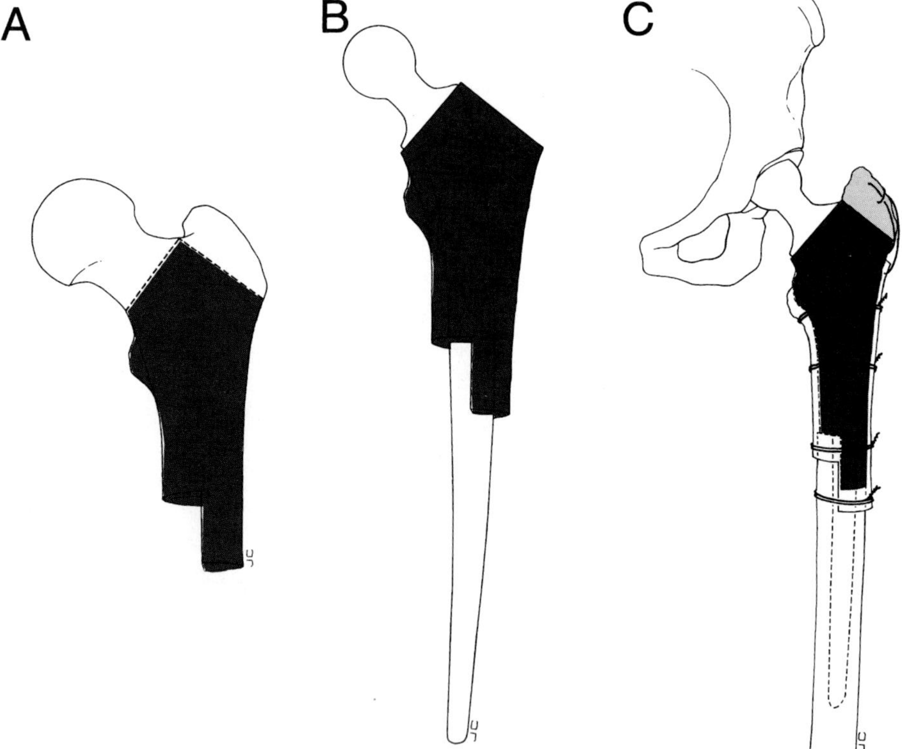

FIGURE 8.

A, Proximal femoral allograft. **B,** allograft cemented to the femoral component. **C,** allograft fixed to the host via a step-cut and cerclage wires. The residual host bone acts as a vascularized bone graft and should be wrapped around host-graft junction to aid in union.

The distal end of the host femur is then reamed gently over a guide wire to assess canal size for the implant rather than to enlarge the canal. When the reamers are at a size that definite reaming is taking place, then the diameter of the implant is selected. The allograft, which is either proximal femur or tibia, is then reamed and broached until a good fit for the implant is achieved. It is important to not over-ream the allograft to get a press-fit of the femoral component into the host. The host canal is always larger than the allograft, and it may therefore be impossible to get a press-fit into the host without over-reaming the allograft, which would weaken it. We therefore cement the implant to the allograft and use a step-cut at the junction of host and allograft to gain stability rather than worry about the press-fit. The length of the allograft necessary is assessed in vivo by placing the femoral implant into the host bone and reducing it into the trial cup. The selected length depends on stability and leg length discrepancy. A Steinmann pin is inserted into the iliac crest, and the distance from it to a fixed point on the femur is measured before dislocation of the hip. A step-cut of about 2 × 2 cm is carried out in the allograft and in the host. Sometimes the host allograft junction is stable without a step-cut. Under these circumstances the step-cut is not necessary. If obtaining stability at the junction is difficult, then cortical strut allografts can be cerclaged around the junction for additional fixation.

When the correct length of allograft is obtained and the stability of the reconstruction is acceptable, the implant is cemented into the allograft after drill holes are made and wires are passed for trochanteric reattachment. It is very important to keep the cement off the interface that will oppose host bone. The allograft with the long-stemmed femoral component cemented in place is inserted into the host, and cerclage wire is used to stabilize the step-cut. The junction of host and allograft is also au-

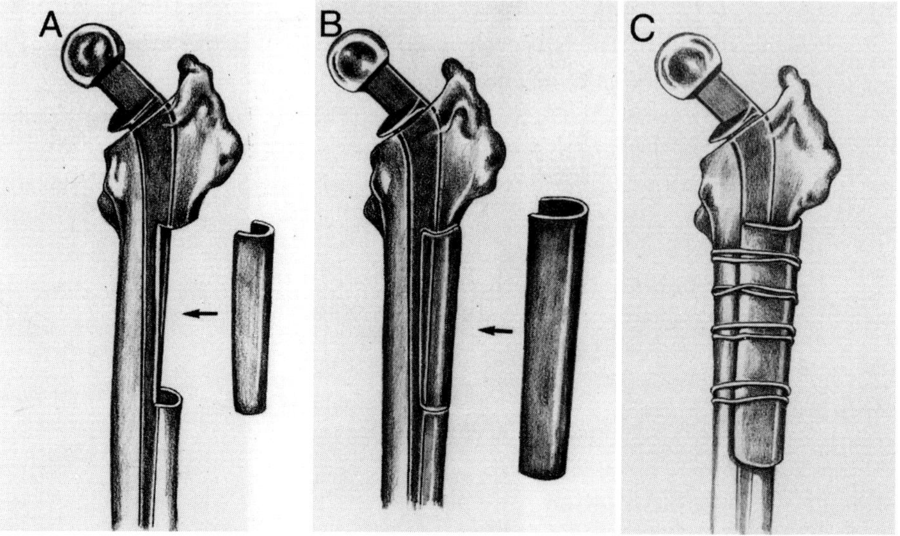

FIGURE 9.

Cortical strut allograft. **A,** a window has been cut in the femur for cement removal. **B,** a cortical strut allograft is used to reinforce the weakened part of the femur. **C,** the cortical strut held in place by cerclage wires.

tografted by bone that was reamed out or by other host bone that is available. The residual host proximal femur is wrapped around the allograft and held by cerclage wires. An attempt is made to bring these vascularized pieces distally to wrap around the osteotomy junction to encourage union.

We attempt to obtain a press-fit of the long-stem femoral component, but this is not crucial for success because once union is achieved at the osteotomy and the implant is cemented to the allograft, the femoral reconstruction is stabilized. It is our opinion that bone ingrowth is impossible to obtain in these multiply revised femoral reconstructions and, therefore, porous coating on the femoral component is not necessary. The implant is always cemented to the allograft (Fig 8). Cortical strut allografts are used to reinforce windows or stress risers or may be used to stabilize osteotomy or allograft host junctions. They are wired into place and if possible their ends are autografted to encourage union to host bone (Fig 9).

PRINCIPLES OF SURGERY FOR FEMORAL GRAFTING (TABLE 3)

1. Use a wide exposure. Trochanteric osteotomy and reflection of the vastus lateralis off the anterior part of the femur offer the best and safest exposure. Do not hesitate to use windows to facilitate cement removal and safe controlled reaming. If a circumferential graft is to be used, the residual host femur should be split and used as a vascularized wrap around the graft to encourage allograft host union and strengthen the allograft. Do not sacrifice or devascularize host bone for this reason.
2. The implant should be cemented into the allograft but not into the host. Cement strengthens the graft and theoretically delays vascularization and membrane formation. Grafts should be longer than 3 cm.
3. Rigid fixation must be achieved between the allograft and host.
4. Autograft the allograft-host junction.
5. Do not use structural circumferential grafts unless necessary, but if necessary, use strong young bone.
6. Do not drill holes into the allograft except for trochanteric attachment.

RESULTS

In an earlier study of our proximal femoral grafts, evaluation was carried out clinically and radiologically.[65] A modified Harris scoring system[63]

TABLE 3.
Femoral Side Defects and Reconstruction

Defect	Reconstruction
Cavitary	Intraluminal graft with a long-stem press-fit femoral component or a cemented femoral component
Structural	*Noncylindrical:* Cortical strut graft
	Cylindrical: Proximal femoral allograft with a cemented femoral component; cement may be used in the allograft but not in the host

(see Table 2) was used, with failure of the procedure being defined as (1) failure to improve the hip score by at least 20 points and (2) the need for any further surgery related to the allograft.

In this study there were 32 calcar grafts (less than 3 cm in length) with an average follow-up of 4.36 years; 16 had uncemented implants and 16 had cemented implants. We found that although these grafts seem to do well clinically, there was an unacceptable rate of implant subsidence (43%) and resorption (over 50%) in 40% of the grafts that had uncemented implants. The calcar grafts did much better when they were cemented, which lessened the incidence of resorption to 10%.[65] We, however, now believe that there is no real indication for a graft less than 3 cm in length because that amount of length can be compensated for by the implant. When, however, short grafts are necessary, they should be cemented by following the same principles as those for long grafts.

The 40 hips in which large-fragment grafts were used had an average preoperative score of 30.5 (range, 6 to 58) and an average postoperative score of 65.8 (range, 21 to 100)—an average improvement of 35.3. The average follow-up was 36.6 months (range, 29 to 83).

The average length of these grafts was 10.4 cm (range, 3.5 to 17).

Radiographic evaluation was possible in only 37 of the 40 hips because 3 failed shortly after surgery. There was evidence of union between the allograft and the host bone in 30 of these 37 hips (81%). Bone bridging across a persistent defect was seen in 3 (8%). Stable nonunion occurred in 1 (3%) and unstable nonunion in 3 (8%).

One 4-cm-long graft fragmented, but resportion was not seen. In 4 hips (11%) there was subsidence ranging from 0.5 to 1.5 cm (average, 1). Gross failure of the construct did not occur.

In the 24 hips that had trochanteric osteotomies, bony radiologic union occurred in 9 (38%) and stable fibrous union in 10 (42%). In 5 hips the trochanter displaced more than 1 cm.

In four hips the score failed to increase postoperatively by 20 points. These included one patient with chronic pain and venous insufficiency who subsequently underwent hip disarticulation and one case of symptomatic nonunion.

Four patients underwent resection arthroplasty, three for deep infection and one for recurrent dislocation. The latter patient had spina bifida and paralytic hip dysplasia.

There was one death caused by laceration of the external iliac vein during acetabular reconstruction.

The overall success rate was 80%. However, if two patients with high postoperative hip scores who also had high preoperative score were regarded as successful, the rate improves to 85% (Fig 10).

Seven cortical strut grafts were also evaluated as part of that study.[65] They all united and remodeled. There was no subsidence of any prosthesis nor any graft structural failure. One patient failed to increase his score by 20 points, for a success rate of 86% (Fig 11).

As of July 1, 1993, 235 proximal femoral allografts have been used for revision arthroplasty of the hip with an average follow-up of 4.36 years (range, 1 to 10). One hundred seventy-six grafts were cylindrical, 51 were cortical struts, and 8 were intraluminal. Of the cylindrical grafts, 32 were calcar grafts (less than 3 cm in length) and 144 were longer than 3 cm in length.

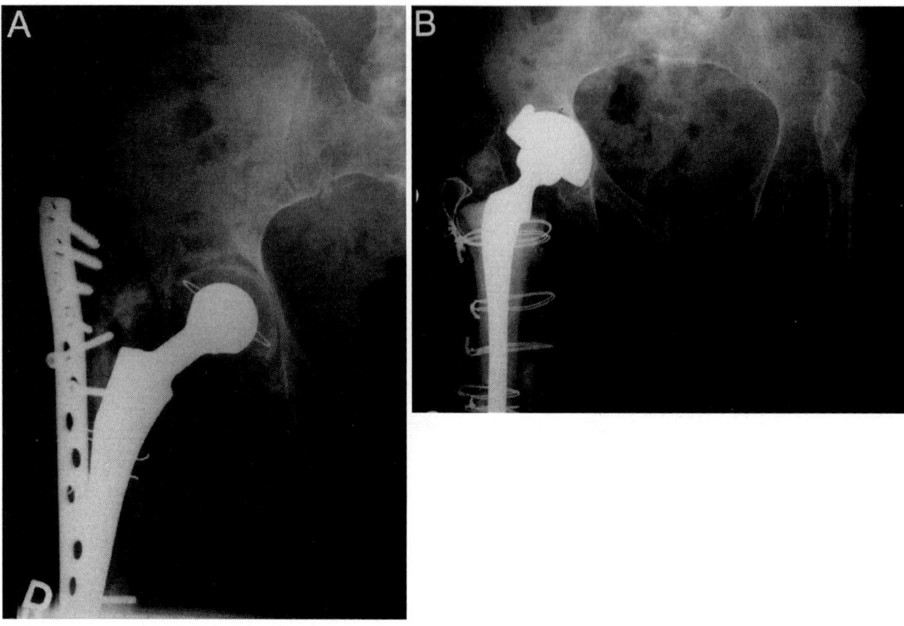

FIGURE 10.
Proximal femoral allograft. **A,** preoperative radiograph of a 55-year-old male with severe loss of proximal femoral bone stock and a loose cemented femoral component. **B,** 7 years after reconstruction of the femur with a proximal femoral allograft. The implant is cemented to the allograft but not to the host. Residual host proximal femur has been wrapped around the allograft, particularly at the junction of the host and allograft. The trochanter has a stable fibrous union.

At present, all of our femoral grafts are longer than 3 cm and are simply called large-fragment proximal femoral allografts. Of the 235 proximal femoral grafts including the calcar grafts, at an average follow-up of 4.36 years there have been 17 revisions for a revision rate of 7%. Four femoral allografts required plating and bone grafting for nonunion (all larger grafts). One calcar graft was revised because of resorption, and 2 calcar grafts required revision for loose implants. Two femoral allografts were revised for infection, 7 for dislocation, and 1 for pain (all large proximal femoral grafts). All revisions were successful.

COMPLICATIONS

As of July 1, 1993, in our entire group of revisions requiring allograft bone (384 hips in 357 patients), the following complications occurred. There were 26 dislocations (6.8%), with 18 requiring further surgery. There have been 10 infections (2.6%), with 3 requiring excision arthroplasty. Two were revised and 5 left with a draining sinus. There have been 4 vascular complications, including 1 intraoperative death. There have been 6 excision arthroplasties, 3 for infection, 1 for recurrent dislocation, and 2 for displacement of pelvic allografts. There have been 5 nerve injuries, with 3 recovering spontaneously, 1 requiring surgical repair, and 1 pending conservative treatment. There have been 5 deaths, 3 unrelated, 1 from an intraoperative external iliac vein laceration, and 1 from intraoperative fat embolism. There has been 1 amputation for pain.

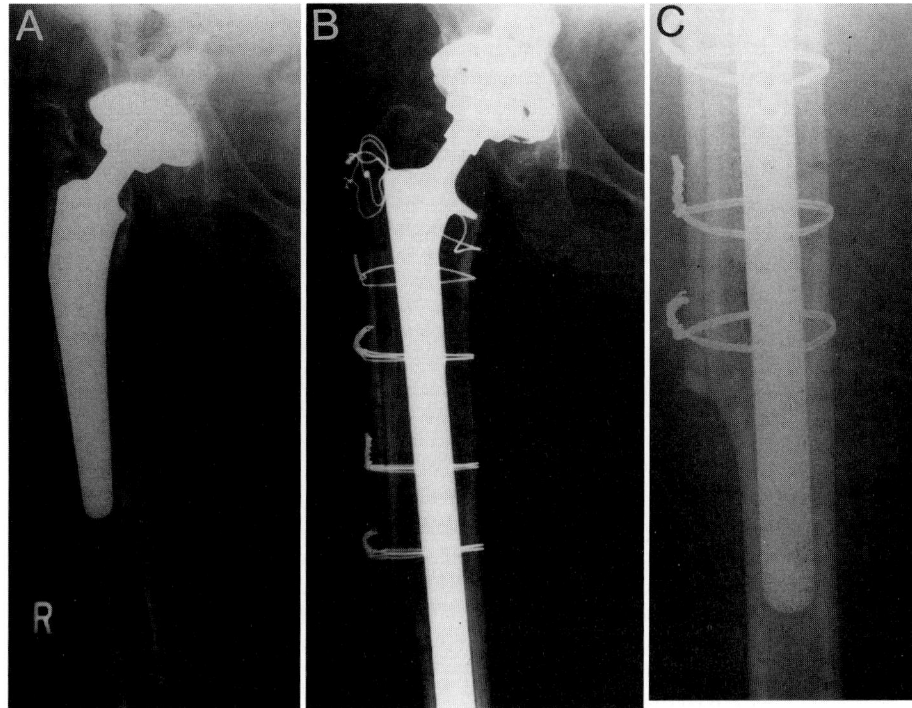

FIGURE 11.

Cortical strut allograft. **A,** preoperative radiograph of a 60-year-old male with a loose cemented femoral component and loss of lateral femoral cortex. **B** and **C,** appearance 3 months postoperatively. The revision was done with a long-stem press fit femoral component and a cortical strut allograft to reinforce the lateral femoral cortex.

CONCLUSIONS

Morsellized autograft and allograft bone should not be used for early primary support of an implant in order to avoid migration and subsidence.

If, however, the graft is protected by surrounding cortical bone (contained cavitary defect) or by an extension of the implant (roof reinforcement ring, collared femoral components), it will remodel and become stronger.

Bulk autografts and allografts used to provide support for acetabular components are very effective if the graft involves less than 50% of the acetabulum (minor column or shelf grafts).

They can be used with cemented or uncemented cups. Fixation should be provided by obliquely to vertically placed screws and supplemented by a flying buttress graft.

Bulk allografts involving more than 50% of the acetabulum (major column grafts) have a high failure rate but restore bone stock and thus make revision possible.

Strong cortical bone and good fixation should improve the long-term results. Cemented cups should be used.

A high hip center is acceptable if good bone stock is available without indiscriminate sacrifice of anatomy and leg length.

Femoral bulk grafts are effective and provide good long-term results.

The femoral implant should be cemented to the allograft but not to the host. Careful attention must be paid to the graft-host junction (rigid fixation via a step-cut and cerclage wire plus an autograft for union).

REFERENCES

1. Freeman MAR, Bradley GW, Revell PA: Observations upon the interface between bone and polymethylmethacrylate cement. *J Bone Joint Surg Br* 64:489, 1982.
2. Goldring SR, Schiller AI, Roelke MS, et al: Formation of a synovial-like membrane at the bone cement interface. *Arthritis Rheum* 29:836, 1986.
3. Goldring SR, Schiller AL, Roelke M, et al: The synovial-like membrane at the bone cement interface in loose total hip replacements and its proposed role in bone lysis. *J Bone Joint Surg Am* 65:575, 1983.
4. Goodman SB, Schatzker J, Summer-Smith G, et al: The effect of polymethylmethacrylate on bone; an experimental study. *Arch Orthop Trauma Surg* 104:150, 1985.
5. Howie D, Oakeshott R, Manthy B, et al: Bone resorption in the presence of polyethylene wear particles. *J Bone Joint Surg Br* 69:165, 1987.
6. Jasty MJ, Floyd WE, Schiller AL, et al: Localized osteolysis in stable, nonseptic total hip replacement. *J Bone Joint Surg Am* 68:912, 1986.
7. Linder L, Lindberg L, Carlsson A: Aseptic loosening of hip prostheses. *Clin Orthop* 175:93, 1983.
8. Pazzaglia UE, Ceciliani L, Wilkinson MJ, et al: Involvement of metal particles in loosening of metal-plastic total hip prostheses. *Arch Orthop Trauma Surg* 104:164, 1985.
9. Revell PA, Weightman B, Freeman MAR, et al: The production and biology of polyethylene wear debris. *Arch Orthop Trauma Surg* 91:167, 1978.
10. Schmalzried P, Jasty M, Harris WH: Periprosthetic bone loss in total hip arthroplasty. *J Bone Joint Surg Am* 74:849–863, 1992.
11. Maloney WJ, Jasty M, Harris WH, et al: Endosteal erosion in association with stable uncemented femoral components. *J Bone Joint Surg Am* 72:1025–1034, 1990.
12. Harris WH, White RE Jr: Resection arthroplasty for non-septic failure of total hip arthroplasty. *Clin Orthop* 171:62, 1982.
13. Grauer JD, Amstutz HC, O'Carroll F, et al: Resection arthroplasty of the hip. *J Bone Joint Surg Am* 71:669–678, 1989.
14. Kostuik J, Alexander D: Arthrodesis for failed arthroplasty of the hip. *Clin Orthop* 188:173–182, 1984.
15. Chao EYS, Sim FH: Composite fixation of salvage prostheses for the hip and the knee. *Clin Orthop* 276:91, 1992.
16. Unwin PS, Cobb JP, Walker PS: Distal femoral arthroplasty using custom-made prostheses: The first 218 cases. *J Arthroplasty* 8:259–268, 1993.
17. Blunn GW, Hua J, Wait ME, et al: Correlation of stress distribution with bony remodelling in retrieved femora with proximal femoral replacement, in Brown K (ed): *Complications of Limb Salvage: Prevention, Management and Outcome.* Montreal, International Society of Limb Salvage, 1991, pp 445–450.
18. Markel MD, Gottsauner-Wolf F, Rock MG, et al: A mechanical comparison of six methods of proximal femoral replacement, in Brown K (ed): *Complications of Limb Salvage.* Montreal, International Society of Limb Salvage, 1991, pp 75–80.
19. Zehr RJ, Heare T, Enneking WF, et al: Allograft prosthesis composite vs. megaprosthesis in proximal femoral reconstruction, in Brown K (ed): *Complications of Limb Salvage.* Montreal, International Society of Limb Salvage, 1991, pp 91–103.

20. Unwin PS, Cobb JP, Walker PS, et al: Loosening in cemented femoral prostheses: A study of 668 tumour cases, in Brown K (ed): *Complications of Limb Salvage*. Montreal, International Society of Limb Salvage, 1991, pp 133–137.
21. Wipperman B, Zwipp H, Sturm J, et al: Complications of endoprosthetic proximal femoral replacement, in Brown K (ed): *Complications of Limb Salvage*. Montreal, International Society of Limb Salvage, 1991, pp 143–146.
22. Mowe JC (ed): *Standards for Tissue Banking*. Arlington, Va, American Association of Tissue Banks, 1984. Revision 1985, 1987, 1988.
23. Jacobs NJ: Establishing a surgical bone bank, in Fawcett KJ, Barr AR (eds): *Tissue Banking*. Arlington, Va, American Association of Tissue Banks, 1987, pp 67–96.
24. Czitrom A, Gross A, Langer F, et al: Bone banks and allografts in community practice. *Instr Course Lect* 37:24–31, 1988.
25. Oakeshott RD, Morgan DAF, Zukor DJ, et al: Revision total hip arthroplasty with osseous allograft reconstruction. *Clin Orthop* 225:37–61, 1987.
26. Oakeshott RD, McAuley JP, Gross AE, et al: Allograft reconstruction in revision total hip surgery, in Aebi M, Regazzoni P (eds): *Bone Transplantation*. Berlin, Springer-Verlag, 1989, pp 265–273.
27. Gustilo RD, Pasternak HS: Revision total hip arthroplasty with a titanium ingrowth prosthesis and bone grafting for failed cemented femoral component loosening. *Clin Orthop* 235:111–119, 1988.
28. D'Antonio JA, Capello WN, Borden LS: Classification and management of acetabular abnormalities in total hip arthroplasty. *Clin Orthop* 243:126–137, 1989.
29. Judet R, Judet J, Letournel E: Fractures of the acetabulum: Classification and surgical approaches for open reduction. *J Bone Joint Surg Am* 46:1615–1646, 1964.
30. Harris WH, Krushell RJ, Galante JO: Results of cementless revisions of total hip arthroplasties using the Harris-Galante prosthesis. *Clin Orthop* 235:120–126, 1988.
31. Estok DM, Harris WH: Long term results of cemented femoral revision using second generation techniques: An average 11% year follow-up evaluation. *Clin Orthop* 299:190–203, 1994.
32. Gross AE, Lavoie MV, McDermott AGP, et al: The use of allograft bone in revision of total hip arthroplasty. *Clin Orthop* 197:115, 1985.
33. Amstutz HC, Ma S, Jinnah RH: Revision of aseptic loose total hip arthroplasties. *Clin Orthop* 170:21–33, 1982.
34. Callaghan JJ, Salvati EA, Pellicci PM, et al: Results of revision for mechanical failure after cemented total hip replacement, 1979 to 1982: A two to five year follow-up. *J Bone Joint Surg Am* 67:1074–1085, 1985.
35. Emerson RH Jr, Head WC, Berklacich FM, et al: Noncemented acetabular revision arthroplasty using allograft bone. *Clin Orthop* 249:30–43, 1989.
36. Engh CA, Glassman AH, Griffin WL, et al: Results of cementless revision for failed cemented total hip arthroplasty. *Clin Orthop* 235:91–110, 1988.
37. Fuchs MD, Salvati EA, Wilson PD Jr, et al: Results of acetabular revisions with newer cement techniques. *Orthop Clin North Am* 19:649–655, 1988.
38. Hedley AK, Gruen TA, Ruoff DP: Revision of failed total hip arthroplasties with uncemented porous-coated anatomic components. *Clin Orthop* 235:75–90, 1988.
39. Hunter GA, Welsh RP, Cameron HU, et al: The results of revision of total hip arthroplasty. *J Bone Joint Surg Br* 61:419–421, 1979.
40. Kavanagh BE, Ilstrup DM, Fitzgerald RH Jr: Revision total hip arthroplasty. *J Bone Joint Surg Am* 67:517–526, 1985.
41. Pellicci PM, Wilson PD Jr, Sledge CB, et al: Revision total hip arthroplasty. *Clin Orthop* 170:34–41, 1982.

42. Pellicci PM, Wilson PD Jr, Sledge CB, et al: Long-term results of revision total hip replacement. A follow-up report. *J Bone Joint Surg Am* 67:513–516, 1985.
43. Wilson-MacDonald J, Morscher E, Masar Z: Cementless uncoated polyethylene acetabular components in total hip replacement. A review of five to 10 year results. *J Bone Joint Surg* 72:423–430, 1990.
44. Pierson JL, Harris WH: Cemented revision for femoral osteolysis in cemented arthroplasties. *J Bone Joint Surg Br* 76:40–44, 1994.
45. Russotti GM, Harris WH: Proximal placement of the acetabular component in total hip arthroplasty. A long-term follow-up study. *J Bone Joint Surg Am* 73:587–592, 1991.
46. Bargar WM: Personal communication, Nov 1993.
47. Gross AE: Revision arthroplasty of the hip using allograft bone, in Czitrom AA, Gross AE (eds): *Allografts in Orthopaedic Practice*. Baltimore, Williams & Wilkins, 1992, pp 147–173.
48. Chao EYS, Ivins JC: The design and application, in *Tumour Prostheses for Bone and Joint Reconstruction*. New York, Thieme-Stratton, 1983, p 335.
49. Barrack RL, Harris WH: The value of aspiration of the hip joint before revision total hip arthroplasty. *J Bone Joint Surg Am* 75:66–76, 1993.
50. Gristina AG, Kolkin J: Current concepts review: Total joint replacement and sepsis. *J Bone Joint Surg Am* 65:128–134, 1983.
51. Johnson JA, Christie MJ, Sandler MP, et al: Detection of occult infection following total joint arthroplasty using sequential technetium-99m HDP bone scintigraphy and indium-111 WBC imaging. *J Nucl Med* 29:1347–1353, 1988.
52. Padgett DE, Kull L, Rosenberg A, et al: Revision of the acetabular component without cement after total hip arthroplasty. *J Bone Joint Surg Am* 75:663–673, 1993.
53. Gie GA, Linder L, Ling RSM, et al: Impacted cancellous allografts and cement for revision total hip arthroplasty. *J Bone Joint Surg Br* 75:14–21, 1993.
54. Gie GA, Linder L, Ling RSM, et al: Contained morsellized allograft in revision total hip arthroplasty: Surgical techniques. *Orthop Clin North Am* 24:717–727, 1993.
55. Bargar WL, Murzic WJ, Taylor JK, et al: Management of bone loss in revision total hip arthroplasty using custom cementless femoral components. *J Arthroplasty* 8:245–252, 1993.
56. Czitrom AA: Immunology of bone and cartilage allografts, in Czitrom AA, Gross AE (eds): *Allografts in Orthopaedic Practice*. Baltimore, Williams & Wilkins, 1992, pp 15–25.
57. Langer F, Czitrom A, Pritzker KP, et al: The immunogenicity of fresh and frozen allogeneic bone. *J Bone Joint Surg Am* 57:216, 1975.
58. Czitrom A, Gross A, Langer F, et al: Bone banks and allografts in community practice. *Instr Course Lect* 37:13–24, 1988.
59. Goldberg VM, Stevenson S: Biology of bone and cartilage allografts, in Czitrom AA, Gross AE (eds): *Allografts in Orthopaedic Practice*. Baltimore, Williams & Wilkins, 1992, pp 1–13.
60. Jasty M, Harris WH: Salvage total hip reconstruction in patients with major acetabular bone deficiency using structural femoral head allografts. *J Bone Joint Surg Br* 72:63, 1990.
61. Hardinge K: The direct lateral approach to the hip. *J Bone Joint Surg Br* 64:17–19, 1982.
62. Allan GD, Butuk D, Gross AE: Morsellized allograft reconstruction of contained cavitary defects in revision total hip arthroplasty. *Orthop Trans* 15:821, 1991.
63. Harris WH: Traumatic arthritis of the hip after dislocation and acetabular frac-

tures: Treatment by mold arthroplasty. An end result study using a new method of result evaluation. *J Bone Joint Surg Am* 51:737, 1969.
64. Gross AE, Allen DG: Revision arthroplasty using allograft bone. *Instr Course Lect* 42:363–380, 1993.
65. Allen DG, Lavoie GJ, McDonald S, et al: Proximal femoral allografts in revision hip arthroplasty. *J Bone Joint Surg Br* 73:235–238, 1991.

Endoprosthetic Reconstruction for Malignant Bone Tumors and Nonmalignant Tumorous Conditions of Bone

Jeffrey J. Eckardt, M.D.
Professor, Department of Orthopaedic Surgery, Chief of Section of Orthopaedic Oncology, University of California, Los Angeles, UCLA School of Medicine, Los Angeles, California

Rong-Sen Yang, M.D., Ph.D.
Visiting International Fellow of Orthopaedic Surgery, Section of Orthopaedic Oncology, University of California, Los Angeles, UCLA School of Medicine, Los Angeles, California

William G. Ward, M.D.
Assistant Professor, Department of Orthopaedic Surgery, Bowman Grey Medical Center, Winston-Salem, North Carolina

Cynthia Kelly, M.D.
Fellow of Orthopaedic Surgery, Section of Orthopaedic Oncology, University of California, Los Angeles, UCLA School of Medicine, Los Angeles, California

Frederick R. Eilber, M.D.
Professor of Surgery, Chief of the Division of Surgical Oncology, University of California, Los Angeles, UCLA School of Medicine, Los Angeles, California

---

Over the past two decades, numerous limb salvage protocols have evolved in conjunction with chemotherapy and radiation therapy adjuvant treatments for malignant bone tumors.[1–16] All of the limb salvage alternatives have been advanced as preferable to amputation as a means of local control of the primary malignant tumor. They have proved to be safe in terms of low risk of local recurrence and are cost-effective as well. Alternative means of extremity reconstruction include resection arthrodesis, allograft, allograft prosthetic composite, endoprosthetic replacement, vascularized autograft reconstruction, rotation-plasty, and in some instances, allograft reconstruction with subsequent Ilizarov leg lengthening.[4–12, 17–41]

The rationale for the use of custom-designed metallic endoprostheses is that they avoid the potential biological hazards of bacterial and viral transmission of disease, they avoid the need for host bone allograft

Advances in Operative Orthopaedics, vol. 3

osteosynthesis, they permit immediate rigorous rehabilitation, and they have proved to provide a durable and functional limb that is relatively complication free within the first 5 to 10 years, during which time a significant number of patients with primary malignant bone tumors will succumb to disease.* Because of the good success seen with endoprosthetic reconstruction in patients with malignant bone tumors, indications have also been defined for their use in selected patients with aggressive or multiply recurrent benign bone tumors, metastatic bone tumors, soft tissues sarcomas involving bone, and occasionally, failed primary joint replacement or chronic nonunions recalcitrant to multiple operative procedures, internal fixation, and bone grafting.[6–9, 11, 18–20, 31, 44]

RATIONALE FOR ENDOPROSTHETIC RECONSTRUCTION IN PATIENTS WITH PRIMARY MALIGNANT BONE TUMORS

Although the survival rate for patients with primary malignant bone tumors has increased greatly over the past two decades secondary to the use of adjuvant and neoadjuvant chemotherapy and radiation therapy protocols, these patients are still at risk for significant mortality within the first 5 to 10 years. Although individual institutions have reported 5-year survival rates for patients with stage IIB osteosarcomas to be as high as 80%, the national average, in reality, is only 50% to 65%.[2, 4, 10–14, 16, 17] Endoprosthetic reconstruction is therefore especially useful in those individuals who ultimately succumb to disease because the reconstructions have proved to have minimal complications during the first 5 to 10 years. Local recurrence, deep wound infections, and soft tissue healing problems are common to all types of limb salvage procedures and are a result of either poor operative planning or poor execution of the operation itself. Major soft tissue healing problems these days should be infrequent with the understanding and the facilities now available with either rotation flaps or free flaps in those instances in which significant soft tissue needs to be removed with the tumor.[9, 42, 45–48] In addition, it has become quite clear that neoadjuvant programs allow us to get closer to the tumor than previously appreciated and that preoperative studies, especially magnetic resonance imaging (MRI), show us the exact level of the tumor within the bone, therefore permitting closer resections. The end result is more retained muscle and bone, which should result in a better long-term functional result.[49–53]

Over the past 20 years there has been an evolution in understanding of the biomechanics and manufacturing techniques for endoprostheses so that now there are modular systems that can be easily modified for each individual situation in both the upper and lower extremity. The basic principles include the following: a rotating hinge knee for distal femoral, proximal tibial, and total femur replacements; a bipolar cup at the hip if at all possible; an anterior bow on femoral stems for proximal femoral replacements and distal femoral replacements; careful attention at the soft tissue reconstruction about the shoulder to prevent dislocation of shoul-

*References 6–9, 11, 18–20, 31, 32, 42, 43.

TABLE 1.
Indications for Endoprosthetic Reconstruction for Musculoskeletal Tumors (Between December 1980 and June 1994, UCLA)*

Indications	Number	Percent
Primary malignant bone tumors	248	73
Primary aggressive benign bone tumors	12	4
Metastatic bone tumors	18	5
Soft tissue sarcoma involving bone	6	2
Failed total joint replacement or endoprosthetic replacement	41	12
Chronic fracture/nonunion, failed open reduction–internal fixation	17	5

*Primary endoprosthetic replacement, 301; revision, 41.

der prostheses and proximal humeral and total humeral endoprostheses; and incorporation of extramedullary porous ingrowth material for soft tissue attachment to not only enhance strength but also seal off the prosthesis-bone junction, which may prevent wear debris from the joint surface from getting to the bone-cement interface and potentially causing osteolysis and radiolucent lines that may go on to aseptic loosening.*

Irrespective of the advances that have been made in the understanding of both endoprosthetic reconstruction and/or allograft reconstruction, the three basic principles and goals of limb salvage should always be kept in mind. The first is that the local recurrence rate with limb salvage procedures should be no greater than that with amputation. The second is that the limb salvage procedure should not in any way delay the administration of additional adjuvant therapy, thereby putting the patient's life in jeopardy. The third is that the reconstruction should be enduring and not be associated with a large number of local complications, thus requiring multiple revisional surgeries and frequent hospitalizations within the first 5 to 10 years.

With the present success of endoprostheses for primary malignant bone tumors involving long bones in the extremities, the indications for endoprosthetic reconstruction have been extended to include the following: special cases of metastatic disease in which conventional means of internal fixation with polymethyl methacrylate may not be satisfactory; unusual or difficult multiply recurrent or late-presenting large stage III benign bone tumors; difficult and recalcitrant nonunions in elderly, osteoporotic patients, especially in the supracondylar area of the femur; and occasional instances in which soft tissues sarcomas abut and/or erode into the bone, thereby necessitating bone resection along with the soft tissue resection (Table 1).[6–9, 11, 18–20, 31, 44]

In general, the longer the patient's life expectancy, the greater attention must be paid to design of the intramedullary stems and preparation

*References 6–9, 11, 18–20, 31, 32, 43, 54, 55.

TABLE 2.
Contraindications to Endoprosthetic Reconstruction for Musculoskeletal Tumors

Contraindications
Pathologic fracture with a huge hematoma extending beyond the compartment boundary
Inappropriately performed biopsy or improperly placed biopsy site
Biopsy site complication: severe infection, large hematoma, etc.
Poor soft tissue condition after chemotherapy or radiation therapy
Encasement of the major neurovascular structure by tumors
Poor responder to adjuvant chemotherapy or radiation therapy

of the medullary canals. This is especially true for patients with parosteal osteosarcomas and those patients with difficult-to-treat and/or multiply recurrent stage III benign tumors of bone. For patients with metastatic disease and recalcitrant nonunion problems, off-the-shelf modular systems may in fact be satisfactory as long as there is an adequate variety of lengths and diameters of intramedullary stems that would include an anterior bow for femoral prostheses.

There are a few situations in which endoprosthetic replacement is contraindicated (Table 2). Endoprosthetic reconstruction is not appropriate for patients with (1) a displaced pathologic fracture and a huge hematoma extending beyond the compartment boundary; (2) inappropriately performed biopsy or biopsy site; (3) biopsy site complication, e.g., severe infection, large hematoma; (4) poor soft tissue condition after chemotherapy or radiation therapy; (5) encasement of the major neurovascular structure by tumor; and (6) poor response to adjuvant chemotherapy or radiation therapy.

PREOPERATIVE PLANNING

Plain radiographs, computed tomography (CT) scans, and MRI of the lesion as well as scanograms of the involved bone are all that is necessary for preoperative planning for reconstruction of the appendicular skeleton once it has been determined that limb salvage surgery is to be undertaken.[49–53] Magnetic resonance imaging is especially useful in showing the soft tissue extension, which ideally will be diminished in size by the neoadjuvant treatments. It will also show quite dramatically the extent of tumor within the bony canal and therefore permit accurate levels of resection that should be several centimeters above and below the lesion. Magnetic resonance imaging may also visualize a skip metastasis[49–52, 56] and can provide continuous follow-up assessment of the tumor bed after adjuvant chemotherapy or radiation therapy or detection of local recurrence after limb salvage surgery.

Computed tomography corroborates this information and also gives information regarding cortical bony destruction. Furthermore, CT can help detect lung metastasis. Multiplanar and three-dimensional CT scans also provide a better evaluation of lesions and help in planning the surgical resection and/or radiation therapy protocols.[53] Scanograms, which are full-length radiographs with a millimeter-for-millimeter reproduction of the anteroposterior and medial-lateral projections of the bone, can then be used to design the prosthesis. Technetium 99 bone scanning should not be forgotten because it will pick up skip metastases as well as the metastatic bony disease seen in both osteosarcoma and Ewing sarcoma of bone.[57]

Biopsy of bone tumor lesions is very important in the differential diagnosis and is usually an essential step for surgical staging and for the development of an appropriate treatment plan.[57–61] The biopsy findings are related to further management of the tumor. An inappropriate biopsy site, poorly performed biopsy, or biopsy-related complications may make the limb salvage procedure infeasible and compromise the survival outcomes of patients. For those patients with lesions that are probably malignant, they should be referred to an experienced musculoskeletal oncologist for biopsy, additional diagnostic studies, and definite treatment.[57–59]

PROSTHETIC DESIGN CONSIDERATIONS

Considerations involved in prosthetic design include the optimal prosthesis size (diameter and length), material for the prosthesis, methods of fixation, manufacturing processing, and the shape of the prosthesis. The requirements for design of a tumor prosthesis are more complex than the conventional ones. An ideal tumor prosthesis must be able to provide adequate range of motion for daily living activities and also be compatible with the remaining soft tissue restraints after wide resection of the tumor. The prosthesis should be easy to revise if failure occurs. In addition, most patients have received chemotherapy and radiation therapy, so adequate wound coverage is an important issue.

The intramedullary stems of the present modular endoprosthetic systems are forged and therefore stronger than the previously made single-piece–cast endoprostheses. However, they still need to maintain a sufficient diameter to avoid fatigue fracture. For distal femoral and proximal femoral replacements, the stems should be 14 to 18 mm in diameter; they should be 125 to 150 mm in length for a distal femur prosthesis and 135 to 200 mm for a proximal femur prosthesis wherever possible. For proximal tibial replacements, the intramedullary stems should be at least 100 to 125 mm in length and 10 to 15 mm in diameter. For a humeral endoprosthesis, although the length may be shortened dramatically depending on the amount of bone stock left, the intramedullary stem should approach 10 to 11 mm in diameter if possible. For the ulnar component of a distal humerus replacement or total humerus replacement, the intramedullary stem should be 70 to 80 mm in length, but the diameter is dependent on the size of the medullary canal. Humeral, tibial, and ulnar stems can be straight, but femoral stems need to be bowed. This allows for better fit and fill. For rare situations with a short stem in the distal femur prosthesis or humerus prosthesis, additional cross-pin fixation is used to secure the fixation and prevent rotation (Table 3). Small stems with large cement mantels can go on to loosen or experience fatigue fracture irrespective of their location, even in the humerus.

TABLE 3.
Principles of Tumor Endoprosthesis Designs

Stem Site	Length, mm	Diameter, mm	Extramedullary Coating	Cross-Pin Fixation	Shape
Proximal femur	135–200	14–18	+	–	Bowed
Distal femur	125–150	14–18	+	+*	Bowed
Proximal tibia	100–125	10–15	+	–	Straight
Humerus	Variable†	10–11	+	+‡	Straight
Ulna of DHR/THR§	70–80	Variable	–	–	Straight

*For a very proximal femoral lesion with a stump 4 cm or less from the lesser trochanter.
†At least 4.5 cm in length.
‡For a very distal humerus lesion with a stem 4.5 cm or less.
§DHR = distal humerus replacement; THR = total humerus replacement.

The size of the humeral head bears special comment. The conventional total shoulder replacement uses a larger humeral head if the rotator cuff is nonexistent or deficient. However, the humeral head of a tumor prosthesis should be smaller because the soft tissue coverage can be difficult. In general, a humeral head 40 mm in diameter permits satisfactory articulation with the glenoid in all adolescent and adult situations. Smaller humeral heads with an expandable endoprosthesis are needed for the pediatric age group.

The design of a scapula prosthesis includes large fenestrations to decrease prosthesis weight and permit better scarring of the underlying serratus anterior and the remnants of subscapularis to the overlying infraspinatus, teres minor, and teres major. The latissimus dorsi can be rotated to give additional soft tissue coverage to maintain stability. The scapula prosthetic design also includes a hooded glenoid component to help with shoulder stability in this unconstrained total shoulder scapular endoprosthesis. There are prosthetic designs that are constrained. Humeral heads come in four sizes, 40, 44, 48, and 52 mm, and are matched to the radius of the hooded glenoid surface. The prosthetic scapula does not have a coracoid process, which would potentially impinge on the brachial plexus, and the scapular spine can be reduced in size or eliminated to permit better soft tissue coverage.

A rotating hinge knee is the desired knee mechanism for distal femoral replacement, proximal tibial replacement, and total femur replacement. Wherever possible, bipolar cups should be used for proximal femoral and total femur replacements because instability can be a significant problem with total hip replacements. In 15 years the authors have not had to convert a bipolar proximal femoral replacement to a total femur replacement because of acetabular wear.

It has become clear that extramedullary porous ingrowth material has multiple functions. At the junction of the segment in the stem, a circumferential 360-degree ring of porous ingrowth material will allow for soft tissue ingrowth and therefore effectively isolate the joint space with the metallic and polyethylene debris and the activated macrophages and ideally avoid loosening and osteolysis of the prosthesis.[55] Porous ingrowth material in the area of the tibial tubercle and the greater trochanter of the hip and over the greater tuberosity of the humerus also enhances soft tissue ingrowth. In general, however, function is quite good because a pseudocapsule forms around the prosthesis and the soft tissues are sutured out to length to their respective fascia. Then they will scar down to the pseudocapsule about the prosthesis, pull through that pseudocapsule, and effectively move the limb through space.[8, 9, 18–20, 55]

It is not necessary to recreate the exact anatomy that has been removed. In general, an endoprosthesis smaller in diameter but exact in length will enhance soft tissue closure without adversely affecting function. The length of the extremity should be the same in order to maintain optimal muscle fiber length. This is especially true at the knee and at the proximal end of the humerus.

The longevity of prostheses about the knee is commonly understood in part to be related to the amount of resection in an inverse manner, i.e., the greater the amount of resection, the greater likelihood that there be a revision because of aseptic loosening or fatigue fracture. For a patient with a large distal femoral replacement in which the osteotomy is above the

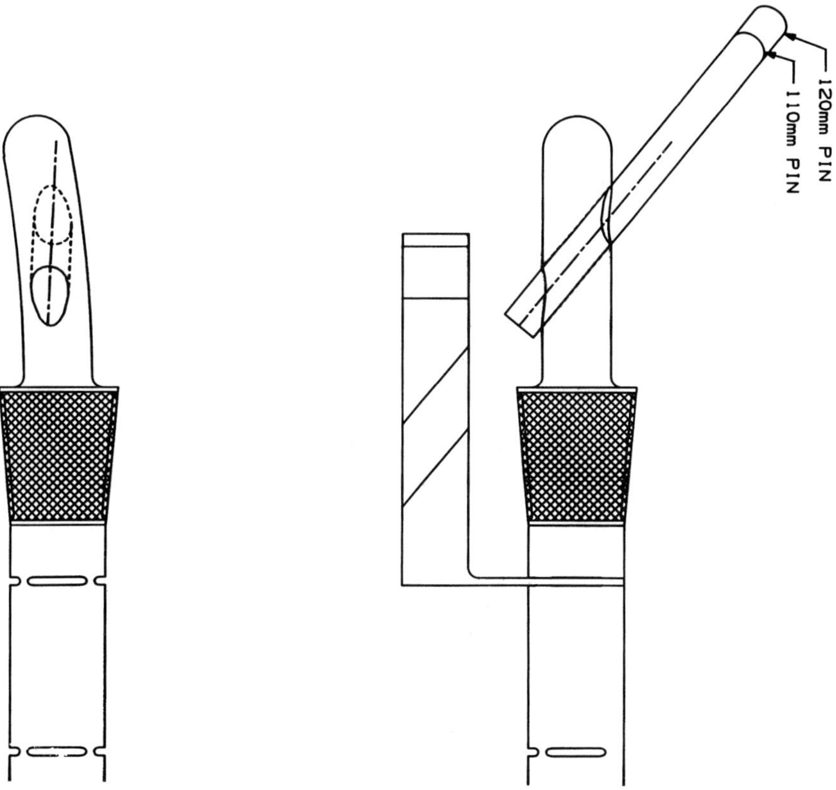

FIGURE 1.
Anteroposterior and lateral views of the cross-pin and guide for a modular distal femoral endoprosthesis.

mid-diaphysis of the femur and/or close to the lesser trochanter, a large, straight intra-medullary or slightly bowed stem with a cross-pin through the stem into the femoral head and neck can add to the rotational stability of the construct (Fig 1). This requires very careful preoperative planning to ensure leg length equality, which should always be within 0.5 cm. This particular technique is also useful for cases needing revision because of aseptic loosening or stem fracture. In general, however, if the patient requires a high osteotomy of the femur, then consideration for initial cross-pin fixation into the femoral neck and head should be considered as part of the initial reconstruction.

SURGICAL APPROACH

The surgical approach for resection to be followed by endoprosthetic reconstruction is similar to that of other limb salvage procedures. Longitudinal incisions are made, and in general, it is our practice to make the incisions along the neurovascular bundles of the extremity.* In the lower extremities it would be a medial incision for distal femoral replacements and proximal tibial replacements. For proximal femoral replacements, the incision starts at the anterior-superior iliac spine and goes to the trochanter and then laterally down the leg. This is the only situation in which neurovascular dissection is not carried out. For upper extremity and scapular incisions, the starting place is at the clavicle, and the incision passes over the coracoid process and down the medial aspect of the arm to the elbow joint, where the brachial vessels and median and ulnar nerves can be easily identified. The vessels of the upper extremity and lower extremity are identified and dissected free, with all the vessels heading toward the involved bone tied before being cut. This not only cuts down on blood loss but also makes the remaining portions of the resection easier. Tourniquets are not generally used in any of the resections. Biopsy sites are ellipsed and kept in continuity with the underlying bone, and if placed laterally on the distal end of the femur, then only skin and subcutaneous tissue can be closed because an attempt to close the fascia will result in lateral subluxation of the patella.[7, 8, 18, 19]

The amount of soft tissue taken with the tumor in part depends on the nature of the tumor and the presumed effectiveness of the neoadjuvant treatment that has been administered. If the patient has had a good clinical response with a decrease in pain, a decrease in size of the mass, and/or calcification of the soft tissue component with decreasing intensity on various types of bone scanning, then one can come quite close to the tumor without fear of getting a local recurrence. If, on the other hand, there has been a poor clinical response and radiograph studies suggest that there has been a poor response, then either a wider resection must be done or an amputation considered. Before the advent of preoperative neoadjuvant chemotherapy, limb salvage surgeons were required out of necessity to take large portions of muscle and/or entire muscle bellies, which is now no longer thought to be necessary.

*References 3–5, 8, 9, 18–20, 32, 44, 54, 55.

For a total scapula and total shoulder replacement, the concept of a shoulder reconstruction is to create a stable shoulder construct to make the arm and forearm more effective so that the patients can get their hand to their face for activities of daily living. By lateralizing the humerus, any retained muscles will function better than if allowed to contract as with a scapulectomy or, even more severely, with a Tikhoff-Linberg type of resection. The muscles are carefully balanced during reconstruction to ensure stability (Fig 2).

For proximal humeral and total humerus replacements, special attention needs to be focused on securing the humeral head and neck to the glenoid area for intra-articular resections. Wherever possible, the glenoid and labrum should be maintained. If adequate rotator cuff is available, then a 5-mm Merseling tape may be used to go circumferentially around the humeral neck and through the labrum to secure it to the glenoid to prevent anterior, posterior, superior, and inferior subluxation. When little rotator cuff remains for soft tissue coverage, then a 40-mm Dacron aortic graft can be used to secure the humeral head. In general, a 40-mm humeral head diameter is all that is necessary to enhance soft tissue closure, and there is no advantage to using a larger head. The largest size of Dacron aortic graft is also 40 mm and can just stretch over a 40-mm endoprosthetic head (Fig 3, A to E).

For total humeral and distal humeral replacements, there are three types of olecranon fixations. The first is to excise the olecranon and cement the ulnar stem directly into the ulnar canal (Fig 4, A). Although this simplifies the operative procedure, patients frequently complain of sensitivity over the area where a bursa forms around the prosthesis. If the olecranon can be retained and excavated so that the ulnar component can be slipped into the proximal end of the ulna, then the olecranon area

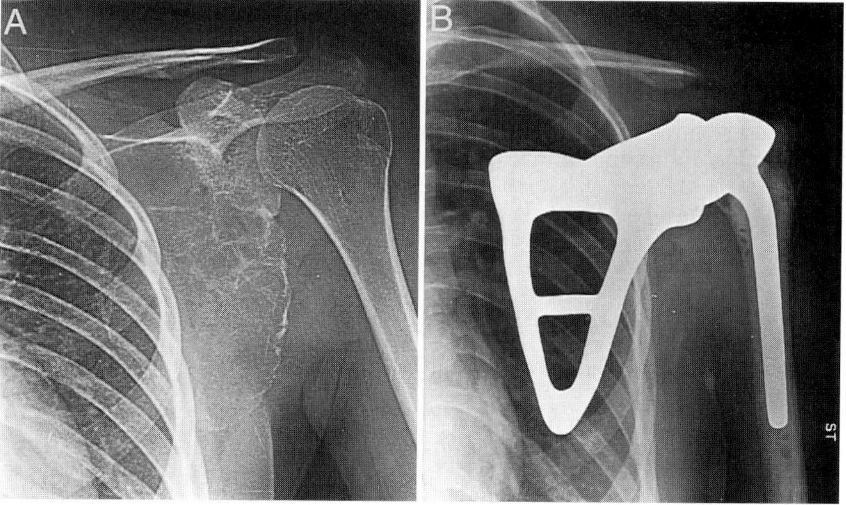

FIGURE 2.

A, anteroposterior radiograph of the left shoulder of a patient with an Ewing sarcoma of the scapula. **B,** anteroposterior radiograph following total scapular replacement.

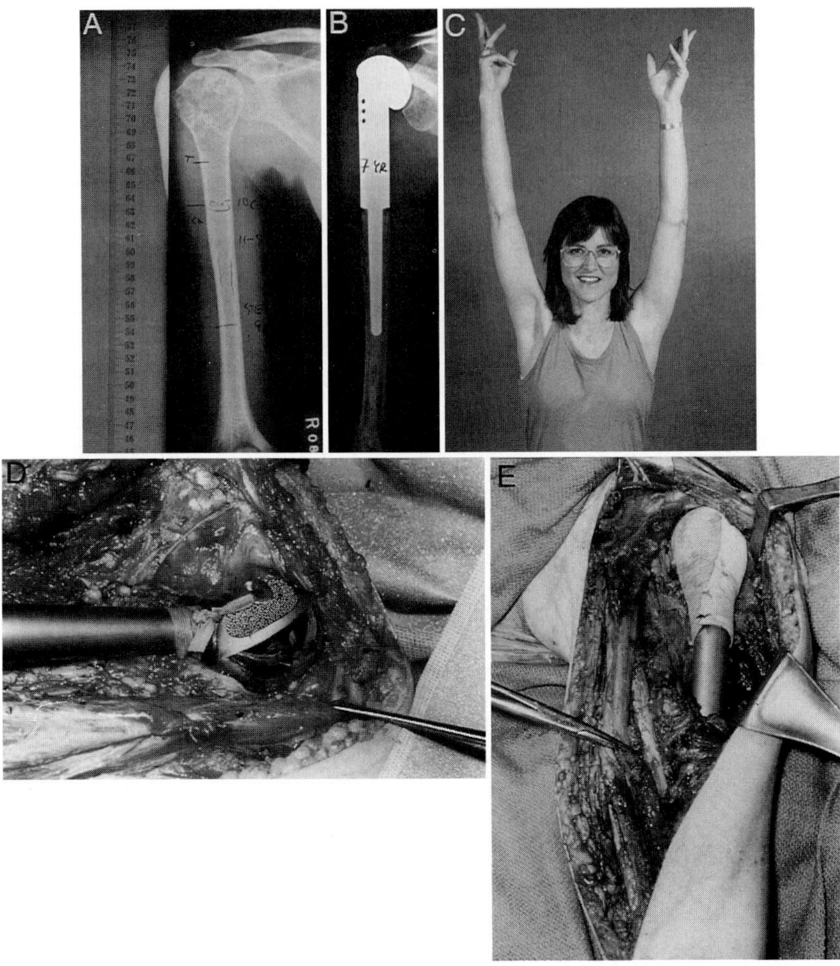

FIGURE 3.

A and **B,** composite anteroposterior scanogram of the proximal portion of the humerus showing the prosthetic design considerations and 7-year follow-up. **C,** the clinical follow-up in this situation is quite good because the rotator cuff and deltoid muscle could be retained. **D,** proximal humeral replacement with a 5-mm Merceling tape wrapped circumferentially through the glenoid and labrum around the neck to prevent subluxation. **E,** a 40-mm Dacron aortic graft sutured to the glenoid and around the proximal portion of the humerus to prevent dislocation in cases in which the rotator cuff is completely removed. This adds stability and prevents dislocation.

is protected and additional strength is maintained by better attachment of the triceps (Fig 4, B). For patients who are skeletally immature, no ulnar component is necessary and a simple condylar design that fits into the patient's olecranon can be stabilized by a pursestring soft tissue closure around it. Prolonged immobilization is unnecessary because this will lead to permanent flexion contracture of the elbow (Fig 4, C).

For a proximal femoral replacement, it is important to ream the femoral canal to maximize fit and fill. Occasionally a cement restrictor can be used, although many times it is not functional because of the distal level

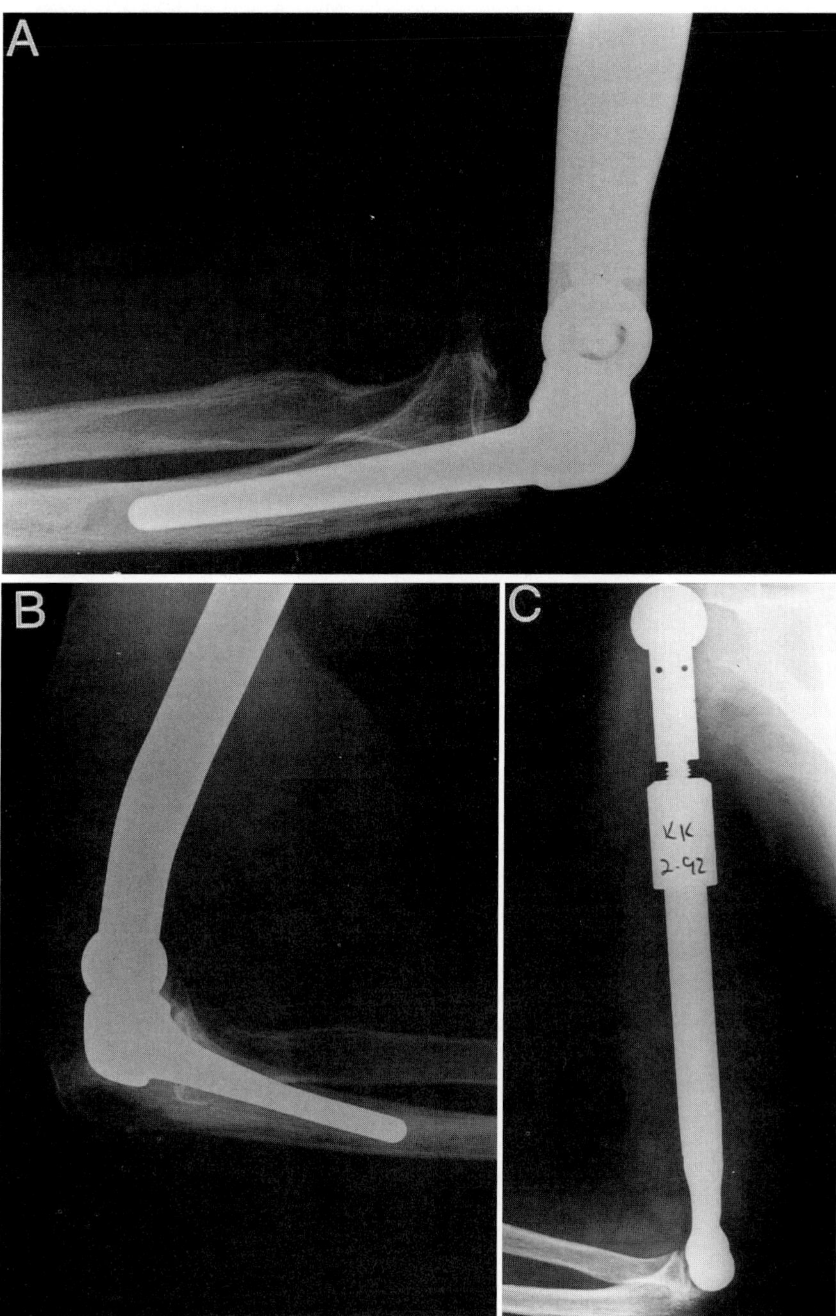

FIGURE 4.

A, distal humeral replacement implanted following resection of the olecranon. This tends to result in a painful bursa over the prosthesis. **B,** anteroposterior and lateral diagrammatic representation of a distal humeral replacement. **C,** distal humeral replacement implanted with retention of the olecranon, which gives better triceps strength and minimal symptoms at the elbow.

of the resection or because the distal tip of the prosthesis is being cemented into the distal metaphysis. The femoral head is sized to accept the appropriate bipolar component. The key to soft tissue reconstruction is to pull all remaining muscles out to length and then suture them to each other and/or their respective fasciae so that they scar in at their normal length and not in a contracted position (Fig 5, A to C).

For a distal femoral replacement, an intra-articular resection can almost always be performed. The tibial and patellar components are cemented first, followed by the femoral component (Fig 6). The rotation of the prosthesis needs to be carefully aligned to avoid excessive external or internal rotation. The soft tissue reconstruction should be carefully done with constant monitoring of the tracking of the patellar tendon. The joint capsule is brought down and sutured to the soft tissues around the proximal end of the tibia and to the mobilized sartorius to get complete muscular closure of the remnants of the vastus medialis to the sartorius medially (Fig 7, A to D).

Total femur and intercalary femoral reconstructions are less frequent than proximal femur and distal femur reconstructions (Fig 8, A and B). Occasionally, the femoral diaphysis is involved with tumor but enough bone remains proximally and distally to allow fixation of the metal prosthesis. Cross-pins through the proximal or distal stem are sometimes necessary to secure rotatory fixation because the stems are short and cemented into the metadiaphyseal areas and, therefore, three-point fixation is not possible. Patients with intercalary femurs will generally have excellent function because the hip and knee are not involved and their motion should be normal except in those instances of Ewing sarcoma where patients receive adjuvant radiation therapy in addition to neoadjuvant chemotherapy, which tends to produce soft tissue fibrosis and limited motion.

For a proximal tibial tumor, medial gastrocnemius muscle flap cov-

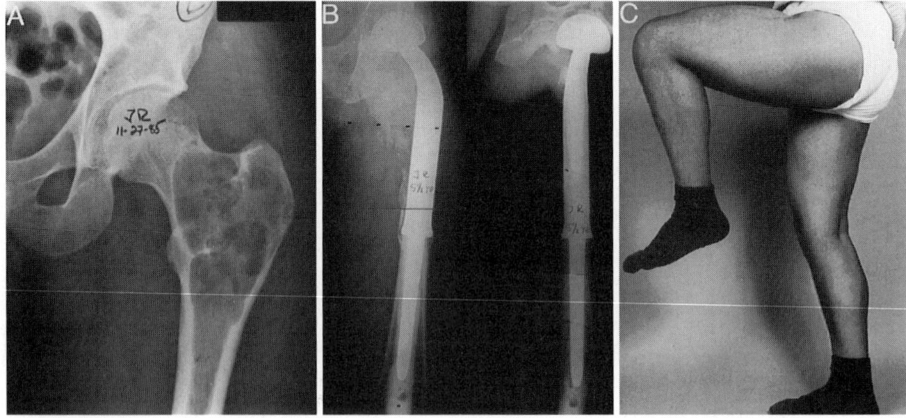

FIGURE 5.

A, anteroposterior radiograph of a chondrosarcoma in the proximal end of the femur. **B,** composite anteroposterior and lateral radiograph 5½ years following proximal femoral replacement with a single-piece proximal femoral replacement. **C,** clinical photograph of the excellent function obtained with proximal femoral replacement. Soft tissue reconstruction must be meticulous in order to achieve this type of functional result.

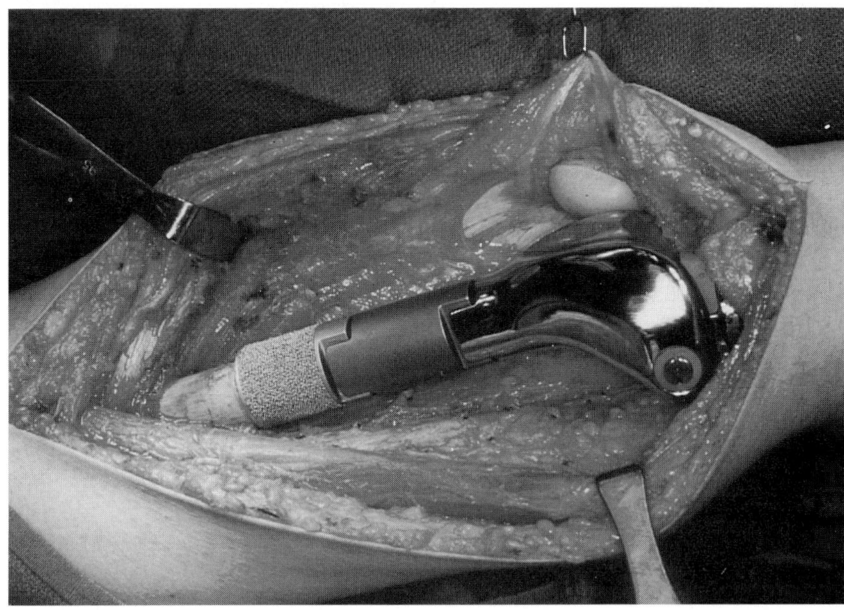

FIGURE 6.

Intraoperative photograph of a new modular distal femoral replacement. The patella and the tibial surfaces are resurfaced with polyethylene components. A circumferential porous ring aids in soft tissue ingrowth to isolate the joint space with the polyethylene and metal debris from reaching the prosthesis-bone-cement interface.

erage technique is very important (Fig 9, A). It is unrealistic to believe that the patellar tendon, even if lengthy, can adhere to a metal prosthesis, although the advent of porous ingrowth material may enhance or permit some direct fixation to the proximal part of the tibia. The transposed medial gastrocnemius flap initially introduced by Jean Dubousset in 1983 has been a great advance permitting proximal tibial reconstruction and limb salvage in many instances that would normally result in amputation.[9, 46, 48] Because the medial gastrocnemius flap is transposed, there is generally larger bulk in the upper part of the leg than before the resection. This necessitates the routine use of a skin graft because of the tissues excised during the biopsy. If the tumor in the proximal portion of the tibia is medial, then the anterior tibial artery along with the proximal part of the fibula can be retained, and dissection on the lateral portion of the tibia can be subperiosteal. On the other hand, if the tumor involves the proximal end of the tibia in a global manner or is laterally placed, then frequently the anterior tibial artery needs to be taken in conjunction with the proximal part of the fibula in order to achieve an oncologic margin (see Fig 9, B and C).

Endoprosthetic replacement of the pelvis has been infrequently done and is generally best limited to tumors involving the immediate periacetabular area. Gradinger[62] has described extensive pelvic constructions. These are technically demanding procedures associated with prolonged operating time, voluminous amounts of blood transfusion, and many perioperative problems. It is not clear that the advantages outweigh the disadvantages, but it is clear that fixation is difficult to achieve because

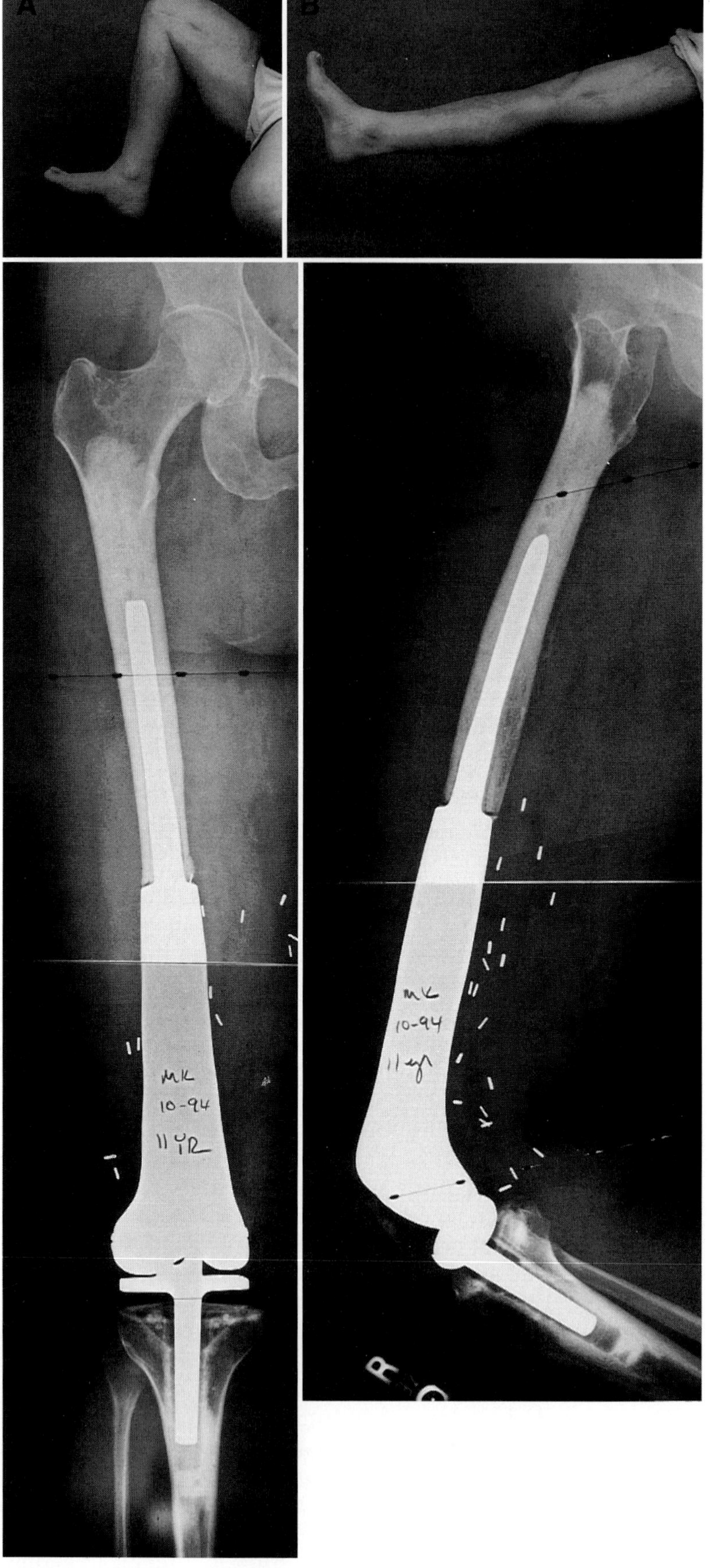
A
B
MK
10-94
11 YR
MK
10-94

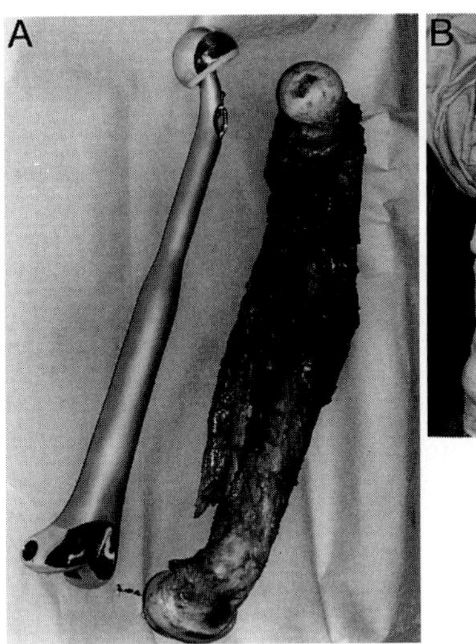

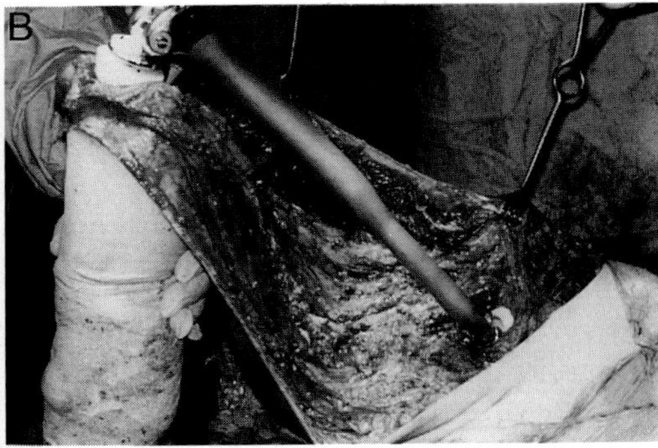

FIGURE 8.

A, intraoperative photograph of a total femur replacement alongside a femur resected for osteosarcoma. **B,** intraoperative view of the total femur replacement in position with a bipolar cup proximally and a rotating hinge knee distally. Function following total femur replacement is more variable because the hip and the knee have to be rehabilitated simultaneously.

most of the rules of rigid internal fixation are violated because of a lack of substantial bone into which to fix screws, plates, or other fixation devices. We have generally been quite pleased with the flail hip or internal hemipelvectomy type of resection for tumors of the hemipelvis. Even when the entire iliac wing is resected and the femur is left articulating to a small portion of acetabulum, function is quite superb and bone graft struts have not been presumed to have been useful.

Patients are treated with prophylactic antibiotics, with the initial dose of cephalosporin given in the operating room before the incision. The patients are continued on a regimen of intravenous antibiotics for approximately 3 to 4 days until the drains are removed. Children and adolescents generally do not receive anticoagulation, although adults and especially those with a predisposing propensity for thrombophlebitis or pulmonary emboli receive anticoagulation with warfarin (Coumadin) postoperatively.

POSTOPERATIVE REGIMEN

SHOULDER

The postoperative regimen varies with the anatomic area. For total scapula, total shoulder, proximal humeral, and total humeral replace-

FIGURE 7.

A–D, clinical photographs and anteroposterior and lateral radiographs of the knee and the total femur of a patient 11 years after distal femoral replacement for chondrosarcoma. There has been no loosening at the bone-cement interface either at the tibia, the femur, or the patella.

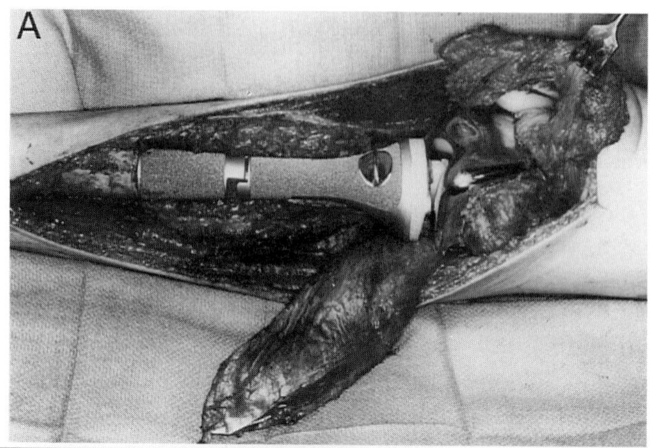

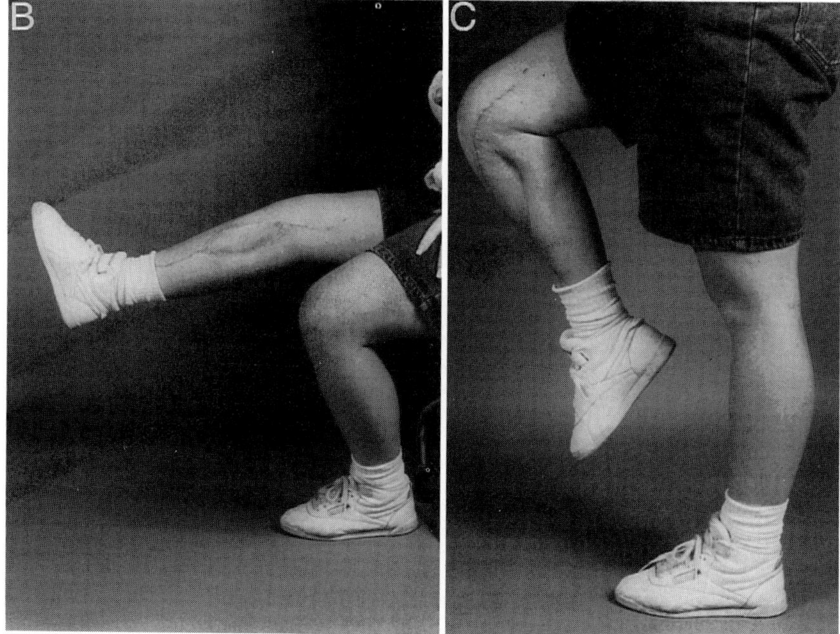

FIGURE 9.
A, intraoperative photograph of a current modular proximal tibial replacement with a medial gastrocnemius flap mobilized for subsequent coverage over the top of the prosthesis, which is then sutured into the patellar tendon and joint capsule. **B** and **C,** anticipated function following proximal tibial replacement. Most patients can achieve nearly full extension, with an average lag of 15 degrees being normal. Note the skin graft.

ments, the patients are kept in an abduction bolster for 3 weeks and then a sling for 3 weeks before commencing range-of-motion exercises of the shoulder. This is done to allow for scarring of the soft tissue reconstructions about the shoulder. Hand, forearm, and elbow range-of-motion exercises and therapy can be begun immediately after surgery. Three weeks following surgery, the patients are switched from an abduction bolster to a sling, where they are kept for an additional 3 weeks. Three weeks from the time of surgery, active and passive range of motion and motor strengthening about the shoulder can be begun. The final Musculoskeletal Tumor Society functional rating for shoulder and proximal humeral reconstructions is totally dependent on the amount of soft tissue resected. If the rotator cuff and the deltoid with the axillary nerve are removed, then the best that can be hoped for is a stable construct that permits good function of the elbow to get the hand to the face for activities of daily living. Occasionally, an excellent result can be obtained if the tumor is totally confined to bone and the majority of the rotator cuff and deltoid can be retained (see Fig 3, C).

The final functional result for total scapula and total shoulder replacement is quite variable, again depending on the amount of muscle resected and the amount of innervated muscle retained. In general, we have been satisfied with a nonconstrained total scapula/total shoulder replacement, which has cosmetic and functional advantages.

ELBOW

Elbow rehabilitation for total and distal humerus replacement is begun immediately. Sling immobilization of the elbow is used only for approximately 3 weeks. Supination, pronation, and hand exercises are begun immediately following surgery, with active elbow flexion and extension permitted at 3 weeks. Prolonged immobilization of the elbow will result in a fixed elbow flexion contracture. Even children who do not have an ulnar component that extends into the proximal part of the ulna but only have an articulating ulnar component can begin therapy at 3 weeks. The soft tissue pursestring closure around the distal humeral component and into the proximal end of the ulna is more than satisfactory at stabilizing the elbow joint.

In general, the Musculoskeletal Tumor Society functional result rating for distal humeral replacements is excellent in that patients can achieve full extension and flexion to 110 degrees or greater and have normal supination and pronation.

HIP

Patients undergoing proximal femoral replacement require 2 to 4 weeks of bed rest in hip abduction to permit the soft tissues to satisfactorily heal. Careful attention needs to be addressed to the soft tissue reconstruction, where all the remaining muscles are pulled out to length and sutured to each other in an effort to obtain complete muscular closure over the prosthesis. Should all the hip abductors need to be resected as part of the reconstruction, then an alternative means of limb salvage reconstruction should be considered because an endoprosthetic reconstruction will be quite unsatisfactory, fair at best and likely to be a poor result. After 2 to 4 weeks of bed rest and hip abduction, the patients are allowed up in a hip abduction brace for possibly a hip-knee-ankle-foot orthosis, depending on the patient's reliability, the amount of soft tissue resected, and the surgeon's feeling on how securely the reconstruction has been accomplished. Rehabilitation of total femoral replacements is prolonged. Patients are required to wear a hip abduction brace for approximately 3 months and will require active organized physical therapy for 6 to 12 months in order to maximize the functional outcome. The great majority of patients, especially younger patients, should be able to ambulate without a cane or a crutch. A Trendelenburg gait or abductor lurch can be seen in some patients, but generally only at the end of the day (see Fig 5, C). Elderly patients will likely require the use of a cane for stability since they are generally unable to rehabilitate themselves to an ambulatory aid–free status.

The Musculoskeletal Tumor Society functional rating for proximal femoral replacements is generally good. This is because some patients will have an abductor gait and/or require an ambulatory aid.

KNEE

Patients with distal femoral replacements are placed in a continuous pressure motion (CPM) machine in the recovery room, with knee flexion to 35 degrees and going to full extension. They are kept in this position for 3 to 4 days, and progressive knee flexion is begun so that by the time patients leave the hospital at 10 days, they have an easy 90 degrees of knee flexion and full passive extension, can perform straight-leg raises 10 times with the knee immobilizer in place, and can ambulate independently on crutches. A soft knee immobilizer is used for ambulation for the first 3 to 4 weeks and then occasionally, a neoprene brace is used, but most individuals can make the transition to just an elastic wrap for several weeks.

The Musculoskeletal Tumor Society functional rating for distal femoral replacements is generally excellent because the great majority of patients achieve 120 degrees of knee flexion and full extension with little or no extensor lag and are ambulatory aid free (see Fig 7, A and B).

Patients with proximal tibial replacements are kept in full extension for a period of 3 to 4 weeks. This is to allow the transferred medial gastrocnemius muscle to heal into the patient's capsule so as to give an anchor for the quadriceps mechanism. Thereafter, the rehabilitation program is the same as that for distal femur replacement.

In general, function following a proximal tibial replacement is good to excellent. Patients generally achieve greater than 90 degrees of flexion, have full passive extension, but may have on average a 15- to 20-degree extensor lag (see Fig 9, B and C). This does not prove to be a significant functional deficit for them, and the patients ambulate quite well. Even a large lag of 70 to 90 degrees is well compensated for by the patient.

When there is minimal proximal and distal femur substance remaining after an oncologic margin taken for a large diaphyseal femoral lesion, then consideration for primary total femur replacement should be entertained. In these instances, the hip and the knee are rehabilitated in much the same way as the proximal and distal portions of the femur as outlined earlier except for the fact that the rehabilitation takes a longer period of time because the patients have to rehabilitate two joints in series. In general, knee function should be good to excellent and hip function should be fair to good. For patients with Ewing sarcoma who received adjuvant radiation therapy in addition to neoadjuvant chemotherapy and were reconstructed with a total femur replacement or intercalary femoral reconstruction, there is generally some stiffness about the knee. However, these patients should be able to achieve 90 degrees of flexion.

DISCUSSION

The experience in this series is based on 342 custom-designed endoprostheses that were implanted into 301 patients at UCLA between December 1980 and June 1994. The location of the reconstruction was the distal end of the femur in 164, the proximal end of the femur in 44, the proximal part of the humerus in 40, the proximal part of the tibia in 29, a total femur in 21, the scapula in 19, a total humerus in 10, an intercalary diaphyseal replacement in 7, the distal end of the humerus including the elbow in 5, and the pelvis in 3. The complications in the UCLA series are shown in Table 4.

Local recurrence of tumor and soft tissue healing problems are the result of either poor operative planning or problems with design of the operative procedure. Deep infection is an operating room contamination problem associated with any limb salvage problem and not particularly inherent in prosthetic reconstructions. The incidence in endoprosthetic reconstruction is presumably less than that with allografts. Endoprostheses do not carry with them the possibility of transmitting bacterial or viral disease unless they are contaminated in the operating theater itself. Transient nerve palsy is occasionally encountered in patients undergoing proximal tibial replacement and distal femoral replacement. All but one have recovered smoothly in this series.

TABLE 4.
Complications of Endoprosthetic Reconstruction for Musculoskeletal Tumors

Complications	Number	Percent
Local recurrence	28/248*	11
Deep infection	13/342†	4
Minor wound dehiscence	10/342	3
Nerve palsy		
Transient	8/342	2.3
Permanent	1/342	0.3
Prosthesis-related complication	39/301‡	13
Aseptic loosening	14/301	5
Prosthetic fatigue fracture	9/301	3
Dislocation/subluxation	9/301	3
Polyethylene failure	7/301	2

*Primary malignant bone tumor: 248.
†Total number of endoprosthetic replacements: primary, 301; revision, 41.
‡Primary endoprosthetic replacement only.

There are, however, a number of problems inherent to endoprosthetic reconstruction, including aseptic loosening, fatigue fracture, dislocation/ subluxation of a component, and mechanical failure including polyethylene failure. Wear debris is a natural phenomenon of all joint replacements and is seen in tumor endoprostheses. The routine use of extramedullary porous ingrowth material may also help prevent wear debris and the activated macrophages that accompany it from getting to the bone prosthesis cement or the bone prosthesis interface and will ideally avoid early osteolysis and loosening. It has been our experience, however, that aseptic loosening and mechanical failure may be corrected by revisional procedures; the patient can return to equal or better function as long as the same reconstructive technique can be employed. Occasionally, patients with failed distal femoral replacements will need their reconstructions to be converted to total femurs, and in that instance, they will experience a decrease in functional ability because they now have a prosthetic proximal femur where before they had their own functioning abductor mechanism and hip. Fatigue fracture has been infrequent in metal components and should be less frequent in the future because of a better understanding of the need for maximizing the diameter of the intramedullary stems and by the use of the forged stems that now accompany most of the modular systems. Dislocation of the hip is an uncommon occurrence with bipolar hip reconstruction as long as careful attention to soft tissue reconstruction is carried out and appropriate protection in the first 3 months following surgery is observed. Dislocation of the proximal humerus reconstruction is again an infrequent occurrence now that standard techniques are available for securing the proximal end of the humerus to the tissues about the glenoid, including 5-mm nonabsorbable tape and 40-mm Dacron aortic grafts.

When used as the means of limb reconstruction for patients with primary malignant bone tumors, endoprostheses have enjoyed good success, and a certain number of these patients will die without needing a major revision in the first 5 to 10 years. Preliminary results show that only about 15% to 20% of prostheses need to be revised during these early years. As more experience is amassed in limb salvage surgeries and a better understanding of the important technical points of the design and implantation of these large metal prostheses is achieved, the long-term results will become better. We have been happy with our past 15-year experience with endoprostheses to the point that alternative reconstructions, including resection arthrodesis, allograft, allograft total joint composites, and rotationplasty, are infrequently done at our institution.

REFERENCES

1. Jaffe N, Frei E III, Traggis D, et al: Adjuvant methotrexate and citrovorum-factor treatment of osteogenic sarcoma. *N Engl J Med* 291:994–997, 1974.
2. Dorfman HD, Czerniak B: Bone cancers. *Cancer* 75(suppl):203–210, 1995.
3. Eilber FR, Eckardt JJ, Morton DL: Advances in the treatment of sarcomas of the extremity: Current status of limb salvage. *Cancer* 54:2695–2701, 1984.
4. Eckardt JJ, Eilber FR, Dorey FJ, et al: The UCLA experience in limb salvage surgery for malignant tumors. *Orthopedics* 8:612–621, 1985.

5. Eckardt JJ, Eilber FR, Grant T, et al: The management of stage IIB osteosarcoma: The experience at the University of California, Los Angeles. *Cancer Treat Symp* 3:117–130, 1985.
6. Eckardt JJ, Eilber FR, Kabo JM, et al: The kinematic rotating hinge knee–distal femoral replacement for tumors of the distal femur. *Orthop Trans* 10:55, 1986.
7. Eckardt JJ, Eilber FR, Kabo JM, et al: Kinematic rotating hinge knee–distal femoral replacement for tumors of the distal femur, in Enneking WF (ed): *The International Symposium on Limb Salvage Surgery and Musculoskeletal Oncology*. New York, Churchill Livingstone, 1987, pp 392–409.
8. Eckardt JJ, Eilber FR, Rosen G, et al: Endoprosthetic replacement for stage IIB osteosarcoma. *Clin Orthop* 270:202–213, 1991.
9. Eckardt JJ, Matthews JG, Eilber FR: Endoprosthetic reconstruction after bone tumor resections of the proximal tibia. *Orthop Clin North Am* 22:149–160, 1991.
10. Bacci G, Picci P, Ferrari S, et al: Primary chemotherapy and delayed surgery for nonmetastatic osteosarcoma of the extremities. Results in 164 patients preoperatively treated with high doses of methotrexate followed by cisplatin and doxorubicin. *Cancer* 72:3227–3238, 1993.
11. Sim FH, Frassica FJ, Miser JS, et al: Current concepts in the evaluation and treatment of osteosarcoma of bone, in Stauffer RN (ed): *Advances in Operative Orthopedics*, vol 1. St Louis, Mosby, 1993, pp 345–366.
12. Winkler K, Bielack SS, Delling G, et al: Treatment of osteosarcoma: Experience of the Cooperative Osteosarcoma Study Group (COSS). *Cancer Treat Res* 62:269–277, 1993.
13. Rosen G, Caparros BI, Huvos AG, et al: Preoperative chemotherapy for osteogenic sarcoma. *Cancer* 49:1221–1230, 1982.
14. Rosen G, Marcove RC, Huvos AG, et al: Primary osteogenic sarcoma: Eight year experience with adjuvant chemotherapy. *J Cancer Res Clin Oncol* 106:55–67, 1983.
15. Eilber FR, Rosen G: Adjuvant chemotherapy for osteosarcoma. *Semin Oncol* 16:312–322, 1989.
16. Tebbi CK, Gaeta J: Osteosarcoma. *Pediatr Ann* 17:285–300, 1988.
17. Delepine N, Delepine G, Desbois JC, et al: Results of multidisciplinary limb salvage in 240 consecutive bone sarcomas. *Biomed Pharmacother* 44:217–224, 1990.
18. Ward WG, Eckardt JJ, Johnston-Jones KS, et al: Five to ten year results of custom endoprosthetic replacement for tumors of the distal femur, in Brown KLB (ed): *Complications of Limb Salvage. The 6th International Symposium on Limb Salvage*. Montreal, ISOLS, 1991, pp 483–491.
19. Ward WG, Eckardt JJ: Endoprosthetic reconstruction of the femur following massive bone reconstructions. *J South Orthop Assoc* 3:108–116, 1994.
20. Ward WG, Dorey FJ, Eckardt JJ: Total femoral endoprosthetic reconstruction. *Clin Orthop* 1995, in press.
21. Cammisa FP, Glasser DB, Phil M, et al: The Van Nes tibial rotationplasty. *J Bone Joint Surg Am* 72:1541–1547, 1990.
22. Van Nes CP: Rotation-plasty for congenital defects of the femur: Making use of the ankle of the shortened limb to control the knee joint of a prosthesis. *J Bone Joint Surg Br* 32:12–16, 1950.
23. Kotz R, Salzer M: Rotation-plasty for childhood osteosarcoma of the distal part of the femur. *J Bone Joint Surg Am* 64:959–969, 1982.
24. Merkel KD, Gebhardt M, Springfield DS: Rotationplasty as a reconstructive operation after tumor resection. *Clin Orthop* 270:231–236, 1991.
25. Gottsauner-Wolf F, Kotz R, Knahr K, et al: Rotationplasty for limb salvage in

the treatment of malignant tumors at the knee. A follow-up study of seventy patients. *J Bone Joint Surg Am* 73:1365–1375, 1991.

26. Krajbich JI: Modified Van Nes rotationplasty in the treatment of neoplasm in the lower extremities of children. *Clin Orthop* 262:74–77, 1991.
27. Mankin HJ, Dopplet S, Tomford WW: The use of frozen cadaveric allografts in the management of patients with bone tumors of the extremities. *Orthop Clin North Am* 18:275–289, 1987.
28. Gebhardt MC, Flugstad DL, Springfield DS, et al: The use of bone allografts for limb salvage in high-grade extremity osteosarcoma. *Clin Orthop* 270:181–196, 1991.
29. Gitelis S, Piasecki P: Allograft prosthetic composite arthroplasty for osteosarcoma and other aggressive bone tumors. *Clin Orthop* 270:197–201, 1991.
30. Alman BA, De Bari A, Krajbich JI: Massive allografts in the treatment of osteosarcoma and Ewing sarcoma in children and adolescents. *J Bone Joint Surg Am* 77:54–63, 1995.
31. Kotz R: Tumor prosthesis in malignant bone tumors. *Orthopade* 22:160–166, 1993.
32. Eckardt JJ, Safran MR, Eilber FR, et al: Expandable endoprosthetic reconstruction of the skeletally immature after malignant bone tumor resection. *Clin Orthop* 297:188–202, 1993.
33. Wood MB, Cooney WP III, Irons GB Jr: Skeletal reconstruction by vascularized bone transfer: Indications and results. *Mayo Clin Proc* 60:729–734, 1985.
34. Sowa DT, Weiland AJ: Clinical applications of vascularized bone autografts. *Orthop Clin North Am* 18:257–273, 1987.
35. Yajima H, Tamai S, Mizumoto S, et al: Vascularized fibular graft for reconstruction after resection of aggressive benign and malignant bone tumors. *Microsurgery* 13:227–233, 1992.
36. Usui M, Ishii S, Naito T, et al: Microsurgical reconstruction in limb-salvage procedures: Comparison between primary and secondary reconstruction. *J Reconstr Microsurg* 9:91–101, 1993.
37. Eilber FR, Morton DL, Eckardt JJ, et al: Limb salvage for skeletal and soft tissue sarcomas—multi-disciplinary preoperative therapy. *Cancer* 53: 2579–2584, 1984.
38. Craig EV, Thompson RC: Management of tumors of the shoulder girdle. *Clin Orthop* 223:94–112, 1987.
39. Sim FH, Beauchamp CP, Chao EY: Reconstruction of musculoskeletal defects about the knee for tumor. *Clin Orthop* 221:188–201, 1987.
40. Malawer MM, Sugarbaker PH, Lampert M, et al: The Tikhoff-Linberg procedures: Report of ten patients and presentation of a modified technique for tumors of the proximal humerus. *Surgery* 97:518–528, 1985.
41. Whitehill R, Wanebo HJ, Mabie KN, et al: Reconstruction after the Tikhoff-Linberg procedure. *Arch Surg* 117:1248–1249, 1982.
42. Horowitz SM, Lane JM, Otis JC, et al: Prosthetic arthroplasty of the knee after resection of sarcoma in the proximal end of the tibia. *J Bone Joint Surg Am* 73:286–293, 1991.
43. Unwin PS, Cobb JP, Walker PS: Distal femoral arthroplasty using custom-made prostheses. The first 218 cases. *J Arthroplasty* 8:259–268, 1993.
44. Freedman EL, Hak DJ, Johnso EE, et al: Total knee replacement including a modular distal femoral component in elderly patients with acute fracture or nonunion. *J Orthop Trauma* 9:231–237, 1995.
45. Quill G, Gitelis S, Morton T, et al: Complications associated with limb salvage for extremity sarcomas and their management. *Clin Orthop* 260: 242–250, 1990.
46. Eckardt JJ, Lesavoy MA, Dubrow TJ, et al: Exposed endoprosthesis: Manage-

ment protocol using muscle and myocutaneous flap coverage. *Clin Orthop* 251:220–229, 1990.

47. Malawer MM, Price WM: Gastrocnemius transposition flap in conjunction with limb-sparing surgery for primary bone sarcoma around the knee. *Plast Reconstr Surg* 73:741–750, 1984.
48. Dubousset J, Missenard G: Reconstruction of quadriceps insertion after proximal tibial replacement in osteogenic sarcoma. Presented at the Second International Workshop on the Design and Application of Tumor Prostheses for Bone and Joint Reconstruction, Vienna, 1983, p 275.
49. Sundaram M, McGuire MH, Herbold DR, et al: Magnetic resonance imaging in planning limb-salvage surgery for primary malignant tumors of bone. *J Bone Joint Surg Am* 68:809–819, 1986.
50. Seeger LL, Eckardt JJ, Bassett LW: Cross-sectional imaging in the evaluation of osteogenic sarcoma: MRI and CT. *Semin Roentgenol* 24:174–184, 1989.
51. Murphy WA: Imaging bone tumors in the 1990s. *Cancer* 67(4 suppl):1169–1176, 1991.
52. Swan JS, Weber DM, Korosec FR, et al: Combined MRI and MRA for limb salvage planning. *J Comput Assist Tomogr* 17:339–342, 1993.
53. Magid D: Two-dimensional and three-dimensional computed tomographic imaging in musculoskeletal tumors. *Radiol Clin North Am* 31:425–447, 1993.
54. Kay RM, Kabo JM, Seeger LL, et al: Hydroxyapatite-coated distal femoral replacements: Preliminary results. *Clin Orthop* 302:92–100, 1994.
55. Ward WG, Johnston KS, Dorey FJ, et al: Extramedullary porous coating to prevent diaphyseal osteolysis and lines around proximal tibial replacements. *J Bone Joint Surg Am* 75:976–987, 1993.
56. Reuther G, Mutschler W: Detection of local recurrent disease in musculoskeletal tumors: Magnetic resonance imaging versus computed tomography. *Skeletal Radiol* 19:85–90, 1990.
57. Simon MA: Current concepts review. Biopsy of musculoskeletal tumors. *J Bone Joint Surg Am* 68:1331–1337, 1986.
58. Simon MA, Biermann JS: Biopsy of bone and soft-tissue lesions. *J Bone Joint Surg Am* 75:616–621, 1993.
59. Simon MA, Finn HA: Diagnostic strategy for bone and soft-tissue tumors. *J Bone Joint Surg Am* 75:622–631, 1993.
60. Enneking WF: Modification of the system for functional evaluation of the surgical management of musculoskeletal tumors, in Enneking WF (ed): *International Symposium on Limb Salvage Surgery and Musculoskeletal Oncology*. New York, Churchill Livingstone, 1987, pp 626–639.
61. Enneking WF: A system of staging musculoskeletal neoplasms. *Clin Orthop* 204:9–24, 1986.
62. Gradinger R, Rechl H, Hipp E: Pelvic osteosarcoma: Resection, reconstruction, local control, and survival statistics. *Clin Orthop* 270:149–157, 1991.

Chondrosarcoma and Its Variants

Michael J. Hejna, M.D., Ph.D.
Department of Orthopaedic Surgery, Rush Medical College of Rush University, Chicago, Illinois

Abid A. Qureshi, M.D.
Department of General Surgery, Rush-Presbyterian-St. Luke's Medical Center, Chicago, Illinois

Joel A. Block, M.D.
Assistant Professor, Departments of Internal Medicine and Biochemistry, Rush Medical College of Rush University, Chicago, Illinois

Steven Gitelis, M.D.
Professor of Orthopaedic Surgery, Director, Section of Orthopaedic Oncology, Department of Orthopaedic Surgery, Rush Medical College of Rush University, Chicago, Illinois

Chondrosarcoma of bone is a rare mesenchymal neoplasm that has been well characterized. There are 500 to 1,000 new cases of chondrosarcoma per year in the United States, and it accounts for between 11%[1] and 14.5%[2] of all malignant bone tumors. Chondrosarcoma is the second most common primary bone tumor, the incidence of osteosarcoma being higher. Although it can occur at any age, it most frequently develops in patients in their fifth and sixth decades. Secondary chondrosarcomas arising within benign enchondromas or osteochondromas usually occur earlier, during the fourth or fifth decades. Chondrosarcomas are distinctly uncommon in children. Those that do occur in children have a relatively poor prognosis.[3–5] The most common sites of occurrence of chondrosarcoma are in the axial skeleton and the proximal portions of the appendicular skeleton. The proximal portions of the femur and humerus, the pelvis, the ribs, and the distal end of the femur are common anatomic locations. More distal locations in the extremities are unusual.

CLINICAL FEATURES

Pain is the most frequent initial complaint in patients with chondrosarcoma of bone. Less commonly the patient may complain of the presence of a mass without pain. Pelvic lesions may become clinically evident as a result of involvement of contiguous nerves, blood vessels, bowel, bladder, or gynecologic structures. Sciatic-type symptoms may be present and result in misdiagnosis if these are assumed to be due to disk pathology. Chondrosarcoma of bone is a relatively slowly growing tumor, and symp-

Advances in Operative Orthopaedics, vol. 3

toms may not arise until late in the course of the disease. The time to clinical symptoms may be prolonged, especially with pelvic lesions, where the tumor can grow to an enormous size before it becomes clinically evident. It is not uncommon that 1 to 2 years may pass before the diagnosis of chondrosarcoma is made.

CLASSIFICATION

CENTRAL CHONDROSARCOMA

Chondrosarcoma of bone is classified according to its location within the bone (central or peripheral) and whether it is a primary or secondary tumor. Primary chondrosarcomas are those that arise de novo within the bone. Secondary chondrosarcomas are those that arise from benign cartilaginous or noncartilaginous lesions. Central chondrosarcomas are generally primary tumors and typically occur in the metaphysis or diaphysis of the long bones and in the pelvis. These tumors tend to be relatively aggressive and are histologically less differentiated than peripheral chondrosarcomas. The bone is frequently expanded with thickening of the surrounding cortex. The tumor may extend within the medullary space well beyond the apparent border on standard radiographs. The tumor may also extend through the cortex into the surrounding soft tissues and make distinction from peripheral chondrosarcoma difficult. Secondary central chondrosarcomas generally result from malignant degeneration of enchondromas, although they have been reported to arise from other benign lesions such as fibrous dysplasia.[6] Malignant degeneration of isolated enchondromas is rare; most secondary central chondrosarcomas occur in the clinical setting of multiple enchondromas. In a series by Dahlin,[7] none of the 59 secondary chondrosarcomas developed in an isolated enchondroma. It has been reported that the risk of malignant transformation in Ollier and Maffucci syndromes is approximately 10% to 20%.[8] Central secondary chondrosarcomas tend to have a good prognosis.[9] Associated epithelial malignancies frequently develop in patients with enchondromatosis.[9]

PERIPHERAL CHONDROSARCOMA

Peripheral (or exostotic) chondrosarcomas are those tumors that arise on the surface of the bone. They are most often secondary malignancies arising from osteochondromas. Osteochondromas are common benign bone tumors that may be seen as isolated lesions or as a hereditary condition of multiple osteochondromas (Fig 1). The lesions may be active during growth of the individual, particularly during adolescence, but typically do not progress after skeletal maturity is reached. The clinical hallmark of malignant degeneration of an osteochondroma is an increase in size of the lesion and the development of pain after skeletal maturity. Thickening of the cartilaginous cap to greater than 1 cm is indicative of malignant degeneration.[10] These tumors tend to be well differentiated and carry a good prognosis. The risk of malignant degeneration of an osteochondroma, whether isolated or in multiple hereditary osteochondromas, is approximately 1% per lesion. In multiple hereditary osteochondromas,

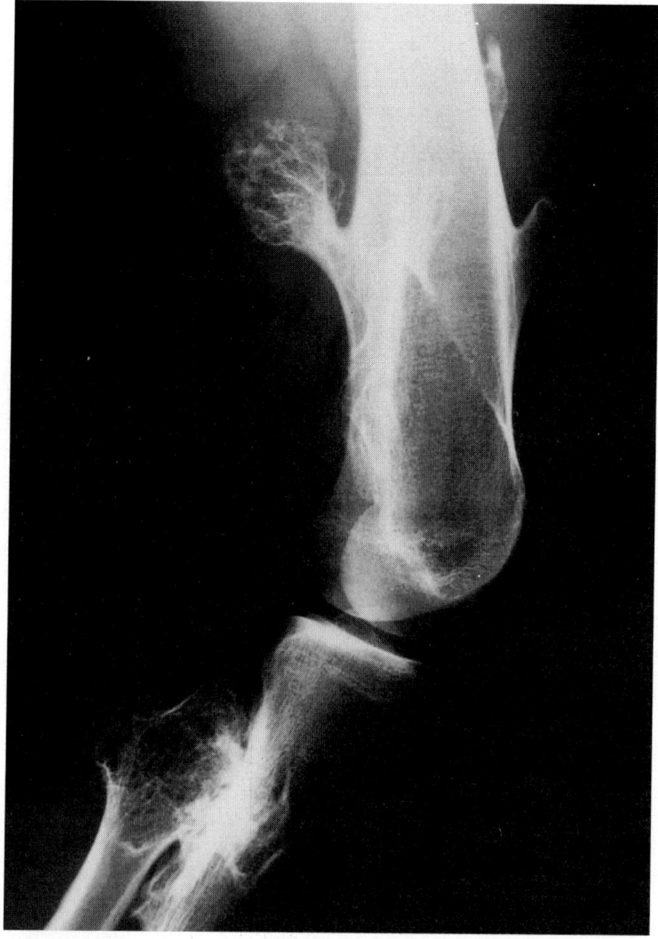

FIGURE 1.

Lateral radiograph of the knee demonstrating multiple hereditary osteochondromas. Note the large pedunculated lesion on the posterior aspect of the distal end of the femur. The development of pain or an increase in size after skeletal maturity suggests malignant degeneration.

where there are usually ten or more lesions, the risk is approximately 10% over the lifetime of the individual. Radiographically, peripheral chondrosarcomas have some features of benign osteochondromas (Fig 2, A to C). They may have an osseous stalk (pedunculated form) or a broad osseous base (sessile form). In both forms a cartilaginous cap exists, and it is the nature of the cap that determines the biology of the sarcoma.

HISTOLOGY AND GRADING

Conventional chondrosarcomas are composed of malignant chondrocytes within an extracellular matrix of type II collagen and aggregating proteoglycan. Histologically, they can be separated into three grades.[2] Histologic grade has been strongly correlated with clinical prognosis.[3, 11] Cytologic features considered in grading chondrosarcomas are overall cellularity,

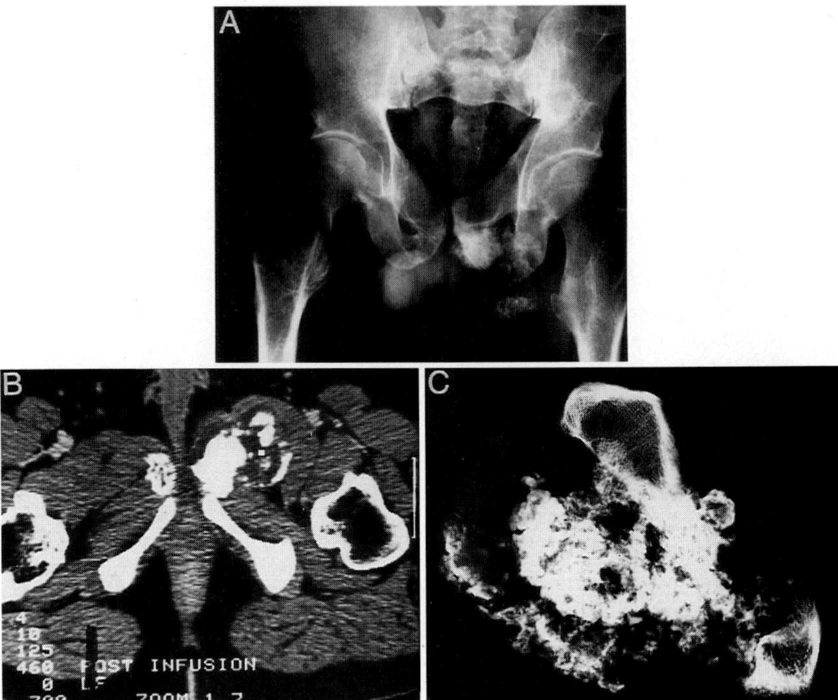

FIGURE 2.

Peripheral chondrosarcoma. **A,** anteroposterior radiograph of the pelvis demonstrating peripheral chondrosarcoma of the ischium. **B,** computed tomographic (CT) scan demonstrating large soft tissue mass on the surface of the ischium with punctate calcification. **C,** specimen radiograph following en bloc resection.

pleomorphism, mitoses, the presence or absence of nucleoli, the presence of binucleate cells, and the degree of myxomatous change.[12, 13] In general, grade 1 chondrosarcomas are extremely well differentiated and contain individual chondrocytes within normal lacunae. Mitotic figures and nuclear pleomorphism are absent. Binucleate cells are rare. The extracellular matrix is abundant and resembles that of normal hyaline cartilage. In contrast, grade 3 chondrosarcomas are hypercellular and demonstrate significant anaplastic features. Mitotic figures may be present but generally do not number greater than three per ten high-power fields. The extracellular matrix may be minimal, and areas of the tumor may be difficult to recognize as cartilaginous. Myxoid areas consisting of stellate cells with interconnecting cell processes within a pale blue–staining background may be present. Grade 2 chondrosarcomas are more cellular and anaplastic than grade 1 tumors but are still fairly well differentiated and recognizable as cartilage.

Histologic evaluation of cartilage-forming tumors is extremely difficult, and the decision as to whether a tumor is benign or malignant should not be made without careful consideration of the clinical features, radiographic characteristics, and gross appearance of the tumor. Periosteal chondromas, which are benign cartilaginous tumors that arise on the surface of long bones, may have cytologic features suggestive of malignancy but have a benign clinical course. Similarly, enchondromas of the hands or feet, especially in Ollier or Maffucci syndromes, may have an aggressive histologic appearance but are clinically benign. In contrast, painful cartilaginous lesions in the upper end of the femur or in the pelvis in adults should be considered malignant until proven otherwise. Central cartilaginous lesions in the metaphysis and diaphysis of a long bone can present a confusing clinical picture. Radiologically these tumors have some osteolysis with matrix mineralization. The mineralization appears as punctate calcification. These are common lesions and represent either a benign enchondroma or low-grade central chondrosarcoma. The distinguishing features include pain and endosteal scalloping on the radiograph. If the tumor is painless and endosteal cortical destruction is not present, then it can be safely followed and assumed to be a benign enchondroma. On the other hand, if the lesion is present in an adult, is painful, and is associated with endosteal scalloping based on either the radiograph or computed tomography, then it usually represents a chondrosarcoma and needs to be dealt with appropriately. Gross appearance may aid in grading the tumor. Low-grade chondrosarcomas typically have a lobulated appearance, whereas high-grade tumors demonstrate less lobulation and may have gelatinous areas that represent a myxomatous component.

CHONDROSARCOMA VARIANTS

Variant forms of chondrosarcoma of bone include mesenchymal chondrosarcoma, dedifferentiated chondrosarcoma, and clear cell chondrosarcoma. These have been well described and are distinct from conventional chondrosarcoma, particularly with respect to their clinical prognoses. Mesenchymal chondrosarcoma and dedifferentiated chondrosarcoma are highly aggressive forms. Both are biphasic tumors histologically consisting of a relatively low-grade cartilaginous component associated with a high-grade noncartilaginous component. Clear cell chondrosarcomas are generally low-grade and carry a favorable prognosis.

DEDIFFERENTIATED CHONDROSARCOMA

Dedifferentiated chondrosarcoma was first described by Dahlin and Beabout in 1971.[14] Dedifferentiated chondrosarcoma histologically consists of well-differentiated or low-grade chondrosarcoma, usually of the central type, combined with a high-grade spindle cell sarcoma.[1, 14, 15] The most common spindle cell pattern has been reported to be that of malignant fibrous histiocytoma[16] or osteosarcoma.[15] Usually the underlying low-grade cartilage tumor remains indolent for years before the tumor becomes aggressive because of the highly anaplastic fibrous tumor. The risk of development of this type of behavior has been reported to be 11%[15] and 6%.[17] The term *dedifferentiated chondrosarcoma* is a misnomer. Most authors do not accept the process of dedifferentiation in the pathogenesis of the high-grade component of this tumor. Rather, the evidence suggests that clonal predominance of a pre-existing high-grade anaplastic clone represents its true oncogenesis.[18]

Approximately 60% of dedifferentiated chondrosarcomas involve the long bones (femur and humerus) and 40% involve the pelvis.[17] Most patients with a dedifferentiated chondrosarcoma are greater than 40 years of age and it is extremely rare in young people. The Enneking stage at the time of initial evaluation is IIB (high-grade, extracompartmental) in the majority of cases.[15] Radiographically there is a mixed picture. Usually the radiographic features of a conventional chondrosarcoma are present along with cortical thickening, bone expansion, and matrix mineralization. In addition, there are areas of either geographic or permeative bone destruction and at times pathologic fracture. Massive soft tissue extension is a frequent finding in dedifferentiated chondrosarcoma (Fig 3, A to F). Dedifferentiated chondrosarcoma has an extremely poor prognosis that is probably related to the poorly differentiated spindle cell sarcoma associated with this tumor. Two-year survival rates of less than 20% have been reported.[17] Attempts at treating this tumor with cytotoxic drugs have been reported, but poor results appear to be inevitable.[16]

MESENCHYMAL CHONDROSARCOMA

Mesenchymal chondrosarcoma is another highly malignant variant of conventional chondrosarcoma. This tumor is extremely rare. In 1982, Christiansen reported on approximately 250 cases representing the total experience in the literature.[19] Approximately one third of these tumors occur in soft tissue.[20] Schajowicz reported on 22 cases. Six of these occurred in the femur, 3 in the tibia, and 2 in vertebrae. Four of his cases arose in soft tissues, 3 in the thigh, and 1 in the leg.[2] Histologically this tumor is composed of well-differentiated low-grade chondrosarcoma mixed with a round cell neoplasm quite reminiscent of Ewing sarcoma. It is the high-grade malignant round cell neoplasm that drives the aggressiveness of this tumor. The malignant round cells frequently have a perivascular arrangement resembling hemangiopericytoma. Huvos subdivided mesenchymal chondrosarcoma into two types: one that was predominantly hemangiopericytoma-like and one that was predominantly a small dark round cell type.[21] The average age when medical attention was first sought according to Huvos was 26 years. Radiologically, when a mesenchymal chondrosarcoma occurs in bone, it typically has a permeative destructive pattern (Fig 4, A and B). The prognosis of this tumor, like that of dedifferentiated chondrosarcoma, is extremely poor. The number of cases, however, is too small to provide any usable statistics. Currently, chemotherapy is being used in the treatment of this tumor, and protocols similar to those used for Ewing sarcoma are frequently applied.

CLEAR CELL CHONDROSARCOMA

The last variant of chondrosarcoma is clear cell chondrosarcoma. Unlike the dedifferentiated and mesenchymal variants, this tumor carries a distinctly better prognosis than conventional chondrosarcoma. It is a rare malignancy, with only 16 cases reported by Unni et al. in 1976.[22] It is a tumor of adults most commonly involving the upper end of the femur, humerus, or tibia. The histologic picture is one of a clear cell tumor that lacks pleomorphism, anaplasia, and other cytologic features of aggressive-

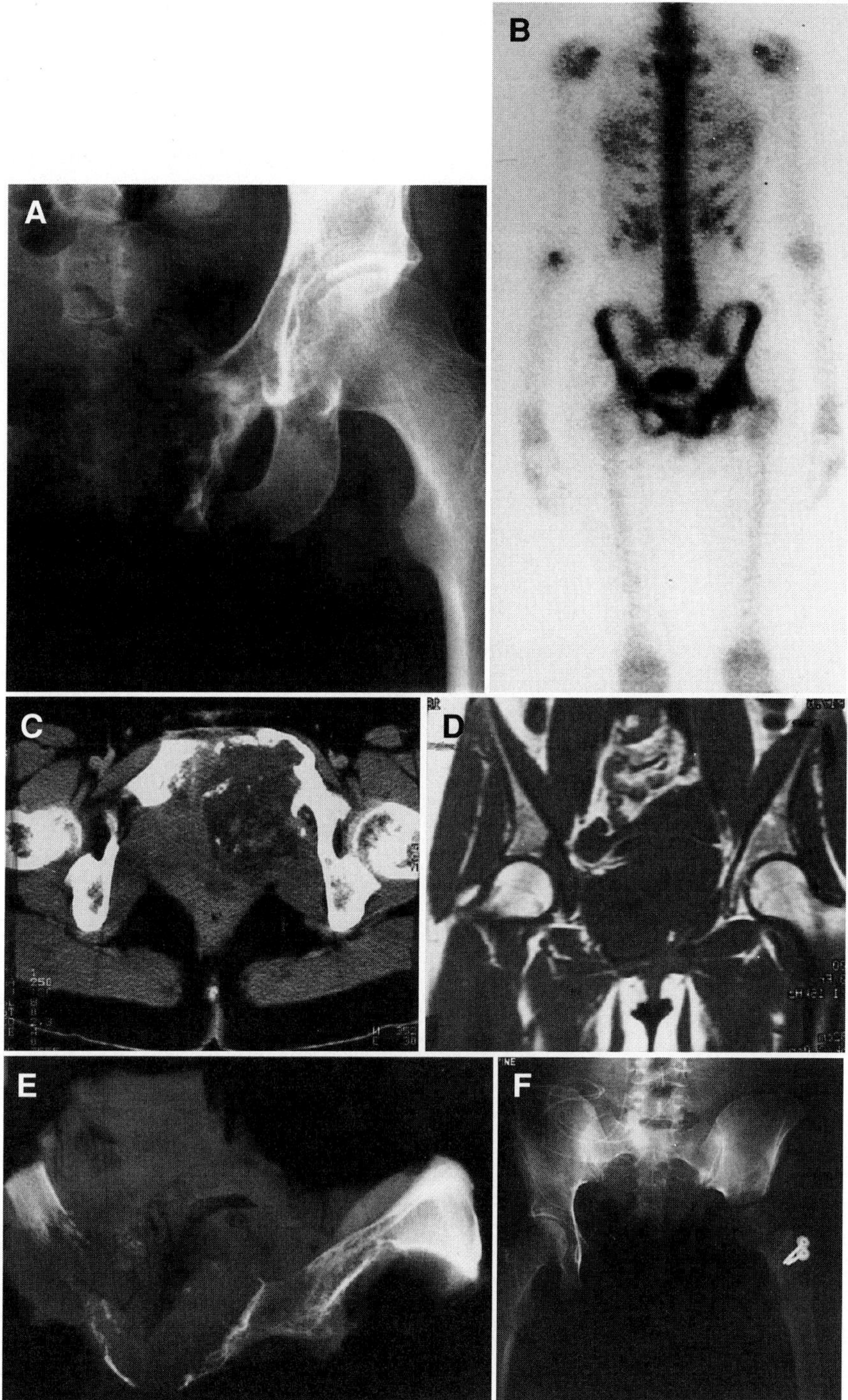

FIGURE 3.

Dedifferentiated chondrosarcoma. **A,** anteroposterior radiograph of the pelvis of a 24-year-old female who was referred for evaluation of a pelvis mass. The radiograph demonstrates a destructive lesion of the pubis. **B,** bone scan demonstrating intense uptake from the left acetabulum to the right superior and inferior pubic rami. **C,** CT scan demonstrating a destructive lesion with a large soft tissue extension. Destructive changes are seen crossing the midline. **D,** MRI scan demonstrating decreased signal intensity in the left acetabulum. **E,** specimen radiograph. **F,** anteroposterior pelvis radiograph following en bloc resection and positioning of the femoral head under the cut surface of the ilium.

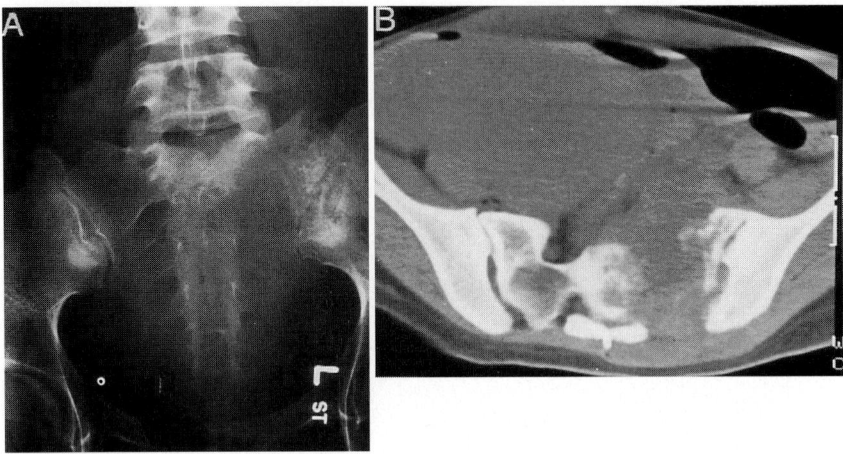

FIGURE 4.

Mesenchymal chondrosarcoma. **A,** anteroposterior radiograph of the pelvis of a 29-year-old female with low back and buttock pain during the third trimester of her pregnancy. **B,** CT scan demonstrating a destructive process in the sacrum.

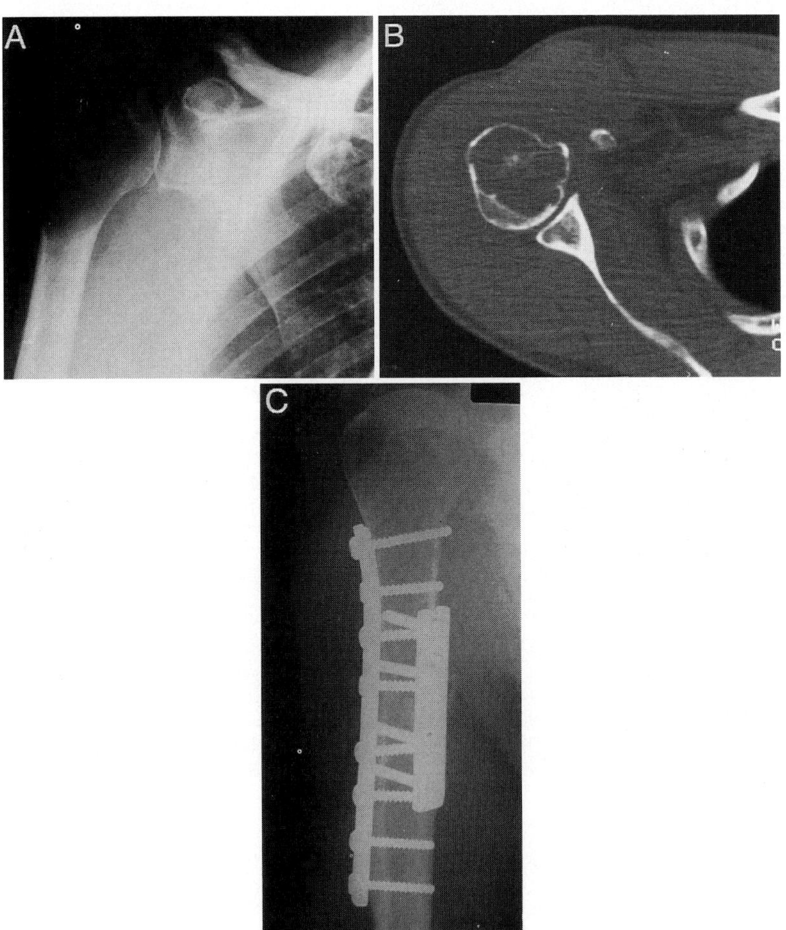

FIGURE 5.

Clear cell chondrosarcoma. **A,** anteroposterior radiograph of the right humerus of a 44-year-old male who was evaluated for pain in the shoulder. **B,** CT scan demonstrating thinning of the cortex and a pathologic fracture. **C,** radiograph demonstrating osteochondral allograft reconstruction.

ness. In approximately 50% of cases, areas of conventional chondrosarcoma are seen. It is somewhat analogous to the pediatric cartilaginous tumor chondroblastoma. It is an epiphyseal tumor that is manifested as a lytic destructive lesion of bone but usually has radiologic features that indicate containment within the bone (Fig 5, A to C). Rarely is matrix mineralization seen in this tumor, which leads one away from the diagnosis of a cartilaginous tumor and more toward giant cell tumor. Unni et al.[22] reported a significant incidence of local recurrence after intralesional excision of this tumor. As a result, they recommended en bloc resection. When treated by this more aggressive surgical procedure, the prognosis is excellent. Bjornsson et al.[23] in 1984 reported an 85% cure rate in 47 patients with clear cell chondrosarcoma. This variant has an excellent prognosis and can generally be controlled by surgical excision.

TREATMENT

Establishment of the diagnosis of chondrosarcoma by open biopsy requires careful consideration and planning because the frequency of spillage of tumor cells at biopsy sites is high. If the radiologic and clinical features are absolutely characteristic of a chondrosarcoma, then wide en bloc resection may be performed without biopsy, thus eliminating the risk of tumor spillage. Should a biopsy be necessary, the incision and dissection should be carried out such that the biopsy site can be resected en bloc with the tumor at the time of definitive treatment. Recurrence of chondrosarcoma has been reported in an arthroscopy portal, so arthroscopy portals should be included in the resection of those chondrosarcomas about the knee that have undergone arthroscopy before diagnosis.

The treatment of conventional chondrosarcoma is surgical.[24–26] Although chemotherapy is used for the aggressive variants dedifferentiated chondrosarcoma and mesenchymal chondrosarcoma, it has not yet proved to be effective for conventional chondrosarcoma.[15, 17] Its use in the variant forms of chondrosarcoma is simply based on the poor prognosis that these tumors carry regardless of treatment. Several authors have shown that if adequate surgery is performed, the prognosis for local control of conventional chondrosarcoma is good. The prognosis appears to be related to both the histologic grade of the tumor and the adequacy of surgical resection.[3, 27, 28] Low-grade chondrosarcomas tend to be slow growing and at times locally aggressive but have a relatively low rate of metastases. If the chondrosarcoma is removed en bloc surgically and if the margins are wide, then local control is usually achieved.[3] These tumors have a relatively good prognosis, with 10-year survival rates reported to be approximately 70% to 80%. High-grade chondrosarcomas, on the other hand, tend to be both locally aggressive and potentially metastatic. The common sites of metastasis reported include the lung and bone. High-grade chondrosarcomas carry a poor prognosis, with survival rates typically below 40%.[29]

Surgical treatment of chondrosarcoma of bone is by wide en bloc resection involving removal of the tumor along with a cuff of normal bone and surrounding soft tissue. When the tumor occurs in the extremities, this usually necessitates complex surgical reconstruction for limb salvage.

When the chondrosarcoma occurs in the pelvis, extensive surgical procedures, either limb sparing or ablative, are necessary.[11, 30, 31] Tumors of the pelvis may involve contiguous structures such as bowel and bladder and may require partial removal of these structures to achieve wide margins. The key issue in surgical management of chondrosarcoma of the pelvis is whether or not the acetabulum is involved. Chondrosarcomas involving only the wing of the ilium or the anterior arch of the pelvis can be treated by wide en bloc resection. Reconstruction is not generally required following resection of tumors in these anatomic sites. Tumors involving the acetabulum, on the other hand, pose a much greater surgical challenge. If the acetabulum needs to be sacrificed by either an intra- or extra-articular resection, some form of complex reconstruction is usually necessary. This is accomplished by either arthroplasty or arthrodesis. With the advent of biological reconstruction as well as improvement in metallic prostheses, more surgical reconstructive options are available. At times, because of massive soft tissue extension, hindquarter amputation may be necessary. Tumors of the humerus and femur tend to be less problematic. In these anatomic sites, wide en bloc resection is usually easier and reconstruction less complicated. Metallic implants and allografts have been used with varying success. There are several anatomic sites where en bloc resection does not require any form of reconstruction. Tumors that occur in expendable bone such as a rib can simply be widely excised without the need for a major reconstructive procedure.

BIOCHEMICAL, MOLECULAR GENETIC, AND CYTOGENETIC ASPECTS OF HUMAN CHONDROSARCOMA

The clinical behavior of human chondrosarcoma is quite variable. In an effort to predict their malignant potential, human chondrosarcomas have been characterized by several parameters. These include histopathologic grading, DNA content, chondrocyte-specific matrix molecules such as type II collagen and proteoglycans, and more recently, molecular genetic and cytogenetic features. Early biochemical analyses of human chondrosarcomas focused on the extracellular matrix; however, these studies did not yield consistent results. Buckwalter identified differences in proteoglycan dimensions among chondrosarcomas but could not correlate these with tumor malignancy.[32] Studies by Mankin et al.[33, 34] and Pal et al.[35] suggested that the size of the keratan sulfate chains of the large aggregating proteoglycan might be inversely related to the histologic grade of the tumor. These findings, however, have not been consistently reproduced in other studies.[36, 37] Human chondrosarcomas have been found to be highly heterogeneous in terms of the biochemical makeup of their extracellular matrices, and there is presently no reliable biochemical marker available to assess the malignant potential of these tumors.

Because of the difficulty in finding reliable biochemical markers of clinical aggressiveness, there has been a more recent emphasis on DNA content and chromosomal aberrations as potential predictors of malignant behavior of human chondrosarcomas. A number of studies have attempted to correlate tumor grade with DNA content. Alho et al.[38] found that 90% of benign cartilage tumor cells were diploid and none were aneuploid whereas only 70% of high-grade chondrosarcoma cells were diploid with 20% being aneuploid. Low-grade chondrosarcoma cells demonstrated 11% tetraploidy and no aneuploidy. Kreicbergs et al.[39] demonstrated a significantly higher survival rate with diploid chondrosarcomas as compared with hyperploid chondrosarcomas. Mankin et al.[40] and Mellin et al.[41] have also shown a correlation between the degree of aneuploidy and clinical aggressiveness of human chondrosarcoma. Despite these studies, the predictive accuracy of this technique remains somewhat limited.

Several studies of the cytogenetic aspects of human chondrosarcomas have shown nonrandom chromosomal aberrations. Reciprocal chromosomal translocations in extraskeletal myxoid chondrosarcomas have been reported by several authors.[42–44] More recently, Jagasia et al. have demonstrated a nonrandom aberration on the short arm of chromosome 9 in cultured human chondrosarcoma cells.[45] This abnormality appears to involve a deletion in the region of the 9p21–22 locus. This deletion may coincide with a recently described tumor suppressor gene, multiple tumor suppressor type 1 (MTS-1), that has been implicated in the pathogenesis of several other malignancies including non–small-cell lung carcinomas, melanomas, ovarian cancer, and acute lymphoblastic leukemia.[46] In conclusion, the search for a molecular biological marker for human chondrosarcoma is ongoing. Should a suitable marker be identified, a more accurate prediction of the clinical behavior of human chondrosarcoma may be possible. More importantly, if the pathogenesis of human chondrosarcoma is related to the deletion of a tumor suppressor gene, then gene therapy may play an important role in the management of this malignancy in the future.

REFERENCES

1. Dahlin DC, Unni KK: *Bone Tumors: General Aspects and Data on 8542 Cases.* Springfield, Ill, Charles C Thomas, 1986.
2. Shajowicz F: *Tumors and Tumorlike Lesions of Bone, Pathology, Radiology, and Treatment*, ed 2. New York, Springer-Verlag, 1994.
3. Gitelis S, Bertoni F, Chieti PP, et al: Chondrosarcoma of bone. The experience at the Istituto Ortopedico Rizzoli. *J Bone Joint Surg Am* 63:1248–1257, 1981.
4. Aprin H, Riseborough EJ, Hall JE: Chondrosarcoma in children and adolescents. *Clin Orthop* 166:226–232, 1982.
5. Huvos AG, Marcove RC: Chondrosarcoma in the young. A clinicopathological analysis of 79 patients younger than 21 years of age. *Am J Surg Pathol* 11:930–942, 1987.
6. Blackwell JB: Mesenchymal chondrosarcoma arising in fibrous dysplasia of the femur. *J Clin Pathol* 46:961–962, 1993.
7. Dahlin DC: *Bone Tumors*, ed 3. Springfield, Ill, Charles C Thomas, 1978.
8. Lewis RJ, Ketcham AS: Maffucci's syndrome: Functional and neoplastic significance. Case report and review of the literature. *J Bone Joint Surg Am* 55:1465–1479, 1973.
9. Schwartz HS, Zimmerman NB, Simon MA, et al: The malignant potential of enchondromatosis. *J Bone Joint Surg Am* 69:269–274, 1987.
10. Lichtenstein L: *Bone Tumors*, ed 5. St Louis, Mosby, 1977.

11. Marcove RC, Mike V, Hutter RVP, et al: Chondrosarcoma of the pelvis and upper end of the femur. An analysis of factors influencing survival time in one hundred and thirteen cases. *J Bone Joint Surg Am* 54:561–572, 1972.
12. Lichtenstein L, Jaffe HL: Chondrosarcoma of bone. *Am J Pathol* 19:553–589, 1943.
13. O'Neal LW, Ackerman LV: Chondrosarcoma of bone. *Cancer* 5:551–577, 1952.
14. Dahlin DC, Beabout JW: Dedifferentiation of low grade chondrosarcoma. *Cancer* 28:461–466, 1971.
15. Frassica FJ, Unni KK, Beabout JW, et al: Dedifferentiated chondrosarcoma: A report of the clinicopathological features and treatment of seventy-eight cases. *J Bone Joint Surg Am* 69:1197–1205, 1986.
16. Johnson S, Tetu B, Ayalo AG, et al: Chondrosarcoma with additional mesenchymal component (dedifferentiated chondrosarcoma): A clinicopathologic study of 26 cases. *Cancer* 58:278–286, 1986.
17. Capanna R, Bertoni F, Betteli G, et al: Dedifferentiated chondrosarcoma. *J Bone Joint Surg Am* 70:60–69, 1988.
18. Gitelis S, Kimura JH, Block JA, et al: Clonal analysis of human chondrosarcoma. *Chir Organi Mov* 75(suppl):11–13, 1990.
19. Christiansen RE Jr: Mesenchymal chondrosarcoma of the jaws. *Oral Surg* 54:197–206, 1982.
20. Enzinger FM, Weiss SW: *Soft Tissue Tumors,* ed 2, St Louis, Mosby, 1988.
21. Huvos AG: *Bone Tumors: Diagnosis, Treatment, Prognosis.* Philadelphia, WB Saunders, 1991.
22. Unni KK, Dahlin DC, Beabout JW, et al: Chondrosarcoma clear cell variant: A report of sixteen cases. *J Bone Joint Surg Am* 58:676–683, 1976.
23. Bjornsson J, Unni KK, Dahlin DC, et al: Clear cell chondrosarcoma of bone: Observations in 47 cases. *Am J Surg Pathol* 8:223–230, 1984.
24. Kaufman JH, Douglass HO Jr, Blake W, et al: The importance of initial presentation and treatment upon the survival of patients with chondrosarcoma. *Surg Gynecol Obstet* 145:357, 1977.
25. Eriksson AI, Schiller A, Mankin HJ: The management of chondrosarcoma of bone. *Clin Orthop* 153:44–66, 1980.
26. Healey JH, Lane JM: Chondrosarcoma. *Clin Orthop* 204:119, 1986.
27. Evans HL, Ayala AG, Romsdahl MM: Prognostic factors in chondrosarcoma of bone. A clinicopathologic analysis with emphasis on histologic grading. *Cancer* 40:818, 1977.
28. Sannerkin NG, Gallagher P: A review of the behaviour of chondrosarcoma of bone. *J Bone Joint Surg Br* 61:395–400, 1979.
29. Henderson ED, Dahlin DC: Chondrosarcoma of bone: A study of 288 cases. *J Bone Joint Surg Am* 45:1450–1458, 1963.
30. Guerra A, Bricolli A, Capanna R, et al: Resection with preservation of the lower limb in chondrosarcoma of the pelvis. *Rev Chir Orthop* 71:493, 1985.
31. Campanacci M, Capanna R: Pelvic resections. The Rizzoli Institute experience. *Orthop Clin North Am* 1:65–86, 1991.
32. Buckwalter JA: The structure of human chondrosarcoma proteoglycans. *J Bone Joint Surg Am* 65:958–974, 1983.
33. Mankin HJ, Cantley KP, Lippiello L, et al: The biology of human chondrosarcoma. I. Description of the cases, grading and biochemical analyses. *J Bone Joint Surg Am* 62:160–176, 1980.
34. Mankin HJ, Cantley KP, Lippiello L, et al: The biology of human chondrosarcoma. II. Variation in chemical composition among types and subtypes of benign and malignant cartilage tumors. *J Bone Joint Surg Am* 62:176–188, 1980.
35. Pal S, Strider W, Margolis G, et al: Isolation and characterization of proteoglycans from human chondrosarcoma. *J Biol Chem* 253:1279–1289, 1978.

36. Thonar EJ-MA, Sweet MBE, Immelman AR, et al: Structural studies on proteoglycans from human chondrosarcomas. *Arch Biochem Biophys* 194:179–189, 1979.
37. Herwig J, Roessner A, Buddecke E: Isolation and characterization of proteoglycans and glycosaminoglycans from human chondrosarcoma. *Exp Mol Pathol* 45:118–127, 1986.
38. Alho A, Skjeldal S, Melvik JE, et al: The clinical importance of DNA synthesis and aneuploidy in bone and soft tissue tumours. *Anticancer Res* 13:2383–2387, 1993.
39. Kreicbergs A, Boquist L, Borssen B, et al: Prognostic factors in chondrosarcoma. A comparative study of cellular DNA content and clinicopathologic features. *Cancer* 50:577–583, 1982.
40. Mankin HJ, Matsuno T, Gebhardt AL, et al: "Flow cytometry in the management of bone tumors," in Unni KK (ed): *Bone Tumors.* New York, Churchill Livingstone 1988, pp 85–106.
41. Mellin W, Dierschauer W, Hiddemann W, et al: Flow cytometric DNA analysis of bone tumors, in Roessner A (ed): *Biological Characterization of Bone Tumors.* Berlin, Springer-Verlag, 1989, pp 115–152.
42. Hinrichs SH, Jaramillo MA, Gumerlock PH, et al: Myxoid chondrosarcoma with a translocation involving chromosome 6 and 22. *Cancer Genet Cytogenet* 14:219–226, 1985.
43. Turc-Carel C, Dal Cin P, Rao U, et al: Recurrent breakpoints at 9q31 and 22q12.2 in extraskeletal myxoid chondrosarcoma. *Cancer Genet Cytogenet* 30:145–150, 1988.
44. Bridge JA, Sanger WG, Neff JR: Translocations involving chromosome 2 and 13 in benign and malignant cartilaginous neoplasms. *Cancer Genet Cytogenet* 38:83–88, 1989.
45. Jagasia AA, Block JA, Diaz M, et al: Molecular and cytogenetic aspects of a myxoid chondrosarcoma. Submitted for publication.
46. Kamb A, Gruis NA, Weaver-Feldhaus J, et al: A cell cycle regulator potentially involved in genesis of many tumor types. *Science* 264:436–440, 1994.

Fibrous Dysplasia of Bone

Pietro Ruggieri, M.D.
Professor of Orthopedics, Department of Orthopedics, University of Bologna, Rizzoli Institute, Bologna, Italy

Frank J. Frassica, M.D.
Associate Professor, Orthopedic Oncology, Chief, Division of Adult and Reconstructive Surgery, Johns Hopkins University, Baltimore, Maryland

Franklin H. Sim, M.D.
Professor of Orthopedic Surgery, Mayo Medical School, Consultant, Department of Orthopedic Oncology, Mayo Clinic, Rochester, Minnesota

HISTORICAL PERSPECTIVE

Fibrous dysplasia is an intraosseous (primarily intramedullary) neoformation of fibrous tissue and bone caused by an anomalous development of mesenchymal tissue that can be monostotic or polyostotic. The term *polyostotic fibrous dysplasia* was used by Lichtenstein in 1938[1] to designate a disease characterized by an anomaly of skeletal development affecting several bones with a tendency toward unilateral involvement of the skeleton. Lichtenstein described eight cases and emphasized the confusion in terminology existing in the literature since similar cases had been described under *osteitis fibrosa*, a term that had been used for other lesions such as hyperparathyroidism, Paget's disease, and giant cell tumor.

In 1942, Lichtenstein and Jaffe[2] reported a series of 86 patients describing the various possible clinical manifestations of fibrous dysplasia. They noted that the disease could be monostotic or polyostotic. Associated extraskeletal manifestations included pigmentation of the skin, premature sexual development, and hyperthyroidism. The association of extraskeletal manifestations with "osteitis fibrosa cystica" had already been described by McCune in 1936[3] and further defined in 1937 by Albright.[4] Albright reported 5 cases of a "syndrome characterized by osteitis fibrosa disseminata, areas of pigmentation, and endocrine dysfunction with precocious puberty in females" and excluded that such a condition could be related to hyperparathyroidism. This syndrome has been variably referred to as Albright syndrome or McCune-Albright syndrome.

Subsequent studies have shown that different forms of endocrine dysfunction may be associated with polyostotic fibrous dysplasia and that precocious puberty can also affect males.[5]

Advances in Operative Orthopaedics, vol. 3

DEMOGRAPHICS

Fibrous dysplasia accounts for about 1% of biopsy-analyzed primary bone tumors.[6] Actually, its incidence is greater since in many cases the radiographic diagnosis is certain, especially for polyostotic fibrous dysplasia. In the series reported by Dahlin and Unni, polyostotic disease represented about one ninth of the cases.[7]

Monostotic fibrous dysplasia is frequent, whereas the polyostotic form is rare.

The disease can be diagnosed at any age. It is often an incidental finding in monostotic forms, whereas polyostotic fibrous dysplasia is usually discovered in the first two decades of age. In 75% of cases, patients are younger than 30 years at diagnosis.[6]

The disease shows a slight predilection for females and can affect any bone. The most frequent sites of monostotic fibrous dysplasia are the femur, tibia, craniofacial bones, and ribs, followed by the humerus, forearm, and pelvis. In Wilner's review,[8] 75% of the solitary lesions were located in the ribs, femurs, tibia, and craniofacial bones, with the same frequency for these three sites, whereas 10% were in the humerus and pelvis. Polyostotic fibrous dysplasia shows a similar skeletal distribution, with a marked tendency to unilaterality of the lesions.

Frequently, polyostotic disease affects two or more areas in a long bone, shows involvement of an entire long bone, or involves two or more adjacent bones (more often the femur and tibia or the ilium, femur, and tibia). Hands and feet are rarely affected by fibrous dysplasia. Rare locations are also represented by the vertebrae, scapula, and clavicle.

The spine and sacrum are rarely involved by polyostotic fibrous dysplasia and are exceptionally the site of monostotic fibrous dysplasia, representing about 0.8% of primary tumors of the axial skeleton other than myeloma.[9] Usually the vertebral body is involved, whereas posterior elements are rarely affected. The thoracic spine is an exceptionally rare site for monostotic fibrous dysplasia.

Nabarro and Giblin in 1994[10] presented a case of fibrous dysplasia of the seventh thoracic vertebra and stated in their review of the literature that they have found only two cases of monostotic disease in the thoracic spine previously reported.[11,12] It is interesting to notice that in Nabarro and Giblin's case, the adjacent rib was involved.

The pelvis is rarely involved by monostotic fibrous dysplasia, whereas it is a frequent site for the polyostotic disease. The ilium is the most common pelvic bone involved. It must be noted that fibrous dysplasia is the most common benign tumor of the ribs. The proximal portion of the femur is by far the most frequent site of monostotic and polyostotic fibrous dysplasia and the location where the most typical and common deformity caused by the disease takes place.

CLINICAL APPEARANCE

Monostotic fibrous dysplasia is often asymptomatic, and in such cases it can be an incidental finding on radiographs (Fig 1) or bone scans obtained for unrelated reasons.

The symptoms of monostotic fibrous dysplasia are essentially caused

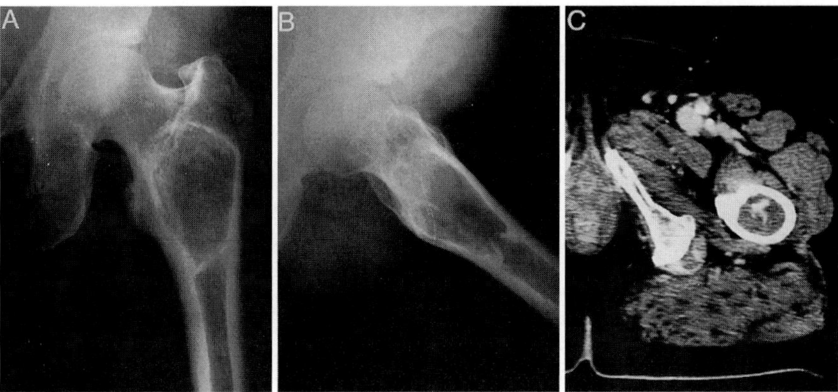

FIGURE 1.

Monostotic fibrous dysplasia in a 68-year-old male (incidental finding on radiographs taken for arthritis of his right hip). Radiographs in the anteroposterior **(A)** and lateral **(B)** views show the typical ground-glass appearance and a rind of sclerosis around the lesion. Computed tomography (CT) **(C)** shows some ossifications within the lesion.

by weakening of the bony structure. In fact, the patient may have pain, usually discontinuous, that is due to microfractures or a frank pathologic fracture. In the case of superficial bones (ribs), swelling with or without pain can be the initial symptom.

The age of the first manifestation of monostotic fibrous dysplasia is extremely variable and is related to the site and the extent of involvement.

Areas of hyperpigmentation of the skin, so-called café au lait spots, are rarely observed in patients with monostotic fibrous dysplasia. When present, they can be useful for diagnosis. Café au lait spots, typical of fibrous dysplasia, are cutaneous spots or patches brown to brownish yellow in pigmentation with irregular borders ("coast of Maine"), as opposed to the regular borders ("coast of California") seen in neurofibromatosis.

Craniofacial fibrous dysplasia, in the absence of other sites of bone involvement, is generally considered monostotic[13] because, uncommonly, just one facial bone is involved and it is difficult to state whether multiple bones were primarily affected or the disease extended from one to another. Craniofacial fibrous dysplasia tends to be manifested early and produces swelling, exophthalmos, or neurologic symptoms caused by obstruction of the foramina of the cranial nerves.

Polyostotic fibrous dysplasia may show a wide variety of initial clinical manifestations. In the classic study by Harris and coworkers[14] reported in 1962, it is well emphasized that both the symptoms and findings at first manifestation and the clinical course of the disease are extremely variable.

Pain, limp, or pathologic fractures were the initial symptoms in 70% of the patients in the study of Harris and coworkers[14]; also variable is the age at onset of symptoms of polyostotic fibrous dysplasia. Usually, the more severe and extended the disease, the earlier the age of first manifestation.

Café au lait spots are a frequent finding in patients with polyostotic fibrous dysplasia; often they can be the first sign prompting attention of the physician and can already be present at birth.[15,16] These pigmented skin areas tend to correspond to the site of bone involvement, although this is not a rule.

In the severe forms of polyostotic fibrous dysplasia, bowing of long bones and repeated pathologic fractures leading to deformities and limb length discrepancy are frequent, especially in the lower limb. The most common of these deformities is coxa vara with a dramatic curvature of the proximal end of the femur known as a "shepherd's crook" deformity. This deformity is caused by repeated fractures and/or microfractures of the proximal portion of the femur.

When the spine is involved, patients may have neurologic symptoms because of nerve root encroachment. Fibrous dysplasia in the spine can also cause severe kyphoscoliosis with secondary compression of the spinal cord.

Swelling of the ribs, tibia, facial bones, and skull is frequently observed with or without pain. Swelling of facial bones can lead to facial disfigurement and tends to cause facial asymmetry with enlargement of one side.

Besides café au lait spots, other extraskeletal manifestations of polyostotic fibrous dysplasia exist. McCune-Albright syndrome classically includes polyostotic fibrous dysplasia, pigmented skin areas, and precocious puberty; in addition, it is seen in about 3% of patients with polyostotic fibrous dysplasia.[6]

Precocious puberty in this syndrome is a form of gonadotropin-independent (gonadotropin releasing hormone–dependent) sexual precocity that can affect both females and males[5] and is usually associated with precocity in growth and premature epiphyseal fusion, which results in a reduced ultimate height.[15]

Other endocrine abnormalities can variably be associated with Albright syndrome, such as acromegaly, hyperthyroidism, hypercortisolism, and phosphaturic osteomalacia.[5]

The possible association of intramuscular myxomas with fibrous dysplasia, usually referred to as Mazabraud syndrome,[17] is rare. Henschen reported the first case of multiple myxomas and "osteitis fibrosa" in 1926,[18] and a similar case was reported by Krogius in 1928.[19] Mazabraud and Girard in 1957[17] described the association of myxomas and fibrous dysplasia. Wirth and coworkers reported two personal cases and reviewed the literature in 1971.[20]

Recent reports of cases of Mazabraud syndrome with a review of the literature[21–23] stated that the most frequent site for myxomas is the lower limb, especially the thigh, and that no defined relationship exists between the number and size of the myxomas and bony lesions. Dahlin and Unni[7] reported 3 such cases in the Mayo Clinic files and Campanacci[24] reported 2 cases in the Rizzoli series. About 20 cases have been described in the literature.

RADIOGRAPHIC APPEARANCE

The typical radiographic feature of fibrous dysplasia is that of a slow-growing process causing an osteolytic lesion that originates in the medullary space of a long bone. Although the lesion tends to expand, it is usually limited by a rind of sclerotic bone (Fig 2). This margination of sclerotic bone may be interrupted. The central lytic portion of the lesion is variably radiolucent and more frequently it has a typical "ground-glass" appearance that is produced by the presence of calcified trabeculae and

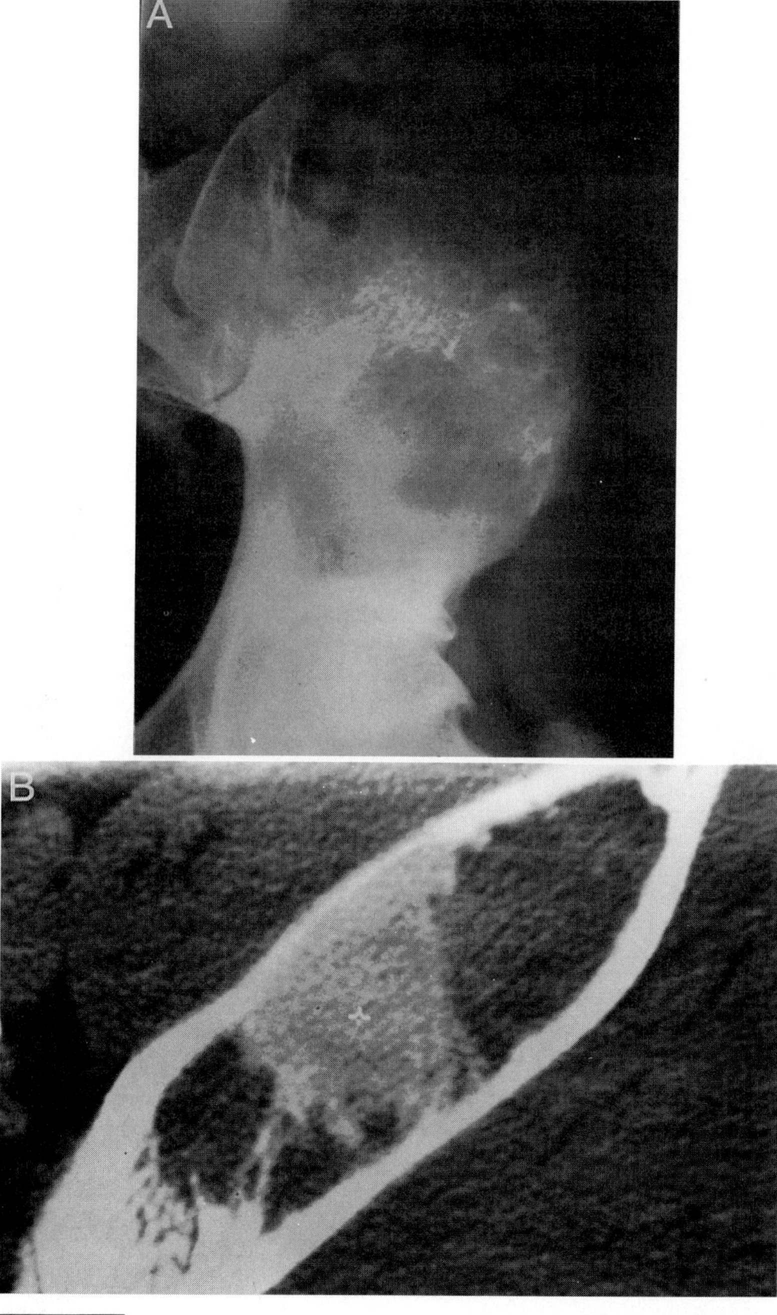

FIGURE 2.
Fibrous dysplasia in the ilium of a 40-year-old female: anteroposterior view **(A)** and CT scan **(B)**.

woven bone within the fibrous tissue (Fig 3). In fact, the radiographic appearance of fibrous dysplasia depends on the quality of the dysplastic tissue and on extension of bone involvement.[15, 24]

This explains the different features that fibrous dysplasia can actually have on radiographs. Sometimes, especially in polyostotic disease, the osteolysis tends to extend longitudinally in a long bone, with a dishomogeneous radiolucency and scarce margination, and spares the epiphysis or just abuts the proximal femoral epiphysis. When the lesion extends to the cortex, this can be eroded or expanded and bowing of the bone can take place.

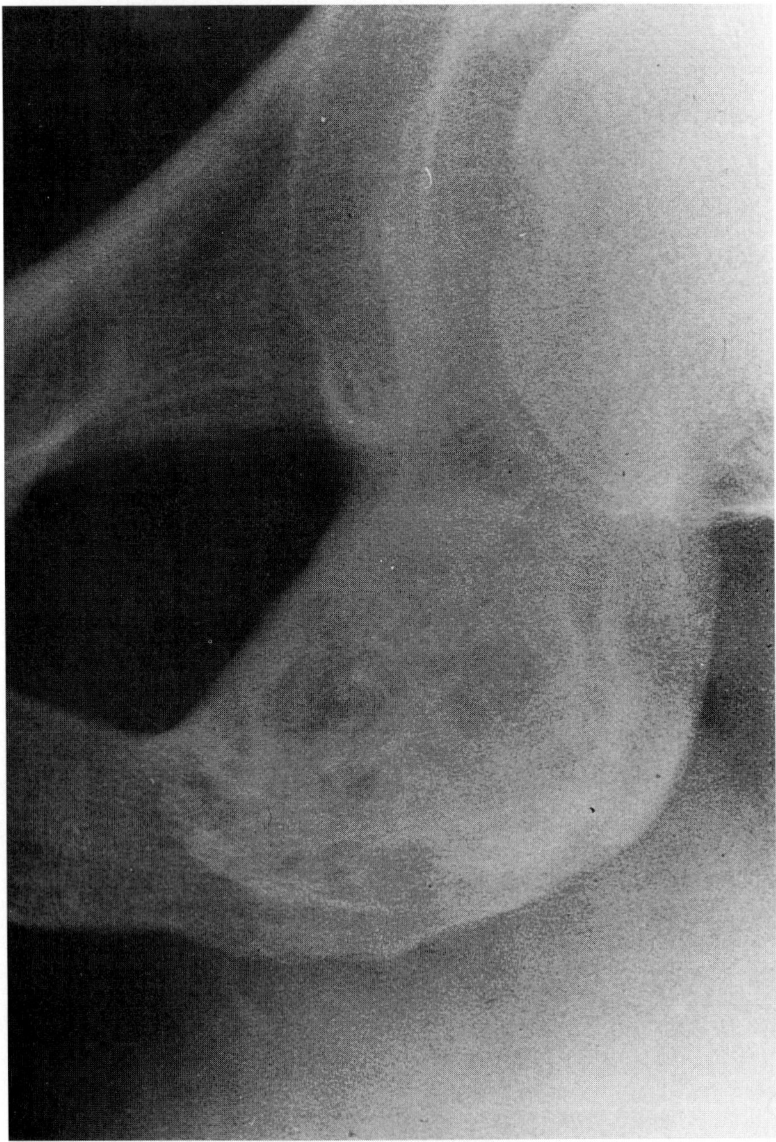

FIGURE 3.
Fibrous dysplasia in the ischium of a 38-year-old male showing the ossification typical of certain cases in the adult age group.

Fatigue fractures and pathologic fractures are frequent and not usually associated with important displacement.

The femur and tibia are the bones most frequently bowed by fibrous dysplasia, and in the proximal end of the femur, repeated microfractures and/or pathologic fractures may lead to the so-called shepherd's crook or hockey stick deformity, which is the most typical and common deformity for fibrous dysplasia. The cortex is reabsorbed on the convex side of the curvature and thickened on the inner side. Sometimes the lytic areas show calcifications inside because of the presence of cartilage lobules, or they may show ossifications and septation. In certain instances, the almost completely fibrous tissues may have the radiographic features of a pure osteolysis that may be similar to a nonossifying fibroma or a giant cell tumor. At other times, the radiolucency is similar to that of a cystic lesion; in lesions extending into a long bone, a "candle flame" appearance may be evident. Mineralization in variable degrees is often noted in older lesions.

Ribs are a frequent location of fibrous dysplasia, often showing expansion and thinning of the cortex, at times with a ground-glass appearance and at other times with a radiolucency similar to that of an aneurysmal bone cyst. Rib lesions may contain calcifications or bone sequestra.

In the pelvis, fibrous dysplasia most frequently involves the ilium and tends to spare the acetabulum. The iliac lesions are usually round or oval-shaped lytic areas with sclerotic margins and a "smudged" appearance or the typical "ground glass"; in older patients, they tend to be more sclerotic.

Skull lesions are characterized by bulging of the outer table and by a typical sclerotic density in the base of the skull.

Wilner[8] has classified the skull lesions into three types: (1) lytic, (2) mixed (localized, regional, and diffuse), and (3) sclerotic. The lytic-blastic mixed type occurs most frequently at 48%.[8]

The radiographic appearance of fibrous dysplasia of the spine is also variable. Usually it is osteolytic, at times with small calcifications or ossifications (Fig 4). Vertebral collapse and kyphoscoliosis can be observed. The presence of a soft tissue mass is also possible.

The bone scan is typically "hot" in fibrous dysplasia lesions; it is due to both the increased vascularity and the continuous bone remodeling. In a study by Machida and coworkers,[25] 93% of the lesions with a ground-glass appearance and 80% of the "cystic" lesions showed increased uptake on bone scans. Also, mechanical factors related to bowing and bone deformities contribute to the increased uptake.

Computed tomography (CT) better shows the typical ground-glass appearance of the matrix in fibrous dysplasia and is especially useful in assessing the extent of the lesion in the craniofacial bones and in the spine. The CT scan may show the fluid-fluid levels in cases of fibrous dysplasia with a cystic component caused by cystic degeneration[26] or, less frequently, a secondary aneurysmal bone cyst.[27–29] Both CT and magnetic resonance imaging (MRI) can show full-thickness cortical destruction in cases where this was not evident on plain radiographs.[30]

An MRI scan is useful in defining the internal architecture of fibrous

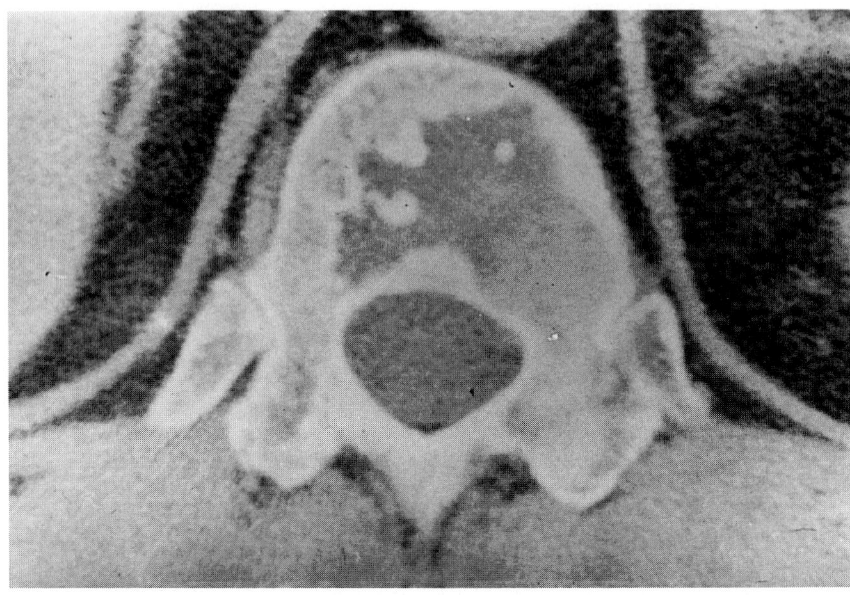

FIGURE 4.
Fibrous dysplasia in a thoracic vertebra of a patient affected by polyostotic fibrous dysplasia.

dysplasia and is the best tool to assess the intraosseous extent of the lesion.[31, 32] The typical abnormal dark gray marrow signal of fibrous tissue on T1-weighted images changes variably on T2-weighted images.[33] The T2 appearance depends on the character of the lesion; calcified and/or ossified portions keep a low T2 signal, whereas an increased T2 signal intensity is detected in cases of cystic areas or pathologic fractures. High signal intensity of T2 sequences has been frequently observed in fibrous dysplasia.[32, 34] In fibrous dysplasia with cystic areas, an MRI scan usually allows the correct diagnosis by showing rind with a low-intensity signal around the lesion.[26]

HISTOLOGY AND GROSS APPEARANCE

The gross appearance of fibrous dysplasia shows a thinned cortex around firm, gritty, whitish to pink tissue. The consistency of this tissue is produced by the osteoid and osseous trabeculae interspersed in the fibrous tissue.

The tissue is generally not richly vascularized, although hypervascularized areas and/or hemorrhagic and cystic lesions can be present. Cysts in fibrous dysplasia may contain either blood or serous fluid, and the cyst wall is lined by a thin, smooth membrane. Foci of cartilage can be observed, usually of small size and peripherally calcified.

The typical histology of fibrous dysplasia is represented by a histiofibroblastic tissue embedding trabeculae of woven bone of variable size and shape (Fig 5). The histiofibroblastic component is composed of spindle cells, at times arranged in whorls with a storiform pattern similar to that of fibrous histiocytoma. The immature trabeculae seems to be

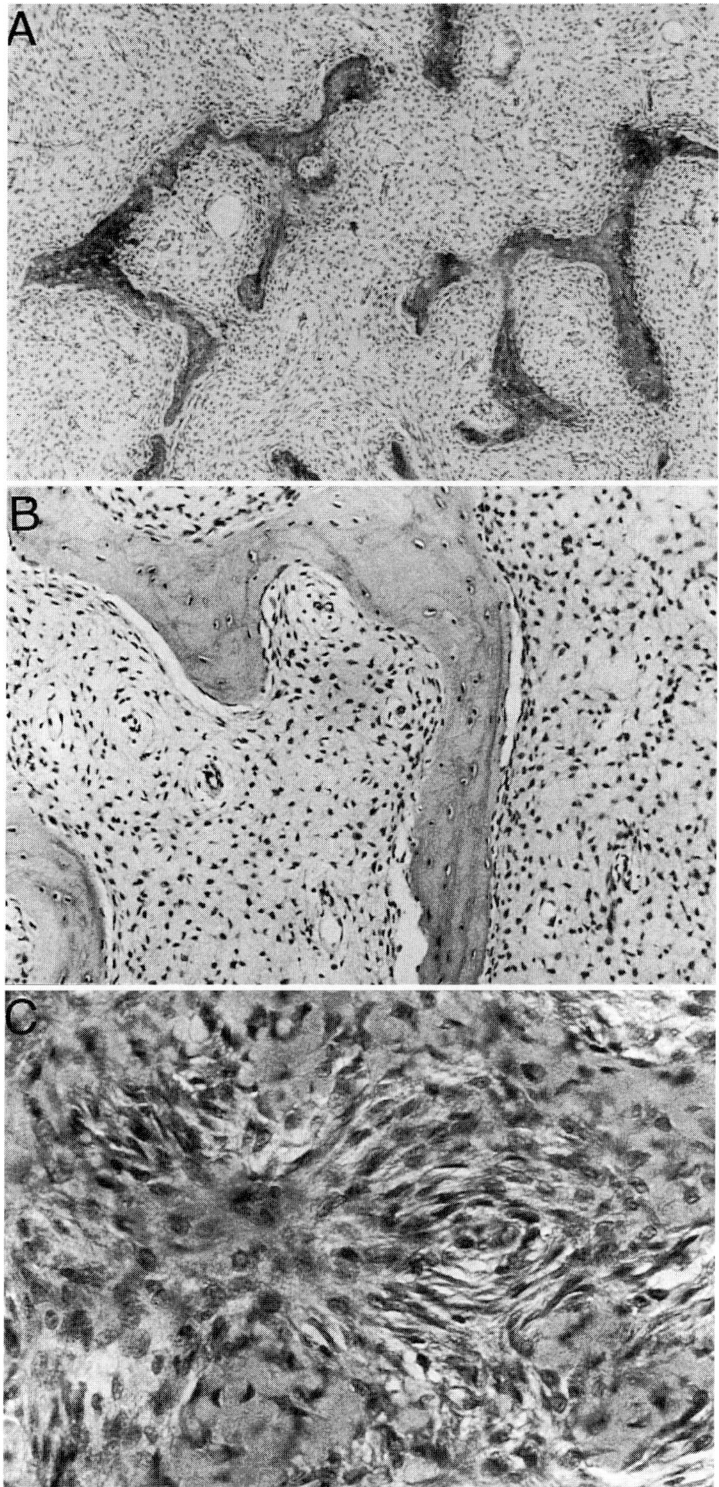

FIGURE 5.

Histology shows the fibrous tissue "embedding" irregular osteoid trabeculae with the typical "alphabet soup" pattern (A, hematoxylin-eosin [HE], ×50; **B,** HE, ×125). At a higher magnification of the histiofibroblastic tissue, some osteoids are evident (**C,** HE, ×300).

produced directly from the spindle cells since they are never lined by active osteoblasts.

A rim of osteoblasts around the trabeculae is an extremely sporadic finding in fibrous dysplasia.[6] The direct formation of woven bone by the spindle cells of the fibrous tissue is usually referred to as "fibro-osseous metaplasia." These dysplastic trabeculae are small and irregular; often they are ovular, round "globs" or are crescent-shaped and tend to have a sort of "alphabet soup" or "Chinese ideogram" pattern. These trabeculae may show reversal lines similar to those of Paget's disease.[7]

The variable amount and maturity of the trabeculae explain both the variable consistency of the gross specimens and the different possible radiographic appearances. The typical ground-glass feature is produced by the presence of many immature trabeculae. The radiolucency of the lesion is predominantly that of fibrous tissue.

Mitotic figures are frequent in the actively proliferating fibrous dysplasia.[7] Areas of degeneration are observed that contain acellular fibrous or myxoid tissue. Nodules of cartilage can be noted; this is hyaline cartilage, similar to that of a physeal plate or a repair callus.[24]

The hypothesis that this cartilage originates from remnants of the growth plate has been variably suggested[6, 15, 24] or denied.[14] Another hypothesis is that the cartilage originates from the repair callus of previous fractures.[6, 14, 24]

Occasionally, fibrous dysplasia may show degenerative foci with benign giant and foam cells.[7, 15] Large confluent cysts derive from the fusion of microcysts and hemorrhagic foci.[15]

In Harris and coworkers' study,[14] repeated biopsies performed in some patients did not show significant changes in time.

The histologic features may show a certain progressive "maturation" in patients of adult age. In fact, a richer cellularity and more immature trabeculae are usually seen in children; in adults, there is decreased cellularity and a denser collagen stroma with more frequent foci of foam cells or cystic degeneration.[24]

The possible observation of the histologic features on an aneurysmal bone cyst in association with fibrous dysplasia has been reported and is referred to as a secondary aneurysmal bone cyst.[27–29]

PATHOGENESIS

Most of the clinical features of fibrous dysplasia such as the associated extraskeletal abnormalities, the age of first manifestation, and the tendency of "maturation" of the tissue seem to indicate a hamartomatous origin. In 1975, Lichtenstein[35] had actually suggested that fibrous dysplasia could have its basis in a genetic defect of development; the newer molecular biology studies in recent years confirm this hypothesis. In fact, all of the hormones involved by the multiple endocrine dysfunctions possibly associated with fibrous dysplasia depend on receptors coupled with the G protein–cyclic adenosine monophosphate (AMP) protein–kinase A–dependent pathway.[5, 36, 37]

Investigation of an activating mutation of the Gs protein (Gs-α) actually showed a mutation in the gene encoding the α subunit of the stimulatory G protein that resulted in constitutive activation of adenylate cyclase in virtually all of the affected tissues of patients with Albright syndrome, including endocrine tissue, skin, and bone.[5, 38–40] This genetic mutation is present in a somatic mosaicism and consequently determines the various clinical manifestations of the disease.[5, 40] A somatic mutation of the Gs-α gene early in embryogenesis could determine the mosaic population of normal and mutant-bearing tissues.[40]

Based on the finding of a discordance for the major signs of McCune-Albright syndrome in monozygotic twins. Endo and coworkers[41] hypothesized a two-hit mutation: an inherited dominant mutation leading to polyostotic fibrous dysplasia and a second mutation in the somatic cells leading to a mosaicism resulting in McCune-Albright syndrome. This finding could possibly be related to the lack of hereditary transmission of the disease.

Recently with a new molecular biology technique, different types of mutations of the Gs-α gene have been identified by Miric and coworkers.[42]

DIAGNOSIS

Polyostotic fibrous dysplasia with the typical clinical manifestations and radiographic findings is easy to diagnose, especially if extraskeletal abnormalities are associated. Monostotic fibrous dysplasia can also be diagnosed by the clinicoradiologic features, but only when there is a typical ground-glass appearance with a sclerotic rim of bone and the lesion is asymptomatic or mildly symptomatic.

Other benign lesions such as a bone cyst, chondroma, giant cell tumor, or histiocystic fibroma may enter into the differential diagnosis with monostotic fibrous dysplasia. The clinical and radiographic findings typical of each of these lesions give a clue to the differential diagnosis. The characteristic radiolucency and a possible "fallen fragment" sign for a unicameral bone cyst, the amount and pattern of cartilage calcification for an enchondroma, the age and epiphyseal involvement for a giant cell tumor, and the eccentric location and cortical defect for a fibrous cortical defect will usually distinguish these lesions from fibrous dysplasia. In some cases when the radiographic findings are not characteristic, a biopsy is necessary for a definitive diagnosis.

Sometimes fibrous dysplasia of the tibia has to be differentiated from osteofibrous dysplasia.[43] As opposed to fibrous dysplasia, osteofibrous dysplasia originates primarily from the cortex and histologically shows lamellar and woven bone trabeculae rimmed by osteoblasts.[24]

One of the most critical problems in the differential diagnosis is presented by low-grade central osteosarcoma. As confirmed by recent reviews from the Mayo Clinic[44] and the Istituto Rizzoli,[45] low-grade central osteosarcoma often has a long duration of symptoms and a radiographic appearance very similar to that of fibrous dysplasia. The clue to the diagnosis is given by the histology; low-grade osteosarcoma constantly shows invasion of bone marrow and periosteum, which is never observed in fibrous dysplasia outside the jaws.[44, 45]

Rarely, Ollier's disease, Paget's disease, and multiple histiocytic fibromas must be considered in the differential diagnosis of polyostotic fibrous dysplasia. The different clinicoradiographic features are usually sufficient, and occasionally a biopsy is required.

Hyperparathyroidism, besides having the radiographic finding of diffuse osteopenia, will easily be differentiated through laboratory tests showing an increase in serum calcium, urinary calcium and phosphorus, and parathyroid hormone.

The only alteration in laboratory test findings in fibrous dysplasia, as first noticed by Lichtenstein in 1938[1] is represented by elevated levels of alkaline phosphatase, which is not a constant finding.

TREATMENT: HISTORICAL PERSPECTIVE

The surgical indications for treatment of fibrous dysplasia have been widely and variably discussed over the past years. As stated by Jaffe,[15] the presence of fibrous dysplasia "is not in itself an indication for treatment." Treatment is indicated for symptomatic lesions, persistent pain, pathologic fracture, or deformity.

In his review of the treatment of fibrous dysplasia, Jaffe suggested curettage and bone grafting for symptomatic lesions of long bones, resection for symptomatic expendable bones (such as ribs), and the use of metal prostheses after correction of severe deformities of the long bones.[15]

Supplementing curettage with a massive autogenous bone graft was also proposed to prevent the possible resorption of bone chips and recurrence[15]; other indications for surgery, according to Jaffe, were for cosmetic purposes in cases of craniofacial bone involvement with disfigurement.[15]

The experience with curettage and bone grafting was reviewed in 1962 by Stewart and associates.[46] These authors affirmed that "early active treatment" by curettage and bone grafting offered good results in monostotic fibrous dysplasia, although the possibility that adult age could have contributed to these good results in their patients was considered.[46] Stewart and associates reported that there was no evidence of the efficacy of radiation therapy in the treatment of fibrous dysplasia and that such treatment involved the risk of growth disturbance and possible postirradiation sarcoma.[46]

The patient's age usually influences the need for surgical treatment. Fibrous dysplasia tends to be less active after puberty, and it is usually manifested as a stage I Enneking lesion in adults, whereas it is most frequently observed in stage II in the prepubertal ages. On occasion, adults will have very active and progressive disease.

Harris and associates[14] studied 50 cases of fibrous dysplasia (13 monostotic and 37 polyostotic) and noticed that progression of the bone involvement was variably observed before and after puberty in their series. They reported three different types of progression: extension of preexisting lesions, the appearance of new lesions, and an increase in deformities.[14] The last was the most frequent type of progression observed in their series.[14]

Harris and coworkers[14] analyzed the repair of 125 fractures in 37 patients with polyostotic fibrous dysplasia—surgical procedures being required in 51 instances. The authors concluded that since nonunion was uncommon (2 cases in over 125 fractures), most pathologic fractures can be treated conservatively; the best indication for curettage and bone grafting is after closure of the epiphyseal plate. In addition, osteotomies with internal fixation are indicated in the treatment of deformities.[14] They also emphasized the hazard of radioinduced malignancies.[14]

In his study of 56 cases of monostotic fibrous dysplasia, Henry[47] reported success in 61% after curettage and bone grafting.[47]

CURRENT TREATMENT AND RECOMMENDATIONS

Many authors agree that operative intervention should be reserved for symptomatic fibrous dysplasia and that curettage in a young age group carries a high risk of recurrence and progression. In recent years, several studies have confirmed this observation.

Stephenson and coworkers[48] analyzed the results of treatment of 65 lesions in 43 patients; good results were obtained in the upper extremities and variable results in the lower extremities. They concluded that nonoperative treatment was sufficient for most symptomatic lesions in the upper extremities whereas internal fixation yielded better results in the lower extremities in patients younger than 18 years since neither nonoperative treatment nor curettage achieved satisfactory results.[48]

Nakashima and associates[49] reported success in six of eight patients treated by curettage and bone grafting. Many authors have reported that early correction of deformities is necessary to prevent progression.[14, 24, 48–51] The most common site of significant deformity is the proximal end of the femur.

Sofield and Millar in 1959 described the correction of proximal femoral deformity in two patients with polyostotic fibrous dysplasia with the use of a custom-made device consisting of an intramedullary rod and a cross-pin in the femoral head and neck.[52]

Connolly in 1977[50] and Freeman et al.[51] later described the use of the Zickel nail[53] following corrective proximal femoral osteotomies in patients with polyostotic fibrous dysplasia; the advantages of this technique are secure intramedullary fixation, decreased stress concentration distally, and excellent fixation of the head and neck. Secure proximal fixation in the femoral head is important because as Harris and coworkers have pointed out, the femoral head itself is not usually involved by the dysplastic bone.

Enneking and Gearen[54] proposed the use of autogenous cortical bone grafts (fibula) in the treatment of fibrous dysplasia in the femoral neck (Fig 6). The advantages of this technique are based on the incomplete creeping substitution of autogenous cortical graft by the host's repair bone, which would decrease the probability of recurrence as compared with the use of autogenous cancellous graft (Fig 7).[54] They reported good results (relief of pain and prevention of deformity) in all 15 patients without curettage or supplemental internal fixation. Bryant and associates reported similar results with fibular strut grafting.[55]

Betz and Knoefel reported the use of an allograft with a blade plate in the treatment of pathologic fractures and large lesions in patients with McCune-Albright syndrome.[56] This technique should be considered in patients with extensive bone loss.

Surgical treatment is rarely necessary in the spine and is reserved for

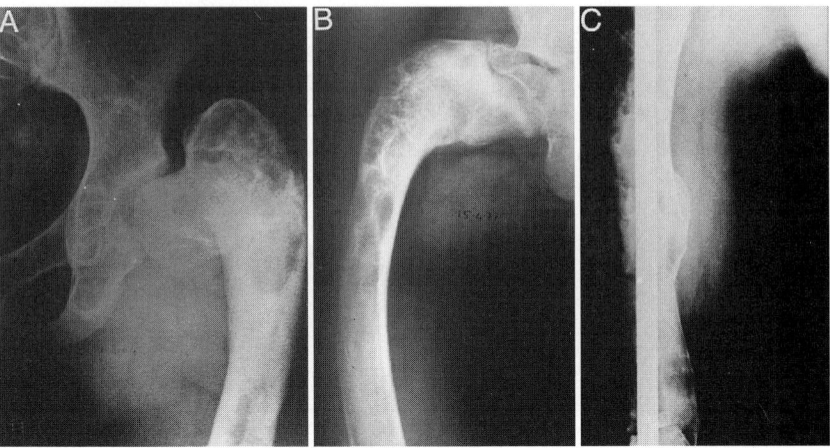

FIGURE 6.
A, "shepherd's crook" deformity of the proximal end of the femur in a patient with polyostotic fibrous dysplasia. **B,** the same type of deformity, in this case treated by osteotomies and internal fixation with an intramedullary rod **(C).**

patients with neurologic compromise or progressive deformity.[10, 57, 58] The goals of surgery are decompression and stabilization by anterior and/or posterior stabilization, as necessary.[57, 58]

Although most authors recommend early correction of deformities to prevent progression, there are numerous difficulties to be overcome to yield successful outcomes. Andrisano et al.[59] reviewed the surgical treatment of 65 patients with infantile fibrous dysplasia. They divided the lesions into "circumscribed" (less than 25% of the bone segment and only one cortex involved) and "extended" (involving more than 25% of the bone segment and both cortices).[59] The results of treatment depended on the extent of the dysplastic lesions: circumscribed lesions require only treatment of complications, whereas early surgical intervention is necessary for extended lesions.[59] They noted a high failure rate with plate fixation and recommended intramedullary fixation.

Recently, the role of medical treatment of fibrous dysplasia has been studied, and encouraging results have been reported with intravenous pamidronate.[60]

In summary, current treatment recommendations can be outlined as follows:

1. Radiation therapy should be avoided because it is ineffective and may potentiate the transition to malignant degeneration.
2. Indications for surgery depend on the clinicoradiographic features, the age of the patient, and the extent of disease.[24]
3. Asymptomatic or mildly symptomatic fibrous dysplasia usually does not require surgery unless there is significant risk of impending fracture. Pathologic fractures can often be treated nonoperatively, especially in the upper extremity.
4. Painful lesions can be safely managed by curettage and bone grafting. Fibular strut grafts (autogenous) are very useful in fibrous dysplasia of the femoral neck, and allografts can be used in some severe pathologic fractures.

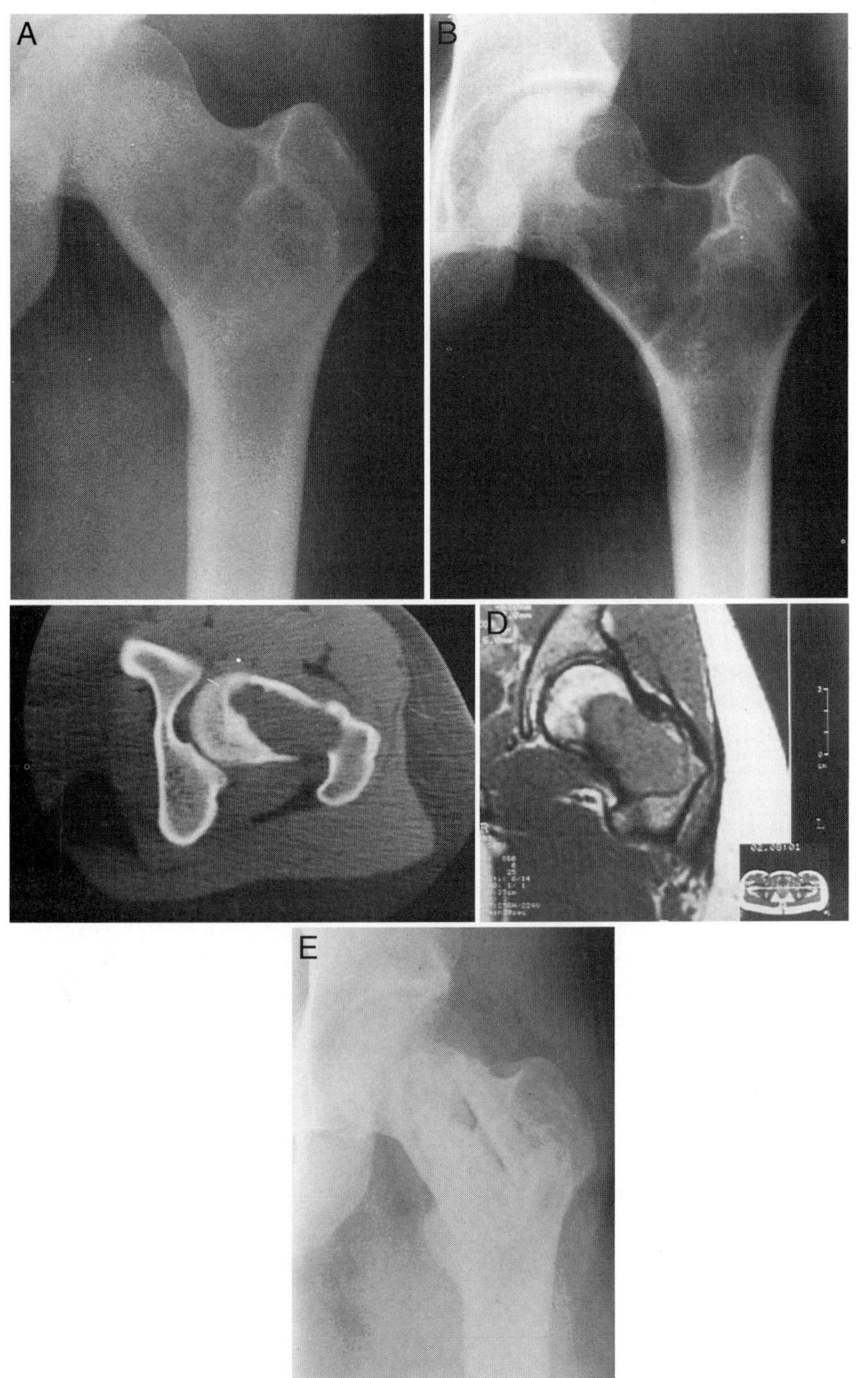

FIGURE 7.

Monostotic fibrous dysplasia of the femoral neck in an 18-year-old female **(A)**. Four months later, a new radiograph showed enlargement of the lytic area **(B)**; the lesion was painful. A CT scan **(C)** and MRI **(D)** clearly document extension of the lesion toward the head of the femur. Curettage and bone grafting with autogenous fibular strut grafts plus autogenous bone chips from the ilium were performed with success **(E)**. The histologic diagnosis was fibrous dysplasia with cartilaginous areas and cystic hemorrhagic foci.

5. Internal fixation, as a rule, is more successfully achieved by intermedullary devices. Early treatment of deformities is highly recommended to prevent further progression. To this aim, osteotomies must be accomplished by rigid internal fixation.[5] Resection of bony segments has rare indications and only for expendable bones (e.g., ribs) if painful and/or for diagnostic purposes.
6. In infantile fibrous dysplasia, "extended" lesions[59] require early surgical correction with adequate intermedullary fixation.

SARCOMAS IN FIBROUS DYSPLASIA

Sarcomas in fibrous dysplasia are rare and can occur in both monostotic and polyostotic fibrous dysplasia at an incidence ranging from 0.5% (in monostotic disease) to 4% (in Albright syndrome).[13] Since the first report by Coley and Stewart in 1945,[61] about 100 cases have been totally described in the literature.

In 1964, Schwartz and Alpert reviewed 26 cases of sarcomas in fibrous dysplasia (2 personal cases and 26 from the literature).[13] Campanacci and coworkers in 1975 reported 6 personal cases.[62] Yabut and associates in 1988 did a careful review of the literature and found 83 cases and added a single case.[63] The most common sarcoma observed in fibrous dysplasia was osteosarcoma, followed by chondrosarcoma and fibrosarcoma.

The role of radiation therapy in the development of sarcoma in fibrous dysplasia has been widely discussed. The two largest series in the literature are that from Memorial Sloan-Kettering (New York) reported by

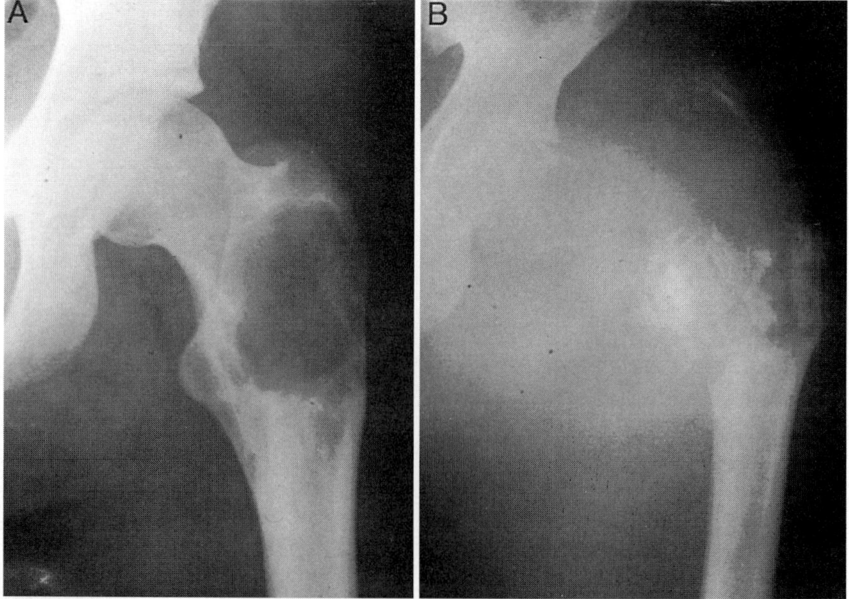

FIGURE 8.
Monostotic fibrous dysplasia in the proximal end of the femur **(A).** Nine years later, a high-grade osteosarcoma developed **(B).**

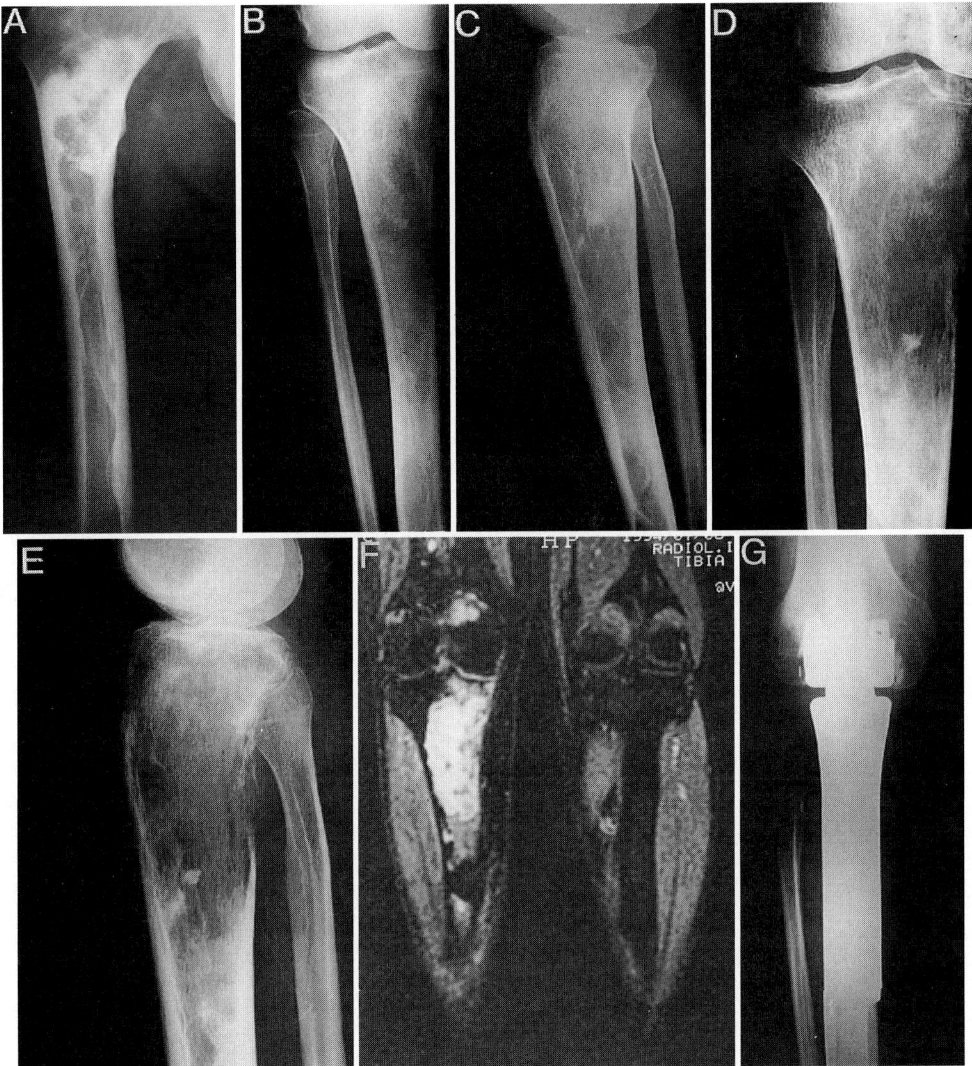

FIGURE 9.
Radiography of the femur **(A)** and tibia **(B** and **C)** in a 42-year-old male in whom polyostotic fibrous dysplasia was diagnosed several years before. One month later, radiographs **(D** and **E)** showed a progression of the lytic lesion with destruction of the posteromedial cortex of the proximal end of the tibia. **F,** T2-weighted image on MRI. Biopsy revealed malignant fibrous histiocytoma in fibrous dysplasia. After preoperative chemotherapy, a wide resection and reconstruction with a prosthesis **(G)** were performed.

Huvos and coworkers in 1972[64] and 1991[65] and that from the Mayo Clinic reported by Ruggieri and coworkers in 1994.[66] In Huvos' series, only 1 of 15 patients had received prior radiation therapy.[65]

In the Mayo Clinic series of 28 sarcomas in fibrous dysplasia, 19 in monostotic and 9 in polyostotic (observed in 1,122 histologically diagnosed cases of fibrous dysplasia), radiation therapy had been previously given in 13 cases (46%).[66] Radiation therapy plays an important role in the occurrence of sarcomas in fibrous dysplasia, but sarcomas do occur in the absence of prior irradiation. These findings confirm that radiation therapy must be avoided in the treatment of fibrous dysplasia. In the Mayo Clinic series of 28 cases, there were 19 osteosarcomas, 5 fibrosarcomas, 3 chondrosarcomas, and 1 malignant fibrous histiocytoma (Fig 8).[66]

In Yabut and associates' review, there were 40 osteosarcomas, 22 fibrosarcomas, 11 chondrosarcomas, and 10 other sarcomas.[63] Low-grade central osteosarcoma, secondary aneurysmal bone cysts in fibrous dysplasia, and cystic degeneration of fibrous dysplasia must be considered in the differential diagnosis of sarcomas in fibrous dysplasia.[66] Computed tomographic and MRI scans are the best tools for the differential diagnosis.

The prognosis of sarcomas in fibrous dysplasia is poor, but the Mayo Clinic data seem to indicate that patients treated more recently with neoadjuvant chemotherapy and adequate surgery have a better prognosis, similar to that of the corresponding primary sarcomas (Fig 9). Current experiences at the Instituto Rizzoli with newly diagnosed and treated cases of sarcomas in fibrous dysplasia seems to confirm this observation. An early diagnosis and adequate treatment are necessary to improve the prognosis of sarcomas in fibrous dysplasia.[66]

REFERENCES

1. Lichtenstein L: Polyostotic fibrous dysplasia. *Arch Surg* 36:874–898, 1938.
2. Lichtenstein L, Jaffe HL: Fibrous dysplasia of bone: Conditions affecting one, several, or many bones; the graver cases of which may present abnormal pigmentation of skin, premature sexual development, hyperthyroidism, or still other extraskeletal abnormalities. *Arch Pathol* 33:777–816, 1942.
3. McCune DJ: Osteitis fibrosa cystica: The case of a nine-year-old girl who also exhibits precocious puberty, multiple pigmentation of the skin and hyperthyroidism. *Am J Dis Child* 52:743-744, 1936.
4. Albright F, Butler AM, Hampton AO, et al: Syndrome characterized by osteitis fibrosa disseminata, areas of pigmentation and endocrine dysfunction with precocious puberty in females: Report of five cases. *N Engl J Med* 216:727–746, 1937.
5. Scully RE, Mark EJ, McNeely WF, et al: Case records of the Massachusetts General Hospital. *N Engl J Med* 328:496–502, 1993.
6. Mirra JM, Picci P, Gold RH: *Bone Tumors, Clinical Radiology, and Pathologic Correlation*, vol 1. Philadelphia, Lea & Febiger, 1989, pp 191–226.
7. Dahlin DC, Unni KK: *Bone Tumors: General Aspects and Data on 8,542 Cases*. Springfield, Ill, Charles C Thomas, 1986, pp 413–420.
8. Wilner D: *Radiology of Bone Tumors and Allied Disorders*, vol 2, Philadelphia, WB Saunders, 1982, pp 1443–1580.
9. Kricun M (ed): *Imaging of Bone Tumors: Tumors of the Spine*. Philadelphia, WB Saunders, 1993, pp 269–270.
10. Nabarro MN, Giblin PE: Monostotic fibrous dysplasia of the thoracic spine. *Spine* 19:461–465, 1994.
11. Rosenblum B, Overby C, Levine M, et al: Monostotic fibrous dysplasia of the thoracic spine. *Spine* 12:939–942, 1987.
12. Singer J, Sundaram M, Merenda GG, et al: Fibrous dysplasia of thoracic vertebra arising de novo: Cheirurogenic in origin? *Orthopedics* 14:855–858, 1991.
13. Schwartz DT, Alpert M: The malignant transformation of fibrous dysplasia. *Am J Med Sci* 247:1–20, 1964.

14. Harris WH, Dudley HR Jr, Barry RJ: The natural history of fibrous dysplasia: An orthopaedic, pathological, and roentgenographic study. *J Bone Joint Surg Am* 44:207–233, 1962.
15. Jaffe HL: *Tumors and Tumorous Conditions of the Bones and Joints.* Philadelphia, Lea & Febiger, 1958, pp 117–142.
16. Korf BR: Diagnostic outcome in children with multiple cafe au lait spots. *Pediatrics* 90:924–927, 1992.
17. Mazabraud A, Girard J: Un cas particulier de dysplasia fibreus a localizations osseuses et tendineuses. *Rev Rhum Ed Fr* 34:652–659, 1957.
18. Henschen F: Fall von ostitis Fibrosa mit multiplen Tumoren in der umgebenden Muskulatur. *Verh Deutsch Ges Pathol* 21:93–97, 1926.
19. Krogius A: Ein Fall von ostitis Fibrosa mit multiplen fibromyxomatosen Muskeltumoren. *Acta Chir Scand* 64:465–471, 1928.
20. Wirth WA, Leavitt D, Enzinger FM: Multiple intramuscular myxomas: Another extraskeletal manifestation of fibrous dysplasia. *Cancer* 27:1167–1173, 1971.
21. Biagini R, Ruggieri P, Boriani S, et al: The Mazabraud syndrome: Case report and review of the literature. *Ital J Orthop Traumatol* 13:105–112, 1987.
22. Gober GA, Nicholas RW: Case report 800. *Skeletal Radiol* 22:452–455, 1993.
23. Prayson MA, Leeson MC: Soft tissue myxomas and fibrous dysplasia of bone: A case report and review of the literature. *Clin Orthop* 291:222–228, 1993.
24. Campanacci M: *Bone and Soft Tissue Tumors.* New York, Springer-Verlag, 1990, pp 391–417.
25. Machida K, Makita K, Nishikawa J, et al: Scintigraphic manifestation of fibrous dysplasia. *Clin Nucl Med* 11:426–429, 1986.
26. Simpson AH, Creasy TS, Williamson DM, et al: Cystic degeneration of fibrous dysplasia masquerading as sarcoma. *J Bone Joint Surg Br* 71:434–436, 1989.
27. Diercks RL, Sauter AJM, Mallens WMC: Aneurysmal bone cyst in association with fibrous dysplasia: A case report. *J Bone Joint Surg Br* 68:144–146, 1986.
28. Martinez V, Sissons HA: Aneurysmal bone cyst: A review of 123 cases including primary lesions and those secondary to other bone pathology. *Cancer* 61:2291–2304, 1988.
29. Wojno KJ, McCarthy EF: Fibro-osseous lesions of the face and skull with aneurysmal bone cyst formation. *Skeletal Radiol* 23:15–18, 1994.
30. Yao L, Eckardt JJ, Seeger LL: Fibrous dysplasia associated with cortical bony destruction: CT and MR findings. *J Comput Assist Tomogr* 18:91–94, 1994.
31. Fisher AJ, Totty WG, Kyriakos M: MR appearance of cystic fibrous dysplasia. *J Comput Assist Tomogr* 18:315–318, 1994.
32. Utz JA, Kransdorf MJ, Jelinek JS, et al: MR appearance of fibrous dysplasia. *J Comput Assist Tomogr* 13:845–851, 1989.
33. Richardson ML, Gillespy T III: Magnetic resonance imaging, in Kricun ME (ed): *Imaging of Bone Tumors.* Philadelphia, WB Saunders, 1993, pp 358–445.
34. Norris MA, Kaplan PA, Pathria M, et al: Fibrous dysplasia: Magnetic resonance imaging appearance at 1.5 tesla. *Clin Imaging* 14:211–215, 1990.
35. Lichtenstein L: *Diseases of Bones and Joints,* ed 2. St Louis, Mosby, 1975, pp 17–24.
36. Lee PA, Van Dop C, Migeon CJ: McCune-Albright syndrome: Long-term follow-up. *JAMA* 256:2980–2984, 1986.
37. Mauras N, Blizzard RM: The McCune Albright syndrome. *Acta Endocrinol Suppl* 279:207–217, 1986.
38. Schwindinger WF, Francomano CA, Levine MA: Identification of a mutation in the gene encoding the alpha subunit of the stimulatory G protein of adenylyl cyclase in McCune-Albright syndrome. *Proc Natl Acad Sci U S A* 89:5152–5156, 1992.

39. Shenker A, Sweet D, Spiegel A, et al: An activating Gs alpha mutation is present in fibrous dysplasia of bone in the McCune-Albright syndrome (abstract). Presented at the 14th Annual Meeting of the American Society for Bone and Mineral Research, Minneapolis, 1992.
40. Weinstein LS, Shenker A, Gejman PV, et al: Activating mutations of the stimulatory G protein in the McCune-Albright syndrome. *N Engl J Med* 325:1688–1695, 1991.
41. Endo M, Yamada Y, Matsuura N, et al: Monozygotic twins discordant for the major signs of McCune-Albright. *Am J Med Genet* 41:216–220, 1991.
42. Miric A, Vechio JD, Levine MA: Heterogeneous mutations in the gene encoding the alpha subunit of the stimulatory G protein of adenylyl cyclase in Albright hereditary osteodystrophy. *J Clin Endocrinol Metab* 6:1560–1568, 1993.
43. Campanacci M, Laus M: Osteofibrous dysplasia of the tibia and fibula. *J Bone Joint Surg Am* 63:367–375, 1981.
44. Sim FH, Kurt AM, McLeod RA, et al: Case report 628. *Skeletal Radiol* 19:457–460, 1990.
45. Bertoni F, Bacchini F, Fabbri N, et al: Osteosarcoma: Low-grade intraosseous-type-osteosarcoma, histologically resembling parosteal osteosarcoma, fibrous dysplasia, and desmoplastic-fibroma. *Cancer* 71:338–345, 1993.
46. Stewart MJ, Gilmer WS Jr, Edmonson AS: Fibrous dysplasia of bone. *J Bone Joint Surg Br* 44:302–318, 1962.
47. Henry A: Monostotic fibrous dysplasia. *J Bone Joint Surg Br* 51:300–306, 1969.
48. Stephenson RB, London MD, Hankin FM, et al: Fibrous dysplasia: An analysis of options for treatment. *J Bone Joint Surg Am* 69:400–409, 1967.
49. Nakashima Y, Kotoura Y, Nagashima T, et al: Monostotic fibrous dysplasia in the femoral neck: A clinicopathologic study. *Clin Orthop* 191:242–248, 1984.
50. Connolly JF: Shepherd's crook deformities of polyostotic fibrous dysplasia treated by osteotomy and Zickel nail fixation. *Clin Orthop* 123:22–24, 1977.
51. Freeman BH, Bray EW, Meyer LC: Multiple osteotomies with Zickel nail fixation for polyostotic fibrous dysplasia involving the proximal part of the femurs. *J Bone Joint Surg Am* 69:691–698, 1987.
52. Sofield HA, Millar EA: Fragmentation, realignment, and intramedullary rod fixation of deformities of the long bones in children: A ten-year appraisal. *J Bone Joint Surg Am* 41:1371–1391, 1959.
53. Zickel RE: A new fixation device for subtrochanteric fracture of the femur: A preliminary report. *Clin Orthop* 54:115–123, 1967.
54. Enneking WF, Gearen PF: Fibrous dysplasia of the femoral neck: Treatment by cortical bone grafting. *J Bone Joint Surg Am* 68:1414–1422, 1986.
55. Bryant DD, Grant RE, Tang D: Fibular strut grafting for fibrous dysplasia of the femoral neck. *J Natl Med Assoc* 84:893–897, 1992.
56. Betz A, Knoefel WT: Pathologic fracture of the femoral neck in a patient with McCune-Albright syndrome. *Orthopedics* 15:743–746, 1992.
57. Ehara S, Kattapuram SV, Rosenberg AE: Fibrous dysplasia of the spine. *Spine* 17:977–979, 1992.
58. Shikata J, Yamamuro T, Shimizo K, et al: Kyphoscoliosis in polyostotic fibrous dypslasia: A case report. *Spine* 17:1534–1539, 1992.
59. Andrisano A, Soncini G, Calderoni PP, et al: Critical review of infantile fibrous dysplasia: Surgical treatment. *J Pediatr Orthop* 11:478–481, 1991.
60. Liens D, Delmas PD, Meunier PJ: Long-term effects of intravenous pamidronate in fibrous dysplasia of bone. *Lancet* 343:953–954, 1994.
61. Coley BL, Stewart FW: Bone sarcoma in polyostotic fibrous dysplasia. *Ann Surg* 121:872–881, 1945.

62. Campanacci M, Bertoni F, Capanna R: Malignant degeneration in fibrous dysplasia: Presentation of 6 cases and review of the literature. *Ital J Orthop Traumatol* 5:373–381, 1975.
63. Yabut SM Jr, Kenan S, Sissons HA, et al: Malignant transformation of fibrous dysplasia: A case report and review of the literature. *Clin Orthop* 228:281–289, 1988.
64. Huvos AG, Higinbotham NL, Miller TR: Bone sarcomas arising in fibrous dysplasia. *J Bone Joint Surg Am* 54:1047–1056, 1972.
65. Huvos AG: *Bone Tumors: Diagnosis, Treatment and Prognosis.* Philadelphia, WB Saunders, 1991, pp 41–48.
66. Ruggieri P, Sim FH, Bond JR, et al: Malignancies in fibrous dysplasia. *Cancer* 73:1411–1424, 1994.

Congenital Pseudarthrosis of the Tibia: Current Concepts of Treatment

Sherman S. Coleman, M.D.
Department of Orthopedics, University of Utah Medical Center, Salt Lake City, Utah

Don A. Coleman, M.D.
Department of Orthopedics, University of Utah Medical Center, Salt Lake City, Utah

Gregory Biddulph, M.D.
Department of Orthopedics, University of Utah Medical Center, Salt Lake City, Utah

Congenital pseudarthrosis of the tibia, although exceedingly uncommon, is one of the most challenging musculoskeletal problems with which the orthopedic surgeon must deal. The reasons are several. First, the etiology has never been well established,[1, 2] and since the exact cause has not been identified, therapeutic programs have been largely based on conceptual considerations as they apply to acquired post-traumatic nonunions. Although frequentiy associated with neurofibromatosis, its direct causal relationship has never been well established and is surely not clearly understood (see later). It is, however, well known that patients with congenital pseudarthrosis of the tibia have a substantially greater incidence of neurofibromatosis as compared with the general population.[3–7]

Second, perhaps one of the most frustrating and disconcerting considerations revolves around the time-proven observation that the well-established and conventional forms of treatment of post-traumatic osseous nonunion are often futile and very often result in failure when applied to the treatment of congenital tibial pseudarthrosis. These failures have resulted in the need for repeated operative procedures, and a multiplicity of therapeutic programs have been proposed in search of the best method of treating this very capricious and challenging problem. These enigmatic issues very often provide a stern test of the willingness of the patient (and the parents) to accept long-term, often unsuccessful surgical ventures that have been employed in search of a predictable cure that will preserve functional use of the limb.

Third, well-established, long-term results of any form of treatment have been rarely reported. Any therapeutic program that in the beginning may show great promise has often subsequently proved to be a failure

Advances in Operative Orthopaedics, vol. 3

after skeletal growth and development. Therefore, any conclusions regarding etiologic factors and therapeutic programs must await the test of time. Currently, there is a notable paucity of any proven long-term end-result studies.[3,4,8–12]

ETIOLOGY, PATHOLOGY, AND PATHOGENESIS

No lesion of the musculoskeletal system has projected more confusion regarding its etiology, pathology, or pathogenesis than congenital pseudarthrosis of the tibia (or fibula). It has been a substantial source of frustration for pathologists as well as surgeons. Much of the explanation for this frustration lies in the fact that there is controversy about the histopathology of the tissues in and about the site of the pseudarthrosis. Analysis of removed tissue specimens from the area of the pseudarthrosis has not been particularly helpful, and because of occasional coexisting lesions, they may be confusing and even counterproductive.

Etiologically, there are several conceptual theories, but none has been unequivocally established. These include the following: (1) localized avascular bone, usually with deformity that often results in fracture with resulting failure of union[13–16]; (2) abnormal bone containing a variety of localized lesions that may (or may not) be etiologically related to the pseudarthrosis[17–19]; some of these lesions have been impossible to classify on a purely histopathologic basis; (3) soft tissue "constriction" bands that emanate from dysplastic or proliferative "hamartomatous tissue"[20,21]; this concept argues that the periosseous tissue is relatively avascular and essentially "squeezes out" the vasculature of the underlying bone; and (4) neurofibromatosis, which although often associated, has a poorly established direct causal relationship to congenital tibial pseudarthrosis. On the other hand, its rather frequent, well-established association with neurofibromatosis is sufficiently evident that the problem may lie in our ineffectiveness in establishing a scientifically proven etiologic relationship.[5–7]

Pathologically, past and current interpretation of the histopathology of the pseudarthrotic area of the tibia (or fibula) has usually focused on nonspecific elements of the lesion. Based on our current knowledge, the following are issues on which there is some consensus: (1) a true neurofibromatotic lesion is uncommon, (2) lesions such as fibrous dysplasia or similarly "dysplastic" fibrous lesions are probably coincidental, and (3) the nondescript "hamartomatous tissue" described by Boyd has not been scientifically proved as a causal factor.[22] Observations that suggest a possible etiologic relationship between a neurofibromatous lesion and congenital pseudarthrosis are those reported by Lloyd-Roberts and Shaw and by Green and Rudo.[3,23] Even their findings suggest more that the pseudarthrosis was the result of a pathologic fracture rather than a neurofibroma eroding the bone. However, Pitt and colleagues[24] have reported that neurofibromatous tissue has been demonstrated as "irritating the periosteum" and that radiolucencies occur in the long bones and are due to proliferation of type 1 neurofibromatosis (NF1) tissue "in the medullary cavity."

The only consistently proven histologic findings that have been observed or reported consist of rather nonspecific observations that include reparative fibrous tissue, healing and reparative cartilaginous callus, and osteoid and osteoblastic elements, all representative of attempts at osseous repair. In brief, with the uncommon exceptions just noted, no helpful histopathologic observations have been identified beyond those found in pseudarthrosis of any long bone irrespective of cause.

We studied several specimens removed at the time of surgery by using electron microscopic techniques and special stains and could find nothing more specific than those observations just noted.[25] We have concluded that irrespective of the numerous efforts made at attempting to identify a proven etiology in congenital tibial pseudarthrosis, its proximate cause and pathogenesis remain obscure. This, of course, confounds any scientifically based efforts at treatment and largely explains the array of therapeutic strategies that have been employed over the years in search of solutions that have often been futile.

CLASSIFICATION

Although any classification of a condition has potential value, it effectively relates only to the manner in which it affects treatment and prognosis. Prior classifications[4, 26–31] of this condition have taken many important issues into account, but they have not been particularly productive, and indeed, they may even be counterproductive. One of the most well accepted classifications heretofore proposed is that of Boyd, who described six types.[22] Even though time honored, his classification has not necessarily influenced methods of treatment, nor does it predict the probable success or failure of any specific treatment program.

The authors have devised a simple classification based on the following: (1) isolated (incidental) prepseudarthrosis or pseudarthrosis unrelated to any other causal localized lesion or syndrome (Fig 1, A), (2) *congenital* pseudarthrosis associated with neurofibromatosis (Fig 2, A), and (3) pseudarthrosis or prepseudarthrosis occurring in the presence of other probable incidental skeletal lesions. This classification also emphasizes the importance of the presence or absence of a fibular pseudarthrosis coexisting with an ipsilateral tibial pseudarthrosis. This seems important because it has been our experience that an isolated tibial lesion has a better rate of successful union than when associated with pseudarthrosis of both bones, especially when they occur at the same level. To this must be added two very important clinical and radiographic findings, namely, the location of the pseudarthrosis and the status of the bone in the area of the pseudarthrosis. If the nonunion is in the distal part of the tibia, fixation across the ankle into the tarsal bones may be required.[32] Also, if the medullary canal and the bone are narrowed or constricted at the prepseudarthrotic (or pseudarthrotic) level, then efforts at gaining union are often less successful.[22]

CLINICAL MANIFESTATIONS AND FINDINGS

From a simplistic point of view, three major scenarios can be encountered most frequently. The first consists of a "prepseudarthrosis" characterized by a congenital anterolateral bowing deformity of the tibia and

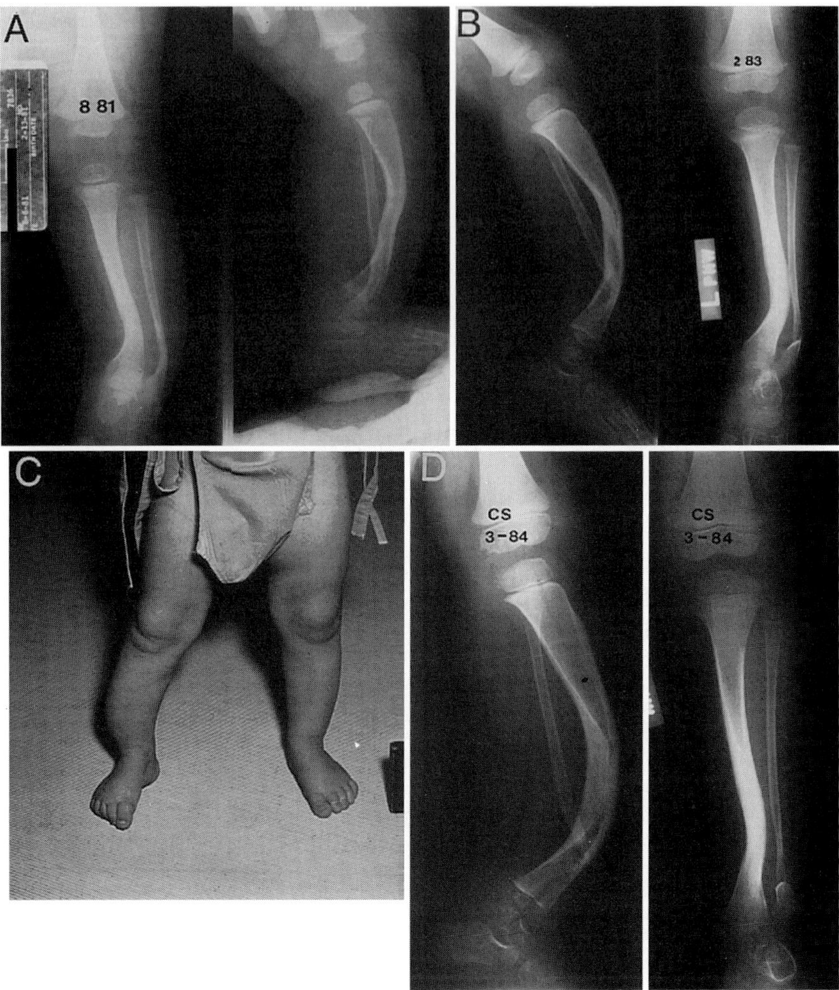

FIGURE 1.

Anteroposterior and lateral radiographs of the leg of a 6-month-old boy **(A)**. Note the anterolateral bowing deformity of both the tibia and fibula. At the age of 2 years, despite bracing, the deformity increased **(B)**. Note the typical anterolateral deformity in the standing photograph **(C)**. One year later the deformity became unacceptable **(D)**.

fibula (Fig 1, A–D). It is often associated with narrowing of the tibia (and fibula) at the site of ultimate fracture or corrective osteotomy. Subsequently, a pathologic fracture results from minimal trauma followed by failure of union, or the deformity increases and necessitates a corrective osteotomy, again followed by failure of union and the development of a pseudarthrosis at the site of the osteotomy (Fig 1, E).

Second, congenital tibial pseudarthrosis may be present at birth (as implied by the name), or it develops during early infancy. It has various radiologic appearances and occurs in varying locations in the tibia. For example, the ends of the fragments may become hyperostotic (favorable prognosis), or they may have a narrowed, atrophic "sucked candy" ap-

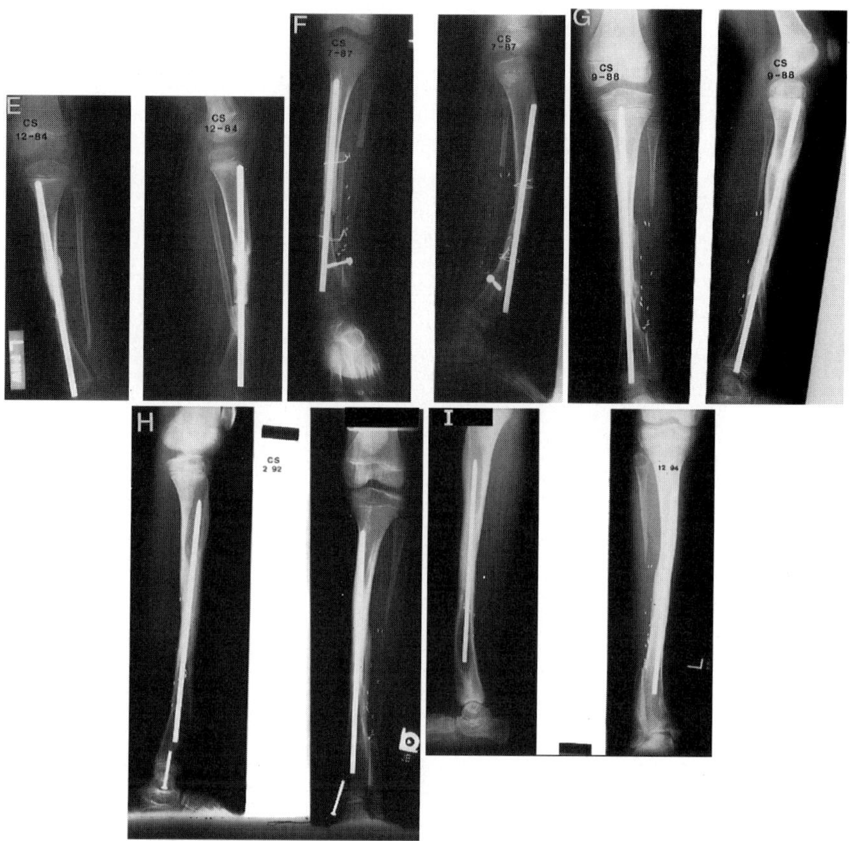

FIGURE 1 (cont.).
Therefore a double tibial osteotomy and intramedullary rodding were accomplished **(E)**. Union occurred at the proximal osteotomy but failed distally. At the age of 7 years a transfer of the ipsilateral fibula was done in addition to synostosis of the distal ends of the tibia and fibula to prevent ankle valgus **(F)**. Union took place, but because of deformity, a new, longer rod was inserted, the deformity corrected, and additional iliac bone graft inserted. Note the tibiofibular synostosis **(G)**. Improved alignment and consolidation of the pseudarthrosis is evident, and a medial malleolar screw has been inserted in an effort to correct the ankle valgus **(H)**. The most recent film at 14 years of age shows good alignment and solid union **(I)**. (From Coleman SS, Coleman DA: *J Pediatr Orthop* 14:156–160, 1994. Used by permission.)

pearance portending an unfavorable prognosis. The fibula is involved more often than not, and a substantial number of cases, as noted earlier, are associated with neurofibromatosis. In this latter situation, the fibula is narrowed and is very often atrophic (see Fig 2, A).[22]

Finally, fracture of the tibia occurs from varying minor degrees of trauma, followed by failure of union and ultimately the development of a true pseudarthrosis. These usually occur in infancy and later childhood and the fibula is rarely if ever involved. We have observed that as a general rule, the prognosis for obtaining union is substantially better than in either of the previous circumstances (Fig 3, A–C).

In all of the aforementioned situations, once the failure of union is

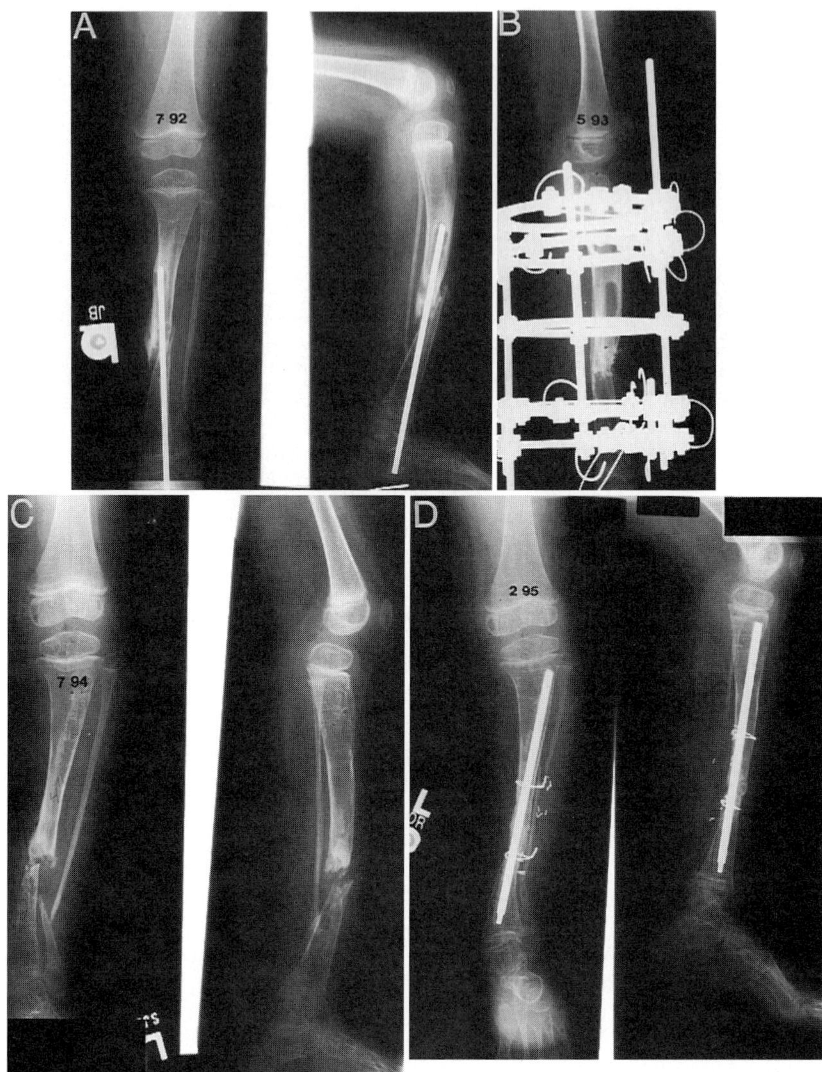

FIGURE 2.
Obvious pseudarthrosis of both the tibia and fibula of a 4-year-old who had previously had his tibia rodded **(A)**. An effort at union by using Ilizarov devices was made **(B)**. Unfortunately union failed **(C)**. As a consequence, an ipsilateral fibular transfer and iliac bone grafting were accomplished. Early union is apparent **(D)**.

identified and a clearly identified pseudarthrosis results, surgical treatment is the only possible reliable means of producing osteosynthesis.[33] This, however, is more easily said than done, as will be underscored in the following historical review of the treatment of this lesion.

HISTORICAL REVIEW OF TREATMENT STRATEGIES

In order to put the complexity of management of this condition into perspective, a brief historical review of the major therapeutic programs that have been attempted in the past, although not complete, is helpful. First

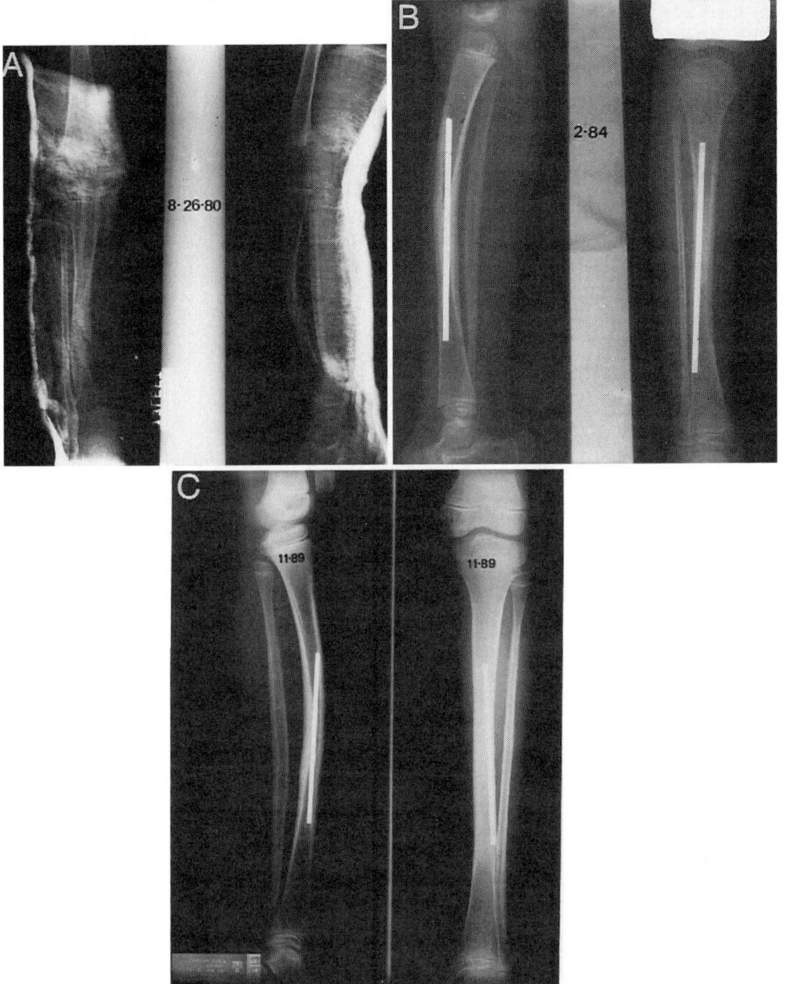

FIGURE 3.
Obvious tibial fracture in a 2-year-old boy with an anterior bowing deformity of the tibia that occurred with minimal trauma. It had been treated in an above-knee cast for 6 months without union. Note the intact fibula **(A)**. Primary osseous union occurred with intramedullary rodding and iliac bone grafting **(B)**. At the age of 11, maintenance of solid union is evident **(C)**.

of all, as noted earlier, all pseudarthroses following the previously described situations require surgical treatment for any likelihood of successful union.[33] However, in the prepseudarthrosis state, usually seen during the first year or two of life, the major problem is an anterolateral bowing deformity of the tibia without fracture (see Fig 1, A–D). For this situation the time-honored and more or less unchallenged therapeutic program involves the use of a custom-made brace that supports the deformed tibia and optimally (although rarely) prevents further deformity or fracture[34] (Fig 4, A and B). The purpose is to delay corrective osteotomy or fracture for as long as possible since osteotomy is most often, if not invariably followed by failure of union. Then a typical pseudarthrosis develops with all of its attendant problems. Few argue with this approach simply be-

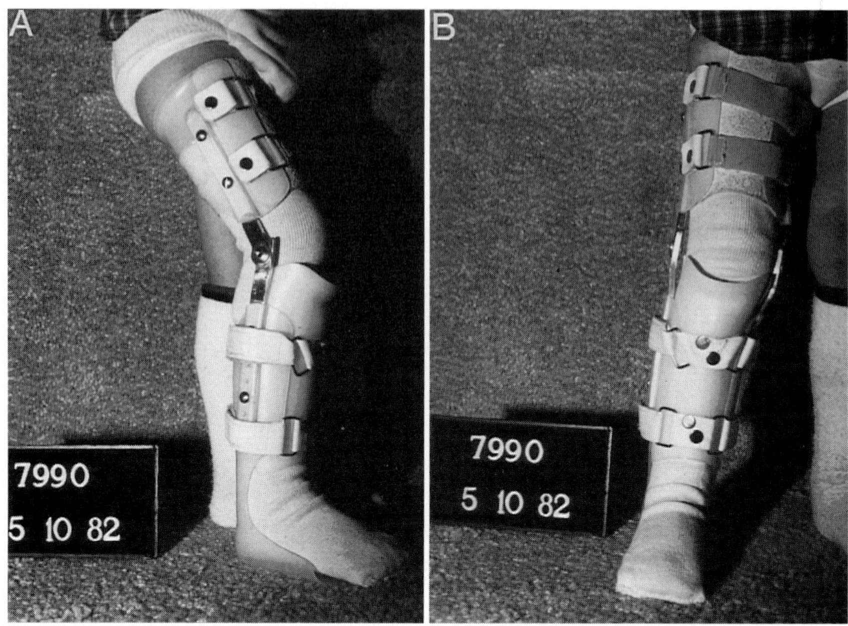

FIGURE 4.
Above-knee brace used both in the anterior bow (prepseudarthrosis) state and following cast removal after surgery **(A** and **B).** Note the solid ankle because the intramedullary rod crossed the ankle joint. This must be a custom-made orthosis. (From Coleman SS, Coleman DA: *J Pediatr Orthop* 14:156–160, 1994. Used by permission.)

cause wearing the brace is rather innocuous and it may rarely produce correction[34]; however, when fracture occurs or osteotomy is accomplished, the brace can and must be used postoperatively after cast removal.

From a surgical standpoint there is a litany of treatment strategies that have been proposed. These are listed as follows:

1. Internal fixation with plates or screws along with an allograft, often being taken from the parents
2. Dual-onlay cortical bone grafts fixed with bicortical screws and using bone oftentimes taken from the bone bank or from a close relative or the parents[35]
3. Autogenous "bypass graft" taken from the patient's opposite tibia[36]
4. A cross-legged vascularized pedicle graft taken from the opposite tibia through a complex program involving the transfer of a bone graft from the donor tibia to the recipient tibia[37]
5. Internal fixation with an intramedullary rod and iliac bone graft[10, 32, 38]; this includes the use of an intramedullary rod that may or may not cross the ankle joint, according to Charnley,[32] depending on the location of the pseudarthrosis in the tibia
6. Double proximal and distal osteotomy followed by complete reversal of the tibial shaft with intramedullary rodding[39]; the concept behind

this approach is that by reversing the entire diaphysis, one is placing healthy bone in the location of the diseased bone

7. Intramedullary rodding and transfer of the vascularized ipsilateral fibula to the tibia accompanied by an autogenous iliac graft[40]
8. Excision of the pseudarthrosis accompanied by "bone transport techniques" using the Ilizarov technique[41]
9. Contralateral microvascular fibular graft preceded at the same operation by excision of the tibial pseudarthrosis[42, 43]
10. Electrical current stimulation of osteogenesis by means of either an internal battery or a transcutaneous electrical field[10]
11. Foot disarticulation or transmedullary amputation prompted by multiple failed surgical efforts and the inability of the parents and/or patient to accept further surgical treatment modalities that have unfortunately resulted in repeated complications and ultimate failure[44, 45]

Many of the aforementioned treatment programs have been discarded, mostly because of their unpredictable performance and resultant failure. For example, the "bypass" graft developed by McFarland,[36] was designed to use a substantial cortical cancellous graft taken from the contralateral tibia. It was placed into the proximal and distal fragments of the affected bone to bridge the pseudarthrosis posteriorly. Thus it served as an osteogenic "strut." Although best employed in cases of anterior tibial bowing (prepseudarthrosis), the success rate was less than desired or expected, and consequently it has largely been abandoned. Two cases attempted by the senior author have failed (Fig 5, A).

Sofield and Millar thought that the basic pathologic problem was the presence of abnormal osseous tissue and poor blood supply at the site of the pseudarthrosis. They therefore proposed that by reversing the entire diaphysis of the tibia (nonvascularized and essentially devascularized), healthy bone in the proximal part of the tibia could be transferred to the area of the pseudarthrosis and somehow stimulate osteogenesis.[39] Even though intramedullary fixation was employed, numerous failures led to its ultimate abandonment. The so-called Sofield "reversal graft" is rarely if ever implemented at this time.

Boyd[9, 22, 35, 46] was one of the leading students of this uncommon, frustrating, but challenging problem. He recognized the great difficulties posed by the pseudarthrosis, which never responded to the usual and conventional methods of treatment of ordinary post-traumatic tibia pseudarthroses. He developed the "dual-onlay" bone graft technique along with its variations.[35] Despite early success in a substantial number of cases, it soon became clear to Boyd himself that failure ultimately occurred in many. The screws produced stress risers, the allografts were often resorbed, and even after promising early union in some cases the pseudarthrosis commonly recurred.

The results of these various "conventional" forms of treatment were so dismal that at one time the amputation rate for congenital pseudarthrosis was upward of 85% (14 of 16 cases in the University of Illinois). Despite this, however, Sofield apprised the American Academy of Ortho-

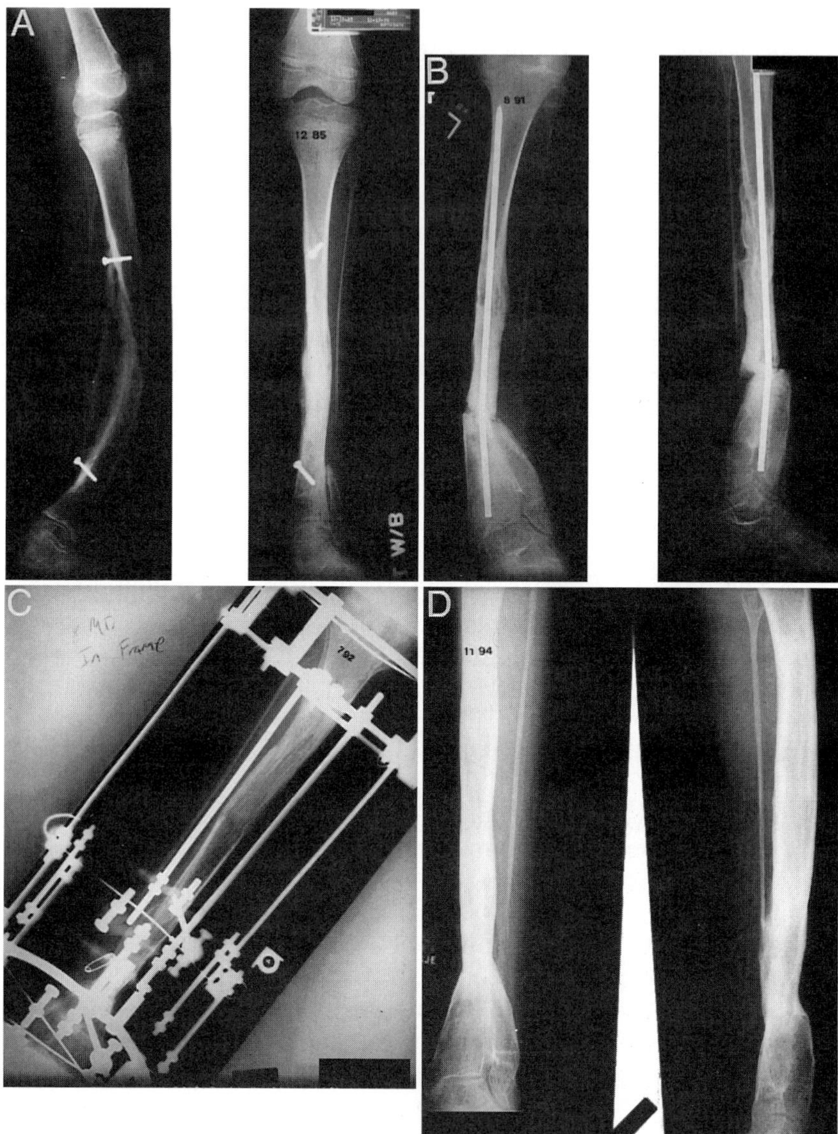

FIGURE 5.
A 9-year-old boy underwent a McFarlane "by-pass" graft 2 years previously **(A)**. The deformity remained and intramedullary rodding and bone grafting were accomplished but resulted in failure **(B)**. A distal tibiofibular synostosis had been accomplished, and final union with correction of alignment was achieved by using the Ilizarov technique **(C)**. Note that patient is now skeletally mature **(D)**. (Courtesy of Dr. Peter F. Armstrong.)

pedic Surgeons at an open meeting that the best approach to this distressing situation was to "keep trying."[1] Nonetheless, the stresses of repeated failures oftentimes mandated a request for amputation by the patient or parents.

In 1952, Farmer proposed transferring a vascularized portion of the contralateral tibia by a cross-legged pedicle technique.[37] The transferred tibial segment maintained its blood supply by anastomosing the donor vessels to the recipient vessels in the involved pseudarthrotic tibia, a technique much the same as employed in microvascular free myocutaneous flaps for major soft tissue defects. The difference was that the donor leg had to be crossed over the recipient leg until satisfactory vascularization of the donor bone took place in its recipient bed. This was rather cumbersome, and even though conceptually attractive, it never became well accepted. In some ways it was a precursor to the microvascularized contralateral fibular transfer currently being promulgated that will be subsequently discussed. As a consequence, the trend has been toward reverting to the more proven and biologically sound programs of pseudarthrosis treatment that have currently evolved. This therefore leads us into the discussion of currently practiced surgical programs.

CURRENTLY PRACTICED SURGICAL MANAGEMENT

With recognition of the abortive efforts of other treatment modalities, it is helpful to discuss in greater detail the current commonly employed therapeutic programs. Each of the technical details will be discussed, illustrative cases will be presented, and then some review of the results of each of these programs will be presented.

PLACEMENT OF AN INTRAMEDULLARY ROD AND ILIAC BONE GRAFTING

This is the one of the most currently accepted initial methods of treatment. This procedure was used and popularized by Charnley.[32] In his cases he thought that purchase of the often short distal tibial fragment was enhanced by passing the rod across the ankle joint into the talus and calcaneus. He reported two successful unions. Because of Charnley's report and based on our own experience, we believe that this is the first operative procedure that should be afforded to these patients.[38, 47] Morrissey agrees with this approach.[48] Because there is nearly always an anterior or anterolateral bowing of the tibia with or without fracture, this must be straightened in order to establish the proper weight-bearing biomechanics of the tibia. It is best maintained in this position by an intramedullary rod, in contrast to screws and plates where stress risers are often created.

The basic concept for use of the intramedullary rod maintains that the bone about the pseudarthrosis is, for whatever reason, pathologic. Therefore the rod serves as a permanent internal splint.[32] The type of intramedullary rod that is used is not crucial, but it must provide firm internal fixation. In the authors' opinion, the rod must therefore extend from the proximal epiphysis to the distal epiphysis, and since the rods used are smooth (nonthreaded), the fact that they cross the physis seems to have no appreciable effect on longitudinal growth.[47] As Charnley has shown,[32] if there is a short distal fragment, then the rod must extend across the ankle and subtalar joints into the calcaneus. Our experience with the rod developed and popularized by Williams suggests that it is the best technical means by which rod implantation can be accomplished. It is well illustrated in appropriate detail by Morrissy (Fig 6, A–D).

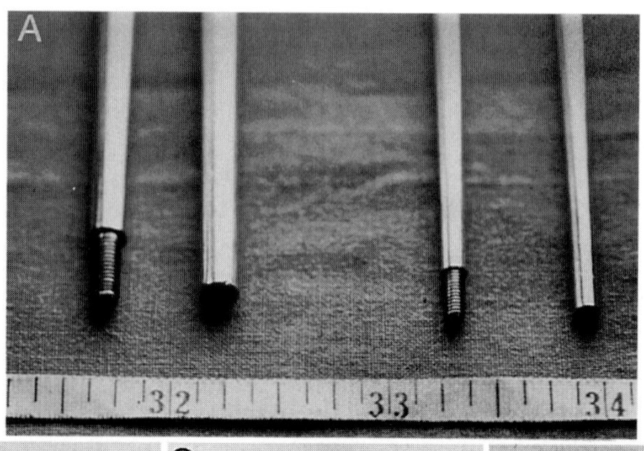

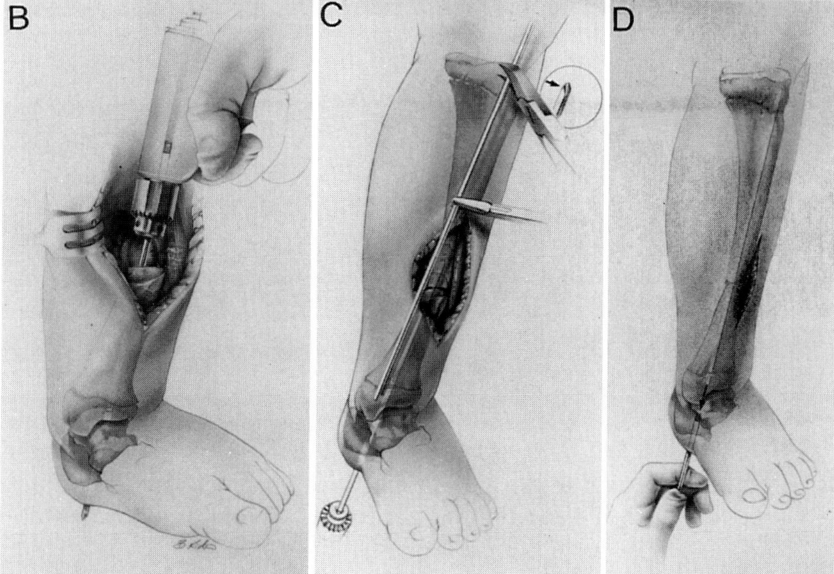

FIGURE 6.
The technique of intramedullary rodding with Williams' rods is illustrated. The male and female ends of the rods are illustrated **(A).** After exposure of the fragments, the proximal fragment is drilled, and then the rod is drilled out through the heel **(B).** After appropriate measurement of length **(C),** the rod is drilled retrogradely into the proximal fragment, and after proper positioning of the rod is achieved, the male portion of the rod is extracted **(D).** (**A** from Coleman SS, Coleman DA: *J Pediatr Orthop* 14:156–160, 1994; **B–D** from *Raymond Morrissy Atlas of Pediatric Orthopedic Surgery*. Philadelphia, JB Lippincott, 1992, pp 517–579. Used by permission.)

After the appropriately sized rod has been placed into the tibia and firm fixation achieved, then cortical-cancellous strips of autogenous iliac bone are placed about the pseudarthrosis and fixed with cerclage wires. This method of fixation of the grafts seems rather important because it provides close, firm approximation of the grafts to the host bone fragments and also permits impaction of the major fragments to occur over the smooth rod.

Occasionally we and Schoenecker et al.[49] have found that the rod may tend to extrude distally. We have used Schoenecker's solution on two occasions. This consists of making a small window in the cortex of the proximal tibial metaphysis and inserting a small plug of methyl methacrylate into the medullary cavity that engages the rod. Although successful to date, long-term results are not available.

Following the intramedullary rod and bone graft procedure, a 1½-hip spica cast is applied in order to prevent the patient from putting weight on the limb. In our experience, most complications such as backing out of the rod or migration of the rod into the knee joint have been the result of the patient having walked on the cast despite having been advised not to do so. The cast remains on for 3 months. It is then removed and the patient is allowed to ambulate in the above-knee brace described previously (see Fig 5). We have found that after 3 months further cast immobilization is not productive because if union has not occurred by that time, then further cast immobilization will not likely be effective.

If the aforementioned procedure succeeds, then the patient is maintained in the above-knee brace until skeletal maturity. In a recent review of 29 personal cases, such a program has succeeded on the first surgical procedure in 13% of the cases.[47] When it has failed, we believe that one more similar effort is justified. Often the patient has outgrown the rod, the rod has penetrated the tibial cortex anteriorly, or a clear-cut pseudarthrosis remains. If so, the procedure is repeated, usually with replacement of the original rod with a larger and longer rod, along with autogenous iliac bone grafts.

One of the important issues that must be faced is the presence of a pseudarthrosis of the fibula, usually at the same level as the tibial pseudarthrosis. Our preference at the original surgery is to rod and graft the fibula at the same time, either through a separate or the same incision.[38] More often than not, the fibular pseudarthrosis does not unite on the initial procedure, and it is our preference at the time of the second operation to perform a synostosis between the distal tibial and fibular fragments[47] (see Fig 1, F). This is done because if the tibia continues to grow and the fibula does not, then with tibial growth the ankle joint becomes canted into valgus, which is usually progressive. Of course if the fibula unites, then this issue becomes less important. However, if the ipsilateral fibula is used for vascularized bone grafting, then distal tibiofibular synostosis is essential.

TRANSFER OF THE IPSILATERAL FIBULA ON ITS VASCULAR PEDICLE

This program consists of placing an intramedullary rod into the tibia and then transferring the ipsilateral fibula on its vascular pedicle as a living graft in order to "bypass" the pseudarthrotic tibia.[40] Supplementary autogenous iliac bone grafts are always added. This has been proposed by the authors in a previous publication and remains our treatment of choice[40] if the earlier described program has failed on at least two occasions.

This is not a new concept since Wilson[50] proposed it for failure of union of congenital tibial pseudarthrosis as well as post-traumatic failures of union of the tibia in 1941. In a similar vein, we have reasoned that the ipsilateral fibula could be readily mobilized distally on its vascular pedicle and easily transferred to the tibia to bridge the pseudarthrosis. The fibula oftentimes has a pseudarthrosis at the same level as the tibia, but even so, the vascularized central segment of the fibula, with careful meticulous dissection, can be effectively displaced distally so as to "bypass" the tibial pseudarthrosis and then be firmly approximated to the tibia by cerclage wires (Fig 7). The adjacent coapting surfaces of the tibia and vascularized fibula are "scarified" in order to enhance close proximation and osteosynthesis. At the same time, if a distal tibiofibular synostosis has not been previously accomplished, it is done so through the same incision. In addition, autogenous iliac cortical cancellous bone

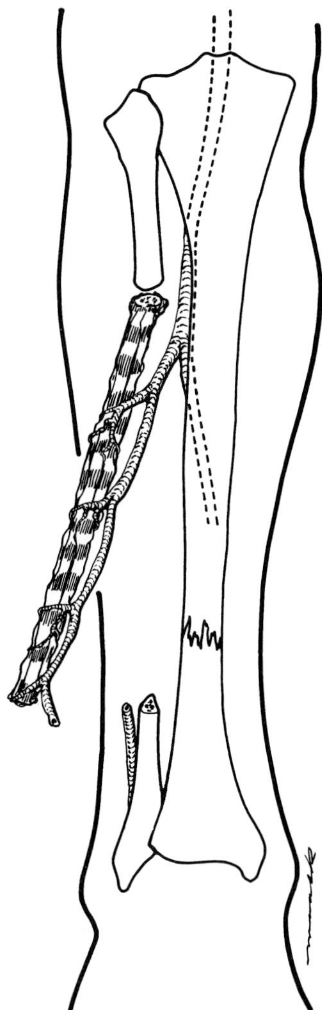

FIGURE 7.
Artist's depiction of the method by which the ipsilateral fibula is transferred while keeping the vascular pedicle in the transferred position. Mobilization of the fibula is made possible by careful dissection of the vascular pedicle. (From Coleman SS, Coleman DA: *J Pediatr Orthop* 14:156–160, 1994. Used by permission.)

grafts are placed both into the trough created between the transferred fibula and tibia and also at the site of the tibiofibular synostosis.[40]

We have performed this "secondary procedure" for the past 6 years, and the success rate, based on the evidence of persistent union and gradual hypertrophy of the transferred graft, is 83% with a minimum of a 2-year follow-up in six cases. No ancillary modalities such as electrical stimulation have been used. Three of the patients have had to have a second autogenous iliac bone graft procedure before final unequivocal union was evident radiographically. Only one apparent clear-cut failure has developed to date, and that occurred in a 5-year-old patient with extensive heritable neurofibromatosis whose transferred fibula simply "melted away."

PSEUDARTHROSIS RESECTION AND MICROVASCULAR TRANSFER OF THE CONTRALATERAL FIBULA

Transfer of the contralateral fibula by microvascular technique and simultaneous resection of the area of the tibial pseudarthrosis have gained some degree of popularity. Although initiated in Shanghai, China, in the Western World the implementation of this procedure for congenital tibial pseudarthrosis has been promulgated by Weiland et al.,[42] who reported on 19 cases with a minimum of 1-year follow-up. The procedure is based on the concept that a normal vascularized portion of the contralateral fibula can be used to replace a resected area of abnormal tibia containing the pseudarthrosis. Vascularization and inherent viability are accompanied by microvascularized anastomosis of the nutrient vessels of the donor fibula to the vessels of the recipient tibia. Rather simple internal fixation is employed (not an intramedullary rod). Osseous union occurs in a substantial number of instances; however, failure of osteosynthesis does occur on occasion at either the distal or proximal anastomosis (Fig 8, B–D). The longest follow-up reported by these authors was 11 years. The union rate at the time of follow-up was 95%.

There is no question about the efficacy of the transfer of the contralateral fibula done with this technique, at least for the short term. However, no long-term protection is provided by means of internal fixation. In addition, the distal fibular fragment of the donor leg is deprived of its normal stimulation, and in a growing child the ankle joint becomes canted into valgus (Fig 8, A). This can be prevented by performing a synostosis of the distal fibular fragment to the tibia as previously described.[47] However, the normal ankle function that requires a mobile fibula is altered, but whether it is meaningful for future years is unknown. Finally, two "one-bone legs" are created by this surgical plan. We believe that the previously described efforts short of foot ablation should be exhausted before this procedure is carried out.

PSEUDARTHROSIS RESECTION AND BONE TRANSPORT

The biological and technological concepts of "bone transport" developed by Ilizarov have been implemented in the treatment of congenital tibial pseudarthrosis. Reports by single individuals and by a multicenter study group have shown promise not only in achieving union but also by si-

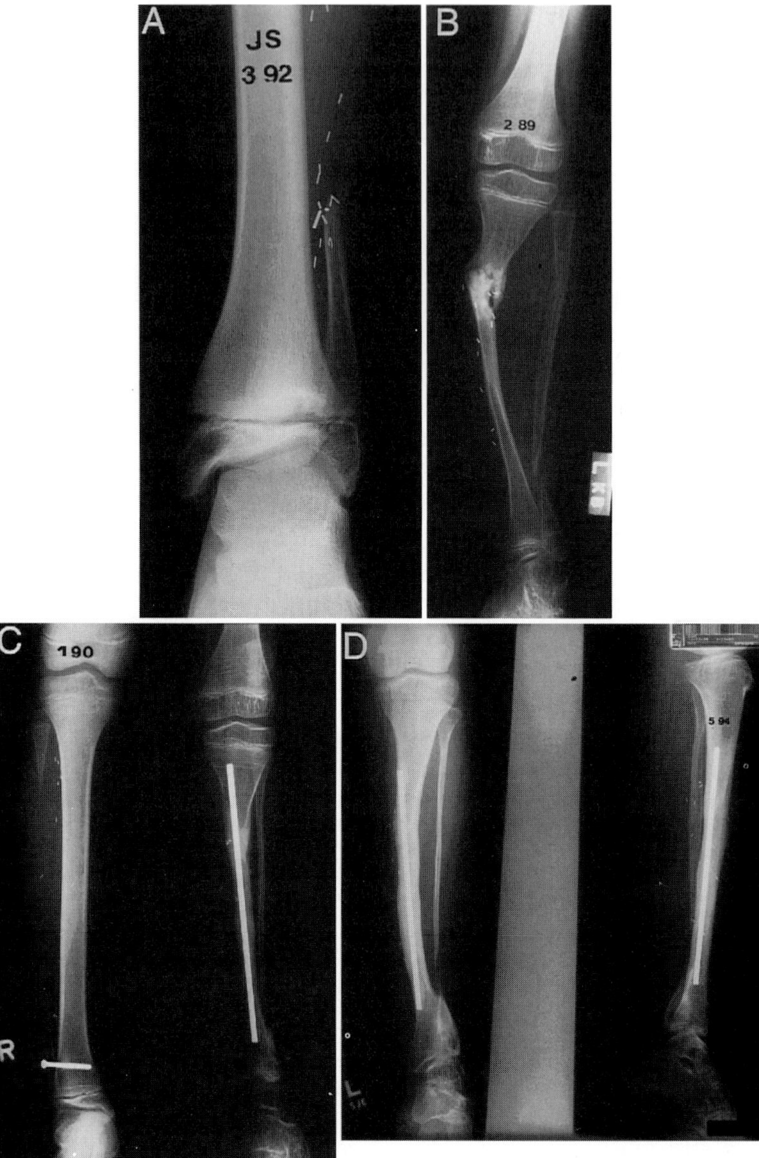

FIGURE 8.
The problem of failure to recognize the ankle problem that can be created in a deficient fibula is demonstrated **(A).** Proximal tibial pseudarthrosis is demonstrated following a *contralateral* fibular transfer **(B).** Successful union followed intramedullary rodding and bone grafting, and a distal tibiofibular synostosis on both ankles was accomplished **(C).** Four years later the tibia is solidly united, as is the synostosis **(D).** (**A** from Coleman SS, Coleman DA: *J Pediatr Orthop* 14:156–160, 1994. Used by permission.)

multaneously managing any limb length inequalities.[41] The program is based on the concept that resection of the pseudarthrosis and an appropriate portion of the adjacent tibia can be replaced by "bone transport." In this technique, the Ilizarov full ring system is applied to the proximal, "middle," and distal tibial fragments. An osteotomy (corticotomy) is made in the proximal fragment, thus creating a "middle" fragment. Then with delayed and slow gradual distraction, the newly created middle fragment is displaced distally. Regenerate bone replaces the proximal distraction gap, and the central tibial fragment gradually approximates the distal fragment. Once the fragments become opposed, continued compression stimulates osseous union in the area of the previous pseudarthrosis (see Fig 5, B–D).

Despite early optimistic results, there are three major potential drawbacks to this program. First, little attention is paid to the fibula, and the same concerns about the ankle mortise apply in this program as were discussed in contralateral fibular transfer. Second, once the pins and the Ilizarov device are removed, there is no residual protection against refracture. Finally, not all efforts are successful, and long-term end results or outcomes are wanting.

During the past year, one of us (D.A.C.) has carried out a transfer of the ipsilateral fibula on two occasions after attempts at the "bone transport" system had failed. The end results of the operations in these two cases have not yet been realized, but the early results are promising (see Fig 2, A–D).

ANCILLARY ELECTRICAL STIMULATION OF OSTEOGENESIS

Ever since Yasuda[51] recognized that an electrical current could exert either an osteogenetic or an osteolytic effect on the behavior of bone repair, clinical application of this modality has been attempted under circumstances designed to enhance bony union.[52] In the usual (posttraumatic) failure of union or failure of union complicated by osteomyelitis, impressive records of success have been recorded by several investigators. Because of the successes in these experiences, both battery-implanted and transcutaneous efforts at transmitting electrical fields have been used in a substantial number of instances of congenital tibial pseudarthrosis.[10] Despite the suggested evidence of promise, this ancillary method of osteogenesis in and of itself has resulted in an unpredictable and questionable degree of long-term success. Even though increased rates of union have been reported, long-term results of union having been maintained are not well recorded. In the currently accepted practice of treatment of congenital tibial pseudarthrosis, the most appropriate place for electrical stimulation appears to be in its ancillary use, added to one of the foregoing surgical programs. Its solitary use is not likely to produce a lasting osteosynthesis in this very complex and unpredictable condition.

TIBIAL PSEUDARTHROSIS AND NEUROFIBROMATOSIS

A currently existing controversy centers about two issues dealing with coexisting neurofibromatosis. The first is the causal relationship of neurofibromatosis to congenital tibial pseudarthrosis. The second has to do with any significance that this relationship has with respect to the prognosis and ultimate success or failure of treatment. Unfortunately, because of the uncommon occurrence of congenital tibial prepseudarthrosis and pseudarthrosis, accurate statistically significant series of their coexistence are difficult to find. Furthermore, it is not always possible to firmly and unequivocally establish the presence or absence of neurofibromatosis. One must therefore propose a well-accepted and reasonably well proven set of diagnostic clinical criteria that support the diagnosis of neurofibromatosis. With the recognition that there may be a controversy even about this issue, it is essential that there be some general acceptance, even though not necessarily a consensus, of the clinical criteria that justify a diagnosis of neurofibromatosis. Most investigators agree that there are two major types of neurofibromatosis.[53] Type 1 (NF1) is the most prevalent form, having an incidence of 1 in 3,500 individuals.

The visceral and somatic lesions currently required to establish the presence of NF1 are as follows[53]: (1) six or more café au lait macules 5 to 15 mm in diameter; (2) two or more neurofibromas of any type; (3) freckling in the axillary or inguinal areas; (4) optic glioma; (5) two or more "Lisch" nodules (iris hamartomas); (6) osseous lesions, specifically, prepseudarthrosis or pseudarthrosis of the tibia; and (7) a first-degree relative with NF1. At least two features should be present in order to make the diagnosis of NF1. Neurofibromatosis type 2 is much less common, having an incidence of 1 per 50,000, and the clinical features differ from those of NF1. Most significantly there is a conspicuous absence of osseous lesions.

The reported incidence of congenital tibial pseudarthrosis in NF1 varies from 1% to 4%.[53] Conversely, when one encounters a patient with congenital tibial prepseudarthrosis or pseudarthrosis, the likelihood of the patient having neurofibromatosis is between 40% and 80%,[3–7] although this figure has been disputed. This, of course, is the "bottom line." It should be emphasized, however, that there are many variations in the manifestations of neurofibromatosis, primarily because of recently introduced genotypes.[53]

The second issue of major importance has to do with the prognosis for successful treatment in patients with congenital pseudarthrosis who have associated neurofibromatosis. This question is difficult to answer because of the multiplicity of therapeutic regimens that have been implemented in the treatment of different series of congenital pseudarthrosis. Although there are reports to the contrary,[22] we have found in our own series that there is not a statistically significant increased number of operative procedures that are required to produce union of the pseudarthrosis in patients with neurofibromatosis as compared with those without neurofibromatosis.[47] Furthermore, the entire course of treatment that is necessary is substantially similar, and usually there is no delay in achieving union in patients with neurofibromatosis as compared with those without. Because of the rather small numbers, our personal statistical results are not very strong. It appears significant, however, that of eight patients with solitary tibial pseudarthroses, only two had neurofibromatosis.

Over the past 34 years, the senior author has personally been involved in the treatment of 29 cases of either prepseudarthrosis (congenital anterolateral bowing) or infantile tibial pseudarthrosis.[47] All were or eventually became established pseudarthroses. Throughout this rather substantial experience, our surgical approach has undergone several modifications, oftentimes based on a failure of previously conceived conventional treatment or because of innovative concepts that have led to more consistent success, even though repeated procedures may have been necessary. Also, despite follow-up evaluation exceeding 33 years, firm conclusions regarding the predictability of success of any specific therapeutic regimen still remain unclear.

Therefore, irrespective of one's enthusiasm for one form of treatment or another, it is evident that the results of surgical strategies for this capricious and frustrating problem must be considered to be preliminary and guarded. No one has enunciated this concept better than Boyd.[22] Our principal reason for clinging to the program we currently practice is based on the fact that our ultimate rate of solid union has been 83%. In some of the younger patients, 3 of these 25 cases of union were considered to have "tenuous" union. Furthermore, only 2 patients during the 34-year period have required or accepted an amputation. One was a 4-year-old boy whose limb was so short and his foot was so small that the parents appropriately requested ablation after multiple operative procedures done elsewhere failed. The other was accomplished on a child whose continued follow-up care was managed elsewhere.

When ablation is considered to be necessary or essential, we have strongly advocated that a Syme-type ankle disarticulation be performed rather than transtibial amputation at or about the pseudarthrosis site.[45] The reasons for this are the following: first, an end-bearing stump is created that is most often very trouble free; second, overgrowth of the tibial amputation site is avoided; and third, the pseudarthrosis usually heals following intramedullary rodding and autogenous bone grafting done before the disarticulation, or it becomes so stable that the prosthesis serves

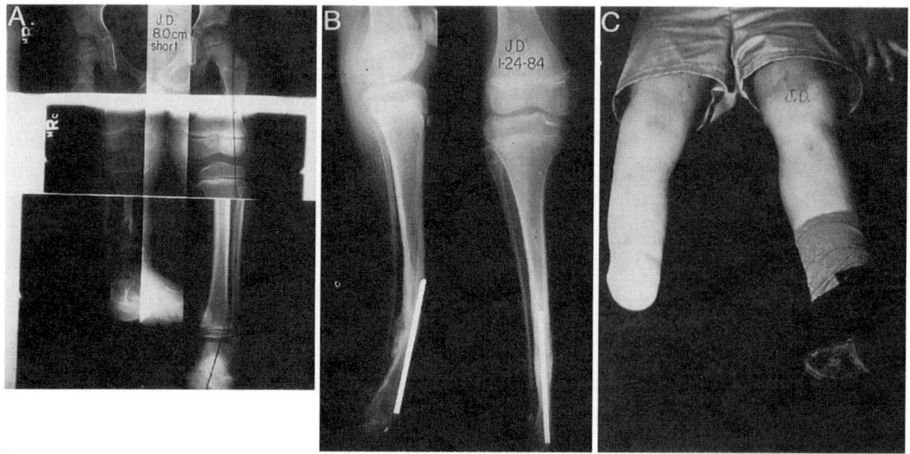

FIGURE 9.
A candidate for foot ablation is seen in this 4-year-old boy who had undergone four previous efforts at union of a tibial pseudarthrosis. Note the extreme shortening and smallness of the foot **(A)**. Following intramedullary rodding, bone grafting, and ankle disarticulation, solid union occurred **(B)**. The clinical photograph shows a functional end-bearing stump **(C)**.

as an external splint permitting relatively vigorous physical activities (Fig 9, A–C). Changes in limb length and foot size are easily accommodated by alterations in the prosthesis.

DISCUSSION AND SUMMARY

It is clear that any discussion of such a complex subject would have to involve a substantial degree of repetition of previously stated information. Therefore, to some degree the discussion must include a summary. To that end, conclusions addressing the main thrust and title of the chapter will also be included.

We hope that this chapter has properly emphasized the historical review of the manifold problems and many frustrating efforts at their solution. Based on the multiplicity of past programs of management, under no circumstances can one conclude that there is any degree of unanimity of opinion on how the various manifestations of congenital prepseudarthrosis and pseudarthrosis of the tibia can or should be managed. Because of the relatively rare occurrence of this lesion, except for Morrissy's report,[8] long-term follow-up studies that encompass a uniform or well-established strategy of surgical treatment are lacking. The issue is complicated by too many pathoanatomic variables scattered among too many different surgical approaches and too many treating surgeons. Even though an ankle disarticulation or transmedullary tibial amputation has eventuated in a substantial number of cases, neither should be looked on as the procedure of choice but rather as a capitulation to the frustrations, failures, and complications of other forms of treatment.

These observations underscore the need for well-controlled prospective studies on how to manage the complications of treatment of this disorder. To date, most information of this nature is largely anecdotal or is based on series of cases too small to have statistical value. Furthermore, as was emphasized early in this chapter, it is difficult to synthesize any therapeutic program for a condition whose etiology is and always has been elusive. In addition, efforts at establishing any consensus regarding the pathogenesis or histopathology have eluded even the most critical observers.

Despite these conceded problems and complexities, the authors have synthesized a program that has been "reasonably" successful and has evolved over a span of 33 years. It may sound very provincial and even parochial. Nonetheless, it is being suggested as a "road map" since it encompasses most of the seemingly long-term successful surgical strategies and excludes those that have had substantially less success. This program therefore represents the summary and conclusions we have reached over this 33-year period of time.

Prepseudarthrosis, which is characterized by congenital anterolateral bowing of the tibia and/or fibula, is treated initially in an above-knee brace that is custom-made and has a free knee and ankle. There is an anterior clam shell that can be tightened as necessary. This is worn until the tibia ultimately almost always fractures or, because of increasing deformity, is osteotomized to achieve correction. The result of the fracture or the osteotomy invariably leads to a pseudarthrosis. Rare instances of this deformity having been corrected by this bracing program have been reported, but they should be considered highly exceptional.[34]

Once the pseudarthrosis develops (or is initially seen), our policy is to place an intramedullary rod of the Williams'[49] variety in the tibia (and the fibula if possible) and place several corticocancellous autogenous iliac bone grafts about the area of pseudarthrosis. These are held by cerclage wires in order to ensure close approximation and some degree of compression. Yet they permit any impaction of the major fragments to take place over the rod. A 1½-hip spica cast is applied in order to immobilize the tibia and prevent (if possible) ambulation by the patient. The cast is left on for 3 months. At that time the pseudarthrosis may or may not have united. Either way, the brace previously described is applied, and if ambulatory, the child is allowed to walk.

More often than not after this initial procedure the pseudarthrosis does not consolidate by the end of 6 months or even a year. The process is then repeated because the rod may have migrated distally or proximally or may have cut through the anterior tibial cortex. The rationale for repeating the same operation is based purely on our experience that for whatever reason the pseudarthrosis not uncommonly consolidates after additional efforts. This may relate to the observation that in our experience union is more likely to take place as the child becomes skeletally mature.

If this program succeeds, then two major concerns face the surgeon: (1) whether the rod remains appropriately aligned and has not migrated and (2) the status of the distal tibiofibular relationships. If the fibula is intact, then the ankle mortise should remain preserved. However, if the fibula has a pseudarthrosis and the tibia unites, then with growth there is an inevitable alteration in the distal tibiofibular relationships leading to a "canting" of the ankle into valgus. Unless this is addressed, a major ankle deformity will result. Our solution to that problem is the creation of a distal tibiofibular synostosis by using a syndesmotic screw and iliac bone grafts just above the tibial and fibular physes. This converts the ankle into a solid mortise and prevents further valgus angulation.

Continued monitoring of the state of union of the tibia must be exercised, especially as it relates to positioning of the rod. It is not uncommon to have to replace the rod because it has been outgrown by the tibia. However, unless the rod tends to erode the anterior tibial cortex or there is a fracture below the rod, continued observation is all that is necessary.

As often as not, the second procedure does not succeed. There is usually no logical explanation for why in one patient the tibia consolidates and in another it does not. Three possible variables may play a role in this scenario. The first is the age of the patient, i.e., the older the patient, the more likely consolidation will occur; the second is the presence of a solid uninvolved fibula. Our experience[47] has shown that union is more likely to occur in patients with an intact fibula. Finally, the presence or absence of neurofibromatosis is a consideration. Although there is considerable controversy about this issue, we have found that patients with proven neurofibromatosis are no less likely to consolidate their pseudarthrosis than those without neurofibromatosis. Irrespective of these controversial issues, our next program of treatment consists of transfer of the ipsilateral fibula on its vascular pedicle to bridge the tibial pseudarthrosis. The technique has been previously described in detail.[40] The concept employs the use of a viable (presumably undiseased) bone graft that can be readily secured to the involved tibia by cerclage wires. The procedure is accompanied by autogenous iliac grafting and the creation of a distal tibiofibular synostosis, if it has not been previously accomplished. The usual 1½-hip spica cast is then applied, and the postoperative and bracing program described earlier is followed.

Our success with this program has been sufficiently good that unless long-term follow-up studies refute this approach as being ineffective, we will continue to employ it. Clearly it is too early to make any long-range predictions with respect to this program, but that is not unusual in this condition. An issue of importance, heretofore not emphasized, is that removal of the intramedullary rod should *not* be done, even in the presence of solid union. The bone must be protected throughout the patient's future.[32]

The employment of some form of electrical stimulation to osteogenesis is controversial in our experience. Surely no harm can occur, and perhaps if it is used in conjunction with the aforementioned program it may be a valuable ancillary part of treatment. As yet, we have had equivocal results with all forms of electrical stimulation; however, other observers have shown that its potential value cannot be disputed or negated.[10, 54–57]

Short of amputation, our approach to further or additional forms of treatment is somewhat uncertain with respect to indications and long-term results. These include the use of transplantation of the contralateral fibula by microvascular surgical technique. Our enthusiasm for this procedure is very guarded, and at the present time its place in our armamentarium is justified only when the previously described protocol has failed and amputation is considered to be the only alternative. Under these circumstances, the creation of two, one-bone legs with resulting questionable, properly functioning ankle joints is justified.

Finally, it is inevitable that the use of the Ilizarov "bone transport" compression program be considered in our currently accepted armamentaria. In our opinion at the present time, however, there is too little follow-up and too few end-result studies to endorse this program as it has been promulgated. There are too many unknowns and uncertainties about the procedure for it to be used with any degree of reliability. Perhaps over the years, long-term proven end-result studies will place this complex procedure into proper perspective, especially when faced with shortening, deformity, and recalcitrant pseudarthrosis. Our local experience, however, has led us to be cautious in implementing it as a primary procedure.

REFERENCES

1. Sofield HA: Congenital pseudarthrosis of the tibia. *Clin Orthop* 76:33–42, 1971.
2. Massermann RL, Peterson HA, Bianco AJ: Congenital pseudarthrosis of the tibia: A review of the literature and 52 cases from the Mayo Clinic. *Clin Orthop* 99:140–145, 1974.

3. Green WT, Rudo N: Pseudarthrosis and neurofibromatosis. *Arch Surg* 46:639–651, 1974.
4. Ducroquet R, Cottard A: A propos des pseudarthrosis et enflexion congenitale du tibia. *Mem Acad Chir* 63:863–868, 1937.
5. Barber CG: Congenital bowing and pseudarthrosis of the lower leg manifestations of Von Recklinghausen's neurofibromatosis. *Surg Gynecol Obstet* 69:618–626, 1939.
6. Madsen ET: Congenital angulation and fractures of the extremities. *Acta Orthop Scand* 25:242–280, 1956.
7. Moore JR: Congenital pseudarthrosis of the tibia. *Instr Course Lec* 14:222–237, 1957.
8. Morrissy RT, Riseborough EJ, Hall JE: Congenital pseudarthrosis of the tibia. *J Bone Joint Surg Br* 63:367–375, 1981.
9. Boyd HB, Sage FP: Congenital pseudarthrosis of the tibia. *J Bone Joint Surg Am* 40:1245–1270, 1958.
10. Paterson D, Simons RB: Electrical stimulation in the treatment of congenital pseudarthrosis of the tibia. *J Bone Joint Surg Br* 68:454–462, 1985.
11. Murray HH, Lovell WW: Congenital pseudarthrosis of the tibia. *Clin Orthop* 166:14–20, 1982.
12. Crossett LS, Beaty JH, Betz RR, et al: Congenital pseudarthrosis of the tibia. *Clin Orthop* 245:16–20, 1989.
13. Codivilla A: On the cure of the congenital pseudarthrosis of the tibia by means of periosteal transplantation. *Am J Orthop Surg* 4:163–169, 1906.
14. Codivilla A: Sulla cura della pseudarthrosis congenita della tibie. *Arch Orthop* 4:163–169, 1907.
15. Bocchi L: Angiografia in uno caso di pseudarthrosi congenitia della tibia. *Chir Organi Mov* 23:154–160, 1937.
16. Camurati M: Le pseudartrosi congenite della tibie. *Chir Organi Mov* 15:1–162, 1930.
17. Inglis K: The pathology of congenital pseudarthrosis of the tibia. *J Coll Surg Aust* 1:194–207, 1928.
18. Compere EL: Localized osteitis fibrosa in the new-born and congenital pseudarthrosis. *J Bone Joint Surg* 18:513–525, 1936.
19. Wade RB: The so-called congenital pseudarthrosis of the tibia. *J Coll Surg Aust* 1:181–186, 1928.
20. McElvenny RT: Congenital pseudarthrosis of the tibia, findings in one case and a suggestion as to possible etiology and treatment. *Q Bull Northwest Univ Med School* 23:413–423, 1949.
21. Aegerter EE, Kirkpatrick JA: *Orthopedic Diseases*. Philadelphia, WB Saunders, 1969, pp 203–210.
22. Boyd HB: Pathology and natural history of congenital pseudarthrosis of the tibia. *Clin Orthop* 166:5–13, 1982.
23. Lloyd-Roberts GC, Shaw NE: The prevention of pseudarthrosis in congenital kyphosis of the tibia. *J Bone Joint Surg Br* 51:100–105, 1969.
24. Pitt MJ, Mosher JF, Edeiken J: Abnormal periostium and bone in neurofibromatosis. *Radiology* 103:143–144, 1972.
25. Coleman SS: Unpublished electron microscope data, 1975.
26. Andersen KS: Operative treatment of congenital pseudarthrosis of the tibia. Factors influencing the primary result. *Acta Orthop Scand* 45:935–944, 1974.
27. Badgley CE, O'Connor SJ, Kudner OF: Congenital kyphoscoliotic tibia. *J Bone Joint Surg Am* 34:349–369, 1952.
28. Bassett CAL, Caulo N, Korte GJ: Congenital "pseudarthrosis" of the tibia; treatment with pulsing electromagnetic fields. *Clin Orthop* 154:136–149, 1981.
29. Hardinge K: Congenital anterior bowing of the tibia. The significance of different types in relation to pseudarthrosis. *Am R Coll Surg Engl* 51:17–30, 1972.

30. McBryde AM Jr, Stelling FH: Infantile pseudarthrosis of the tibia. *J Bone Joint Surg Am* 54:1354–1355, 1972.
31. Nicoll EA: Infantile pseudarthrosis of the tibia. *J Bone Joint Surg Br* 51:589–592, 1969.
32. Charnley J: Congenital pseudarthrosis of the tibia treated by the intramedullary nail. *J Bone Joint Surg Am* 38:283–290, 1956.
33. VanNess CP: Congenital pseudarthrosis of the leg. *J Bone Joint Surg Am* 48:1467–1483, 1966.
34. Tuncay IC, Johnston CE II, Birch JG: Spontaneous resolution of congenital pseudarthrosis or bowing of the tibia. *Pediatr Orthop* 14:599–602, 1994.
35. Boyd HB: Congenital pseudarthrosis: Treatment by dual bone grafts. *J Bone Joint Surg* 23:497–515, 1941.
36. McFarland B: Pseudarthrosis of the tibia in childhood. *J Bone Joint Surg Br* 33:36–46, 1951.
37. Farmer AW: The use of composite pedicle graft for pseudarthrosis of the tibia. *J Bone Joint Surg Am* 34:591–600, 1952.
38. Umber JS, Moss SW, Coleman SS: Surgical treatment of congenital pseudarthrosis of the tibia. *Clin Orthop* 166:28–33, 1982.
39. Sofield HA, Millar EA: Fragmentation realignment and intramedullary rod fixation of deformities of the long bones in children. *J Bone Joint Surg Am* 41:1371–1391, 1959.
40. Coleman SS, Coleman DA: Congenital pseudarthrosis of the tibia: Treatment by transfer of the ipsilateral fibula with vascular pedicle. *J Pediatr Orthop* 14:156–160, 1994.
41. Paley D, Catagni M, Argnani F, et al: Treatment of congenital pseudarthrosis of the tibia using the Ilizarov technique. *Clin Orthop* 280:81–93, 1992.
42. Weiland AJ, Weiss APC, Moore JR, et al: Vascularized fibular grafts in the treatment of congenital pseudarthrosis of the tibia. *J Bone Joint Surg Am* 72:654–662, 1990.
43. Pho RWH, Levack B, Satku K, et al: Free vascularized fibular graft in the treatment of congenital pseudarthrosis of the tibia. *J Bone Joint Surg Br* 67:64–70, 1985.
44. McCarthy RE: Amputation for congenital pseudarthrosis of the tibia. *Clin Orthop* 166:58–61, 1982.
45. Jacobsen ST, Crawford AH, Millar EA, et al: The Syme amputation in patients with congenital pseudarthrosis of the tibia. *J Bone Joint Surg Am* 65:533–537, 1983.
46. Boyd HB, Fox KW: Congenital pseudarthrosis: Follow-up study after massive bone grafting. *J Bone Joint Surg Am* 30:274–283, 1948.
47. Biddulph GE, Coleman SS, Beane J: Unpublished data.
48. Morrissy RT: Personal communication, 1994.
49. Anderson PJ, Schoenecker, PL, Rich MM: The use of the Peter Williams intramedullary rod in treatment of congenital pseudarthrosis of the tibia. *Orthop Trans* 14:638–705, 1990.
50. Wilson PD: A simple method of two-stage transplantation of the fibula for use in cases of congenital pseudarthrosis of the tibia. *J Bone Joint Surg* 23:2–39, 1941.
51. Yasuda L: On the piezoelectric activity of bone. *J Jpn Orthop Surg* 28:267–271, 1954.
52. Bassett CAL, Becker RO: Generation of electrical potentials by bone in response to mechanical stress. *Science* 137:1063–1068, 1962.
53. *National Institutes of Health Consumers Development Conference Statement.* 6(12):1–7, 1987.
54. Langenskiold A: Pseudarthrosis of the fibula and progressive valgus defor-

mity of the ankle in children: Treatment by fusion of the distal tibial and fibular metaphysis. *J Bone Joint Surg Am* 49:463–470, 1967.

55. Sutcliffe ML, Goldberg MB: The treatment of congenital pseudarthrosis of the tibia with pulsing electromagnetic fields: A survey of 52 cases. *Clin Orthop* 166:45–57, 1982.
56. Brighton CT, Friedenberg ZB, Zemsky LM, et al: Direct current stimulation of non-union and congenital pseudarthrosis. *J Bone Joint Surg Am* 57:368–377, 1975.
57. Bassett CAL, Pilla AA, Pawluk RJ: A nonoperative salvage of surgically-resistant pseudarthrosis and non-unions by pulsing electromagnetic fields: A preliminary report. *Clin Orthop* 124:128–143, 1977.

The Role of Minimally Invasive Surgery in Spinal Disorders

Parviz Kambin, M.D.
Clinical Associate Professor, University of Pennsylvania School of Medicine; Chief, Division of Spinal Surgery, Department of Orthopaedic Surgery, Graduate Hospital; Director, Disk Treatment and Research Center, Graduate Hospital, Philadelphia, Pennsylvania

Laminectomy with direct decompression of a compromised nerve root[1, 2] is a traditional and effective treatment method, but at times it is associated with a number of serious complications.[3–6] Nuclear debulking for indirect decompression of herniated disks, either by mechanical nucleotomy,[7, 8] laser nuclear vaporization,[9–12] or chemonucleolysis,[13] does not always result in the alleviation of clinical symptoms or neurologic deficits[14, 15] and can also cause serious complications.[16–21] Although mechanical nuclear extraction and annular fenestration are associated with a reduction in intradiscal pressure,[22–24] no credible evidence has been presented to demonstrate a major reduction in the contour of the annulus fibrosus following this operative procedure. Symptoms are generally produced by posterior or posterolateral herniated fragments. The failure of chemonucleolysis to relieve pain and neurologic symptoms has been attributed to the inability of the enzyme to digest these collagenized posterior herniated fragments.[25, 26]

This author attempted mechanical nuclear decompression through a Craig cannula[27] inserted dorsolaterally into the intervertebral disk.[28–31] In order to observe the effect of nucleotomy on the external contour of the annulus at the site of disk herniation, posterolateral nuclear resection was combined with a laminotomy in a number of our patients. In the mid 1970s, an additional 20 patients with symptomatic lumbar disk herniation were subjected to partial nucleotomy through a Craig cannula with the aid of micropituitary-type forceps.

In the late 1970s, our suboptimal clinical outcome with central nucleotomy led us to develop technology to access posterior and posterolateral herniated disk fragments.[28] Enlargement of the diameter of the access cannula to allow passage of upbiting forceps and the introduction of high negative pressure to dislodge the herniated fragments were the first steps in the right direction to access the offending compressive disk fragments. By 1983 it became apparent that it was impossible to extract posterior herniated fragments without articulating instruments.[22]

In March 1983 we attempted our first percutaneous interbody fusion

Advances in Operative Orthopaedics, vol. 3

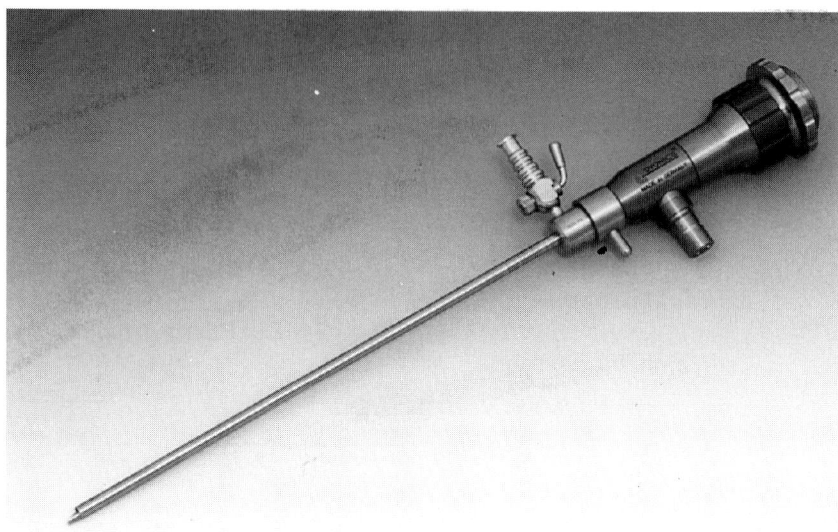

FIGURE 1.
Arthroscope with an irrigation sheath assembly for the inflow of saline solution.

at the L4–5 level by using biportal access and a 30-degree arthroscope. The utilization of articulating and decorticating instruments demanded visual control and the introduction of arthroscopic visualization. The subsequent availability of small-caliber 30- and 70-degree rigid scopes permitted the development of an arthroscope with an irrigation sheath–cannula assembly (Fig 1) that permitted visualization and fluid management through a single portal.[32–36]

Our efforts toward the development of a multichannel working scope that permitted the deflection of inserted instruments was unsuccessful. The lack of depth perception that is an inherent limitation of all uniportal-access instruments combined with the large diameter of a multichannel deflecting working scope prevented its development and use for intradis-

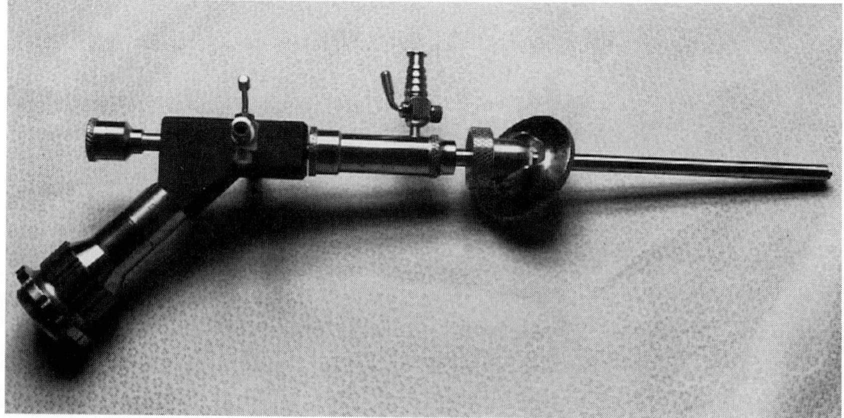

FIGURE 2.
Working channel arthroscope inserted into a universal-access cannula and the cannula stopper.

cal surgery. However, a simple working scope (Fig 2) that provides channels for fluid management and an instrument is currently being used for periannular or intradiscal surgery.

In 1975 Hijikata et al.[37, 38] independently used forceps and a series of cannulas for nucleotomy. Schreiber and Suezawa adapted Hijikata's technique and reported satisfactory outcomes following nuclear debulking procedures. These authors later reported on their biportal access to the lumbar intervertebral disk and their use of the arthroscope for visualization and extraction of nuclear tissue.[39, 40] However, their technique did not use articulating instruments or a means to remove the offending posterior herniated fragments.

INSTRUMENTS

Currently, two essentially different instruments and techniques are being used for minimally invasive disk surgery through posterolateral access. Straight or slightly maneuverable instruments[7, 11, 12] that are used with or without an accompanying arthroscope through uniportal access are only capable of resecting non–symptom-producing nuclear tissue that is located at a distance from the herniation site. In contrast to this, arthroscopic microdiscectomy instruments provide access to the symptom-producing posterior and posterolateral herniated fragments. These instruments may be used through a single portal or through dual portals.

The inherent limitation of mechanical[7, 8] or laser-assisted[9–12] nucleotomy instruments that are inserted through a single small-caliber cannula are as follows.

1. The inability to establish adequate inflow and outflow of saline solution leads to poor visibility.
2. A lack of depth perception is invariably necessary when the operating surgeon is working in the area adjacent to the dura and the neural structures.

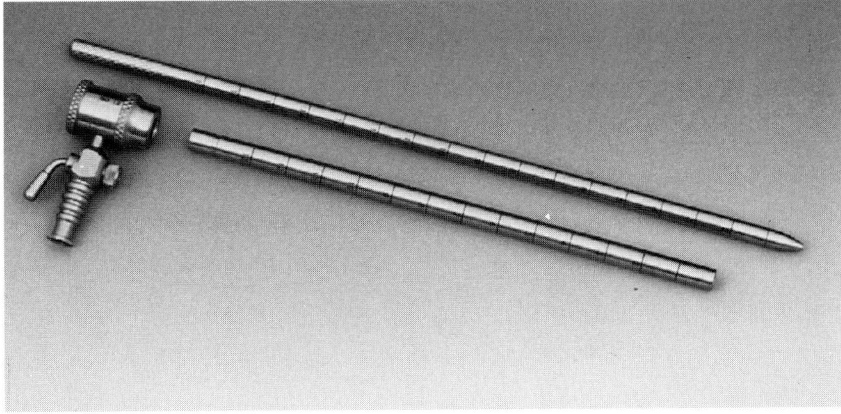

FIGURE 3.
Top, blunt-ended cannulated obturator. *Bottom*, universal-access cannula with a suction-irrigation valve.

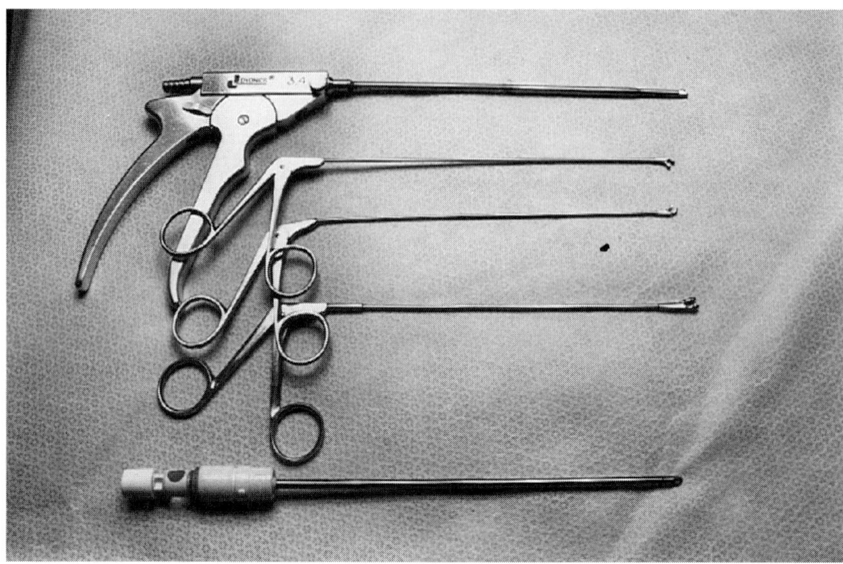

FIGURE 4.
From top to bottom: suction punch forceps; downbiting, upbiting, and flexible-tipped forceps; trimmer blade.

3. The inability to determine exactly where the cutting end of the maneuverable instrument is located results in a wide and indiscriminate nuclear resection. It should be noted that plain fluoroscopic examinations that are routinely performed during surgery are also inadequate for detecting the position of the tips of the instruments.
4. The existing flexible scopes that are used in conjunction with mechanical or laser nucleotomes limit instrument flexibility. The wide arc of deflection prevents the necessary intradiscal maneuvering.
5. Use of a heat-producing laser adjacent to the neural structures is potentially hazardous.
6. The efficacy of nucleotomy for the treatment of lumbar root compression associated with posterior and posterolateral herniated disk frag-

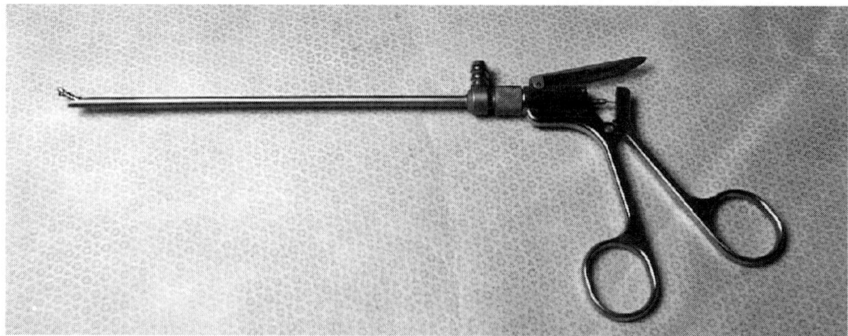

FIGURE 5.
Deflecting suction forceps that permits 120-degree dorsal angulation of the tip in order to access posterior and posterolateral herniated fragments.

Moving?

I'd like to receive my ***Advances in Operative Orthopaedics*** without interruption.
Please note the following change of address, effective:

Name: ______________________

New Address: ______________________

____

City: ______________ State: ________ Zip: ________

Old Address: ______________________

____

City: ______________ State: ________ Zip: ________

Reservation Card

Yes, I would like my own copy of ***Advances in Operative Orthopaedics.*** Please begin my subscription with the current edition according to the terms described below.* I understand that I will have 30 days to examine each annual edition. If satisfied, I will pay just $74.95 plus sales tax, postage and handling (price subject to change without notice).

Name: ______________________

Address: ______________________

City: ______________ State: ________ Zip: ________

Method of Payment

❍ Visa ❍ Mastercard ❍ AmEx ❍ Bill me ❍ Check (in US dollars, payable to Mosby, Inc.)

Card number: ______________ Exp date: ________

Signature: ______________________

LS-0909

*Your *Advances* Service Guarantee:

When you subscribe to *Advances*, we'll send you an advance notice of future volumes about two months before they publish. This automatic notice system is designed to take up as little of your time as possible. If you do not want *Advances*, the advance notice makes it quick and easy for you to let us know your decision, and you will always have at least 20 days to decide. If we don't hear from you, we'll send you the new volume as soon as it's available. And, of course, *Advances* is yours to examine free of charge for 30 days (postage, handling and applicable sales tax are added to each shipment.).

NO POSTAGE
NECESSARY
IF MAILED
IN THE
UNITED STATES

BUSINESS REPLY MAIL
FIRST CLASS MAIL PERMIT No. 762 CHICAGO, IL

POSTAGE WILL BE PAID BY ADDRESSEE

Chris Hughes
Mosby-Year Book, Inc.
200 N. LaSalle Street
Suite 2600
Chicago, IL 60601-9981

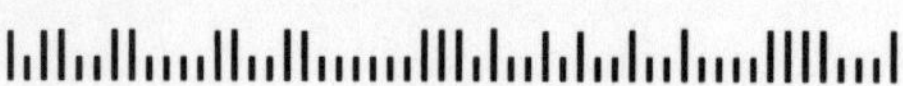

NO POSTAGE
NECESSARY
IF MAILED
IN THE
UNITED STATES

BUSINESS REPLY MAIL
FIRST CLASS MAIL PERMIT No. 762 CHICAGO, IL

POSTAGE WILL BE PAID BY ADDRESSEE

Chris Hughes
Mosby-Year Book, Inc.
200 N. LaSalle Street
Suite 2600
Chicago, IL 60601-9981

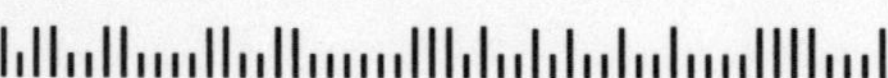

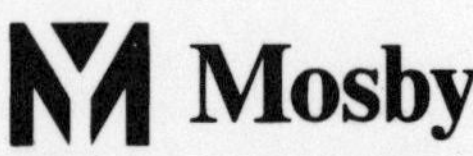

Dedicated to publishing excellence

ments has not been established.[14, 15] Castro et al. in an experimental study have demonstrated that reduction of the height of the intervertebral disk following central nucleotomy may lead to an increased radial bulge of the annulus, potentially increasing compression on the nerve root.[41, 42]

Instruments for arthroscopic microdiscectomy (Figs 3 to 5) may be used for the diagnosis or treatment of spine-related disorders.

POSTEROLATERAL APPROACH AND INSERTION OF INSTRUMENTS

Since a posterolateral approach is employed in all of the procedures that will be described, it will be detailed here and any modifications will be indicated with the relevant procedure.

The patient is placed in the prone position on an operating or frac-

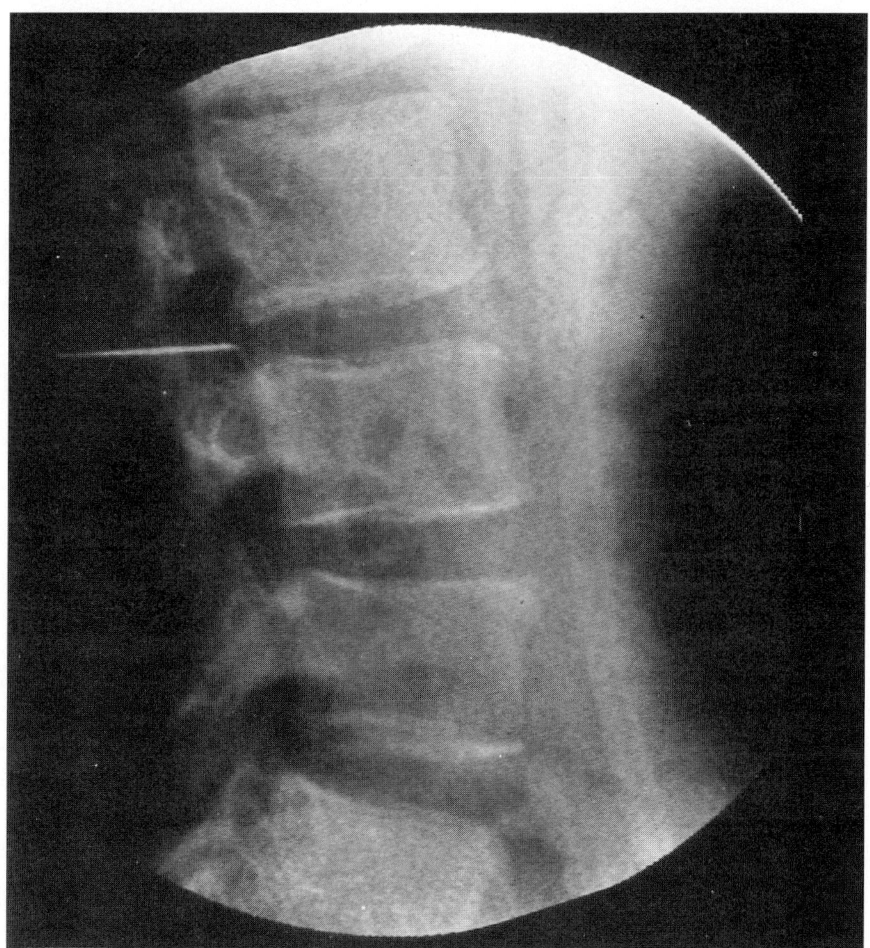

FIGURE 6.

Appropriate position of the needle at the L2–3 intervertebral disk space. In the lateral view, the tip of the needle is seen in alignment with the posterior border of the proximal and distal vertebrae.

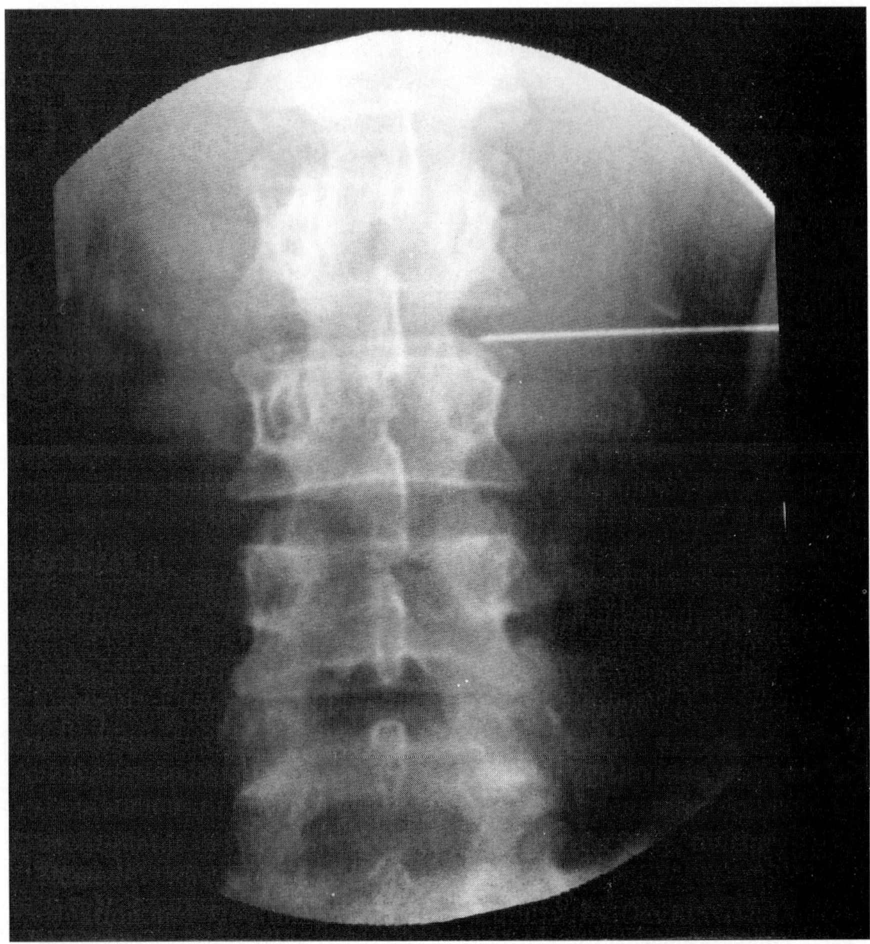

FIGURE 7.
Intraoperative fluoroscopic examination in the anteroposterior projection. The tip of the needle is properly positioned in alignment with the midpedicular line.

ture table with a radiolucent top. An adjustable radiolucent frame is used to hold the hips in flexion and flatten the lumbar lordosis. This position provides paramedial access to the intervertebral disk from both the left and right side of the spine. A fracture table is preferred because it is narrow and does not interfere with rotation of the C-arm.

There is well-founded concern about causing injury to the spinal nerve during insertion of instruments through the posterolateral approach. However, as the spinal nerve descends, it passes distally, anteriorly, and laterally from the foramina. It is then positioned anterior to the transverse process of the lower lumbar segment. Thus it is possible to insert the instruments into a triangular working zone[32, 34, 43] bordered by the spinal nerve anteriorly, the proximal plate of the distal segment inferiorly, the proximal articular process of the lower vertebra posteriorly, and the traversing nerve root medially. The iliac arteries and vein are located anteriorly and are not usually in the path of the instruments. To provide an extra margin of safety, the instruments have been designed so

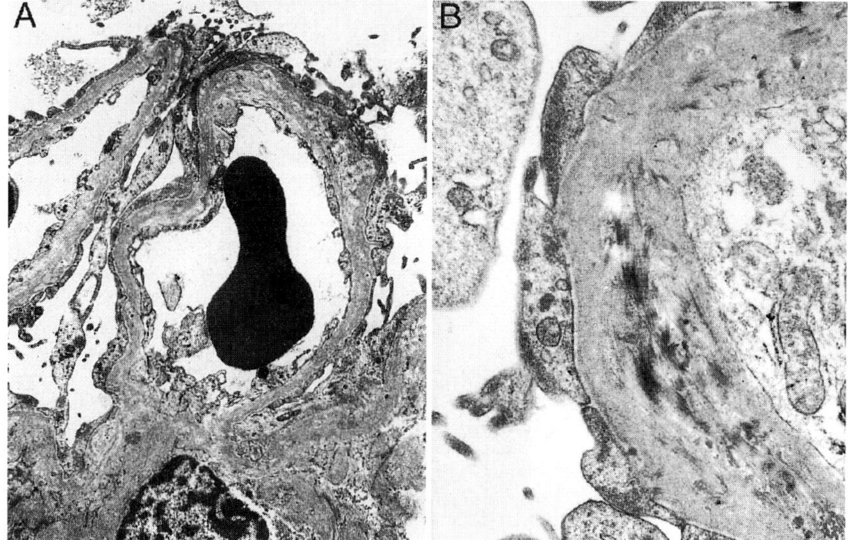

FIG 6.
The glomerular basement membrane (GBM) in nail-patella syndrome. The GBM is irregularly thickened by lucent areas **(A)** in which there are fibers that can be demonstrated to consist of collagen with regular structure and periodicity **(B).** (Electron micrographs: **A,** × 6,250; **B,** phosphotungstic acid impregnation, × 12,000.) (From Kissane JM, Bernstein J: Hereditary nephritis, in Edelmann CM Jr: *Pediatric Kidney Disease,* ed 2. Boston, Little, Brown, 1992, pp 1159–1170. Used by permission.)

months.[126, 127] No treatment is known to be effective in preventing the progression of the renal disease in this disorder.

The antigenicity of the GBM in NPS has been found to be variable when it has been studied with a mouse monoclonal antibody (MCA-P1) directed toward the Goodpasture antigenic determinant. Noel et al.[128] found normal fixation. A later study, however, reported complete absence of binding of MCA-P1 in two of three patients with the nephropathy of NPS. This was taken to mean that the NPS may represent a disorder of collagen.[129] Nevertheless, the findings of Sutcliff et al.[129] and Noel et al.[128] show that loss of Goodpasture antigenicity is not invariably present.

Genetics

NPS is inherited as an autosomal dominant. The gene is carried on the long arm of chromosome 9 where it is genetically linked to the gene for ABO blood groups and adenylate cyclase.[120] The recent demonstration that the gene for type V collagen (COL5A1) maps to the q34.2 → q34.3 region of chromosome 9, near the lo-

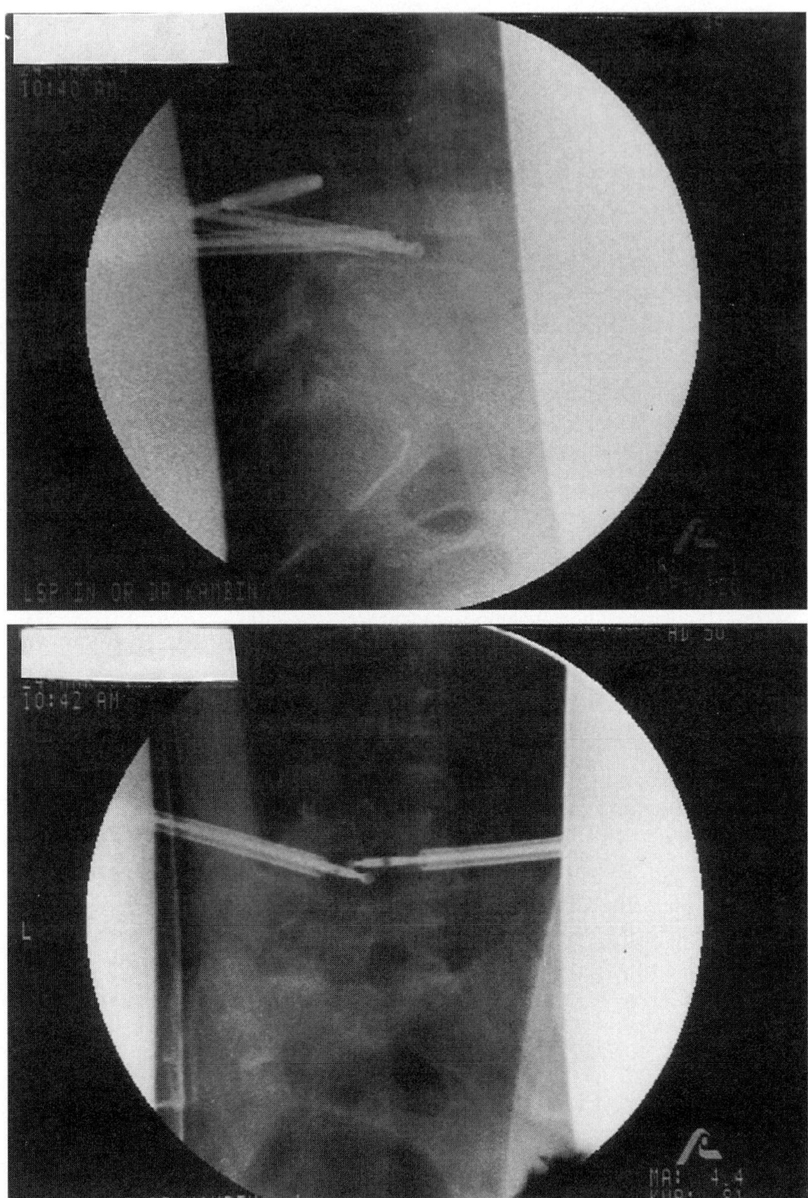

FIGURE 9.

Intraoperative fluoroscopic examination. Anteroposterior and lateral roentgenograms show biportal access to the L4–5 intervertebral disk. Note the engagement of the universal-access cannulas into the annular fibers and the contact between the arthroscope and the instrument that is introduced through the opposite portal.

eodiscoscope is inserted through the access cannula for thorough inspection of the annulotomy site.

The annulus is fenestrated, first with a 3-mm and then with a 5-mm trephine. The nucleus is extracted, usually with powered trimmer blades. Straight and upbiting forceps are used to remove herniated fragments that are located adjacent to the open end of the access cannula. A biportal approach is generally used for large central subligamentous herniations or nonmigrated extraligamentous herniations. Deflectable forceps are used to remove these fragments under arthroscopic control. Instruments may be inserted either through the same portal alternately with the scope or through a separate portal from the opposite side so that the procedure can be performed under constant (Fig 9) visualization.

DIAGNOSTIC SPINAL ARTHROSCOPY

PERIANNULAR INSPECTIONS

Inspection of annulus and the contents of the triangular working zone is essential and should be conducted at the onset of all arthroscopic surgical procedures on the spine. The loosely woven adipose tissue that invariably covers the surface of the annulus (Fig 10) should be extracted to permit clear visualization of the annular surface (Fig 11). An abnormal communication between the spinal nerves or conjoined nerve roots may be diagnosed and properly protected throughout the operative procedure.

FORAMINAL AND EPIDURAL ARTHROSCOPY

Kambin has described the arthroscopic appearance of the annulotomy site, spinal nerve, and foramina.[32, 36, 43] The access cannula may be passed under the pars interarticularis for inspection of the contents of the foramina and the spinal canal. The videodiscoscope cannula assembly or the working-channel discoscope may be used to accomplish this (Fig 12).

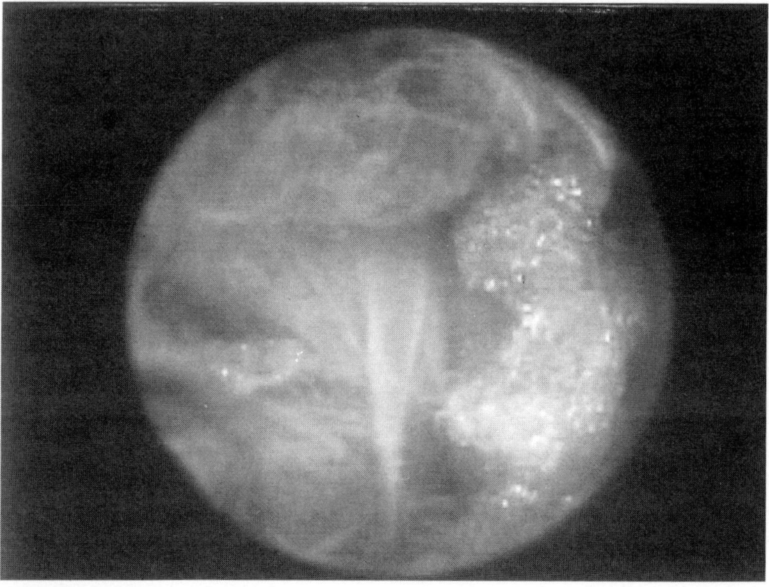

FIGURE 10.

Arthroscopic view of the triangular working zone. Note the loosely woven fatty tissue in the periphery that extends from 6 to 10 o'clock.

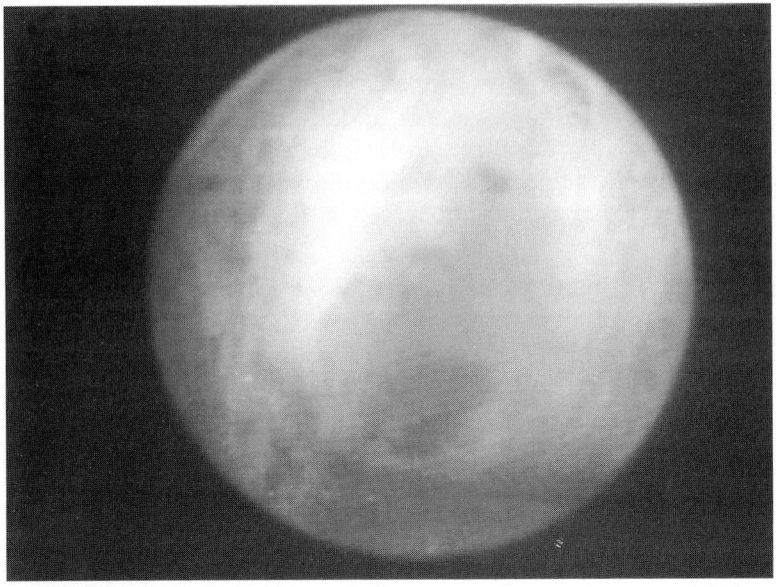

FIGURE 11.
The smooth surface of the annulus is visualized following extraction of the adipose tissue.

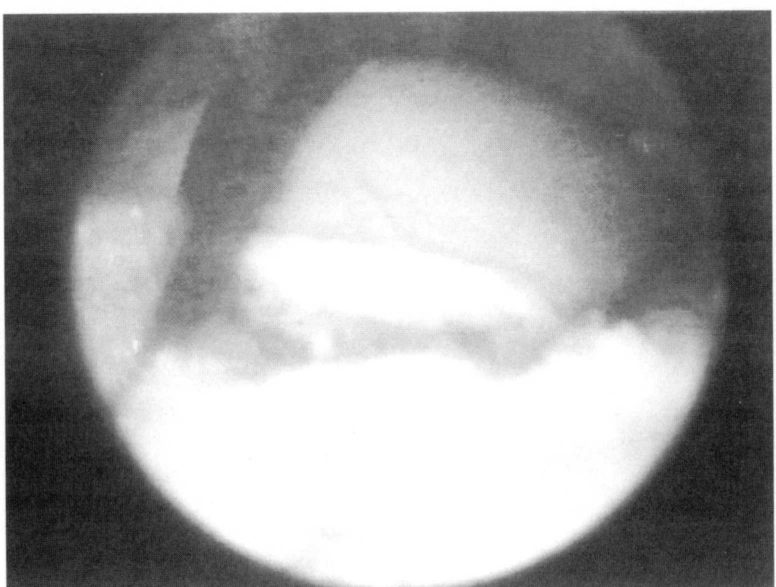

FIGURE 12.
Arthroscopic view of the spinal canal via a 30-degree arthroscope. The intervertebral disk is seen in the foreground and the dura in the background.

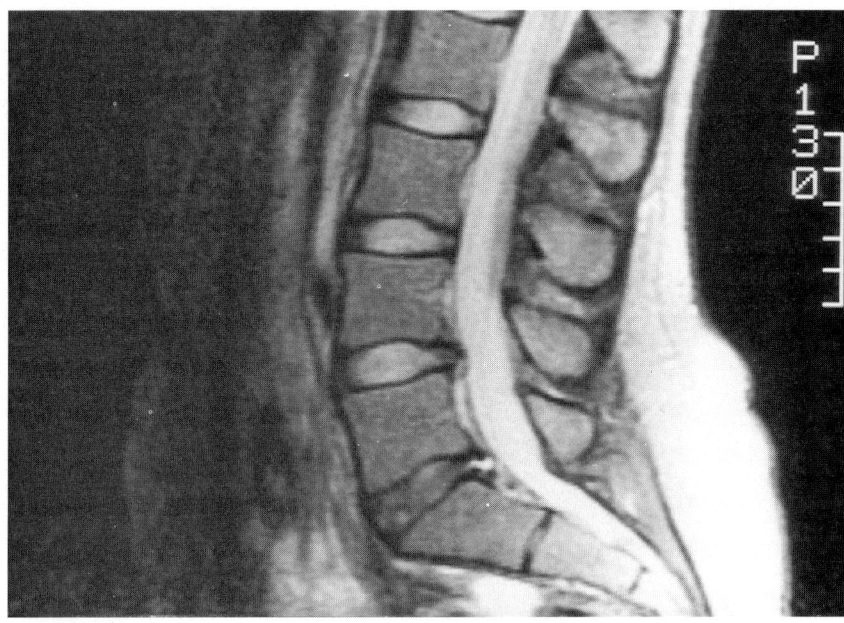

FIGURE 13.
Preoperative MRI study demonstrating an area of high intensity under the posterior longitudinal ligament in T2 MRI images at the L5–S1 level.

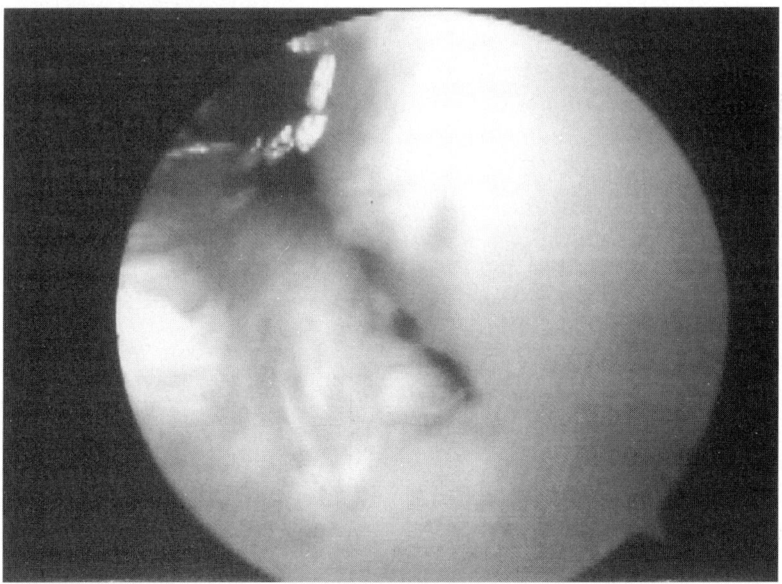

FIGURE 14.
Intraoperative arthroscopic view of an annular rim defect and ingrowth of granulation tissue.

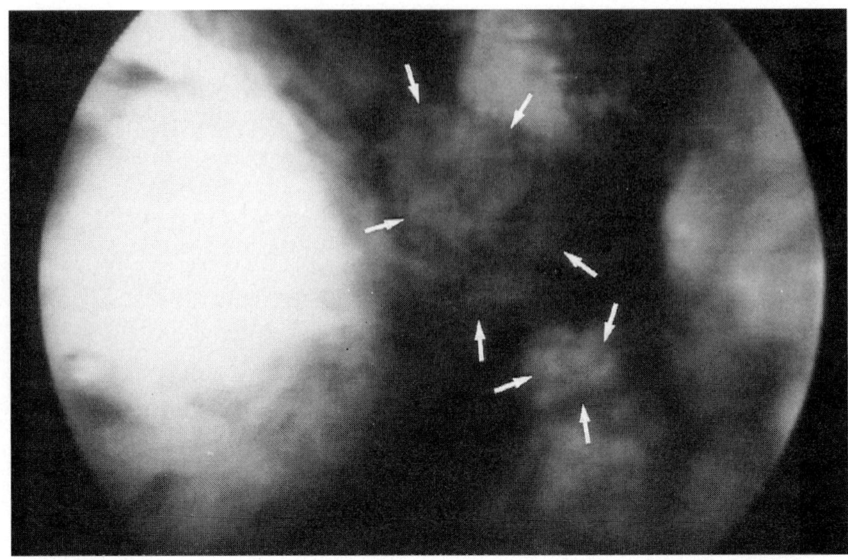

FIGURE 15.
Arthroscopic view of a free fragment inside the intervertebral disk (internal disk sequestration).

ANNULAR RIM LESIONS

The presence of a defect in the outer annular attachment secondary to mechanical stress has been implicated as a cause of recurrent back pain.[44] However, in a given clinical setting, the diagnosis of this pathologic condition may be difficult. Discography may or may not show communication between the detached annulus and the nucleus pulposus. This peripheral annular defect is usually associated with ingrowth of granulation tissue that may be demonstrated as an area of high intensity under the posterior longitudinal ligament in T2 magnetic resonance imaging (MRI) studies (Fig 13). The annular rim lesion may be diagnosed via intradiscal arthroscopic examination (Fig 14).

INTERNAL DISK SEQUESTRATION

We have previously reported on the pathophysiology of intradiscal collagenized nuclear fragments and their role in the production of low back and sciatic pain. These intradiscal fragments are readily diagnosed through arthroscopic intradiscal examination (Fig 15).

We have hypothesized that periodic migration of these collagenized fragments toward the superficial layer of the annulus and the posterior

FIGURE 16.
A, lateral extension roentgenogram demonstrating retrolisthesis at L3–4 associated with severe back pain and subjective numbness of the anterior aspect of the thigh and an intact neurologic examination. **B,** postoperative roentgenographic evaluation demonstrating reduction of the spondylolisthesis and temporary stabilization of the L3–4 segments via removable pedicular bolts and subcutaneous plates.

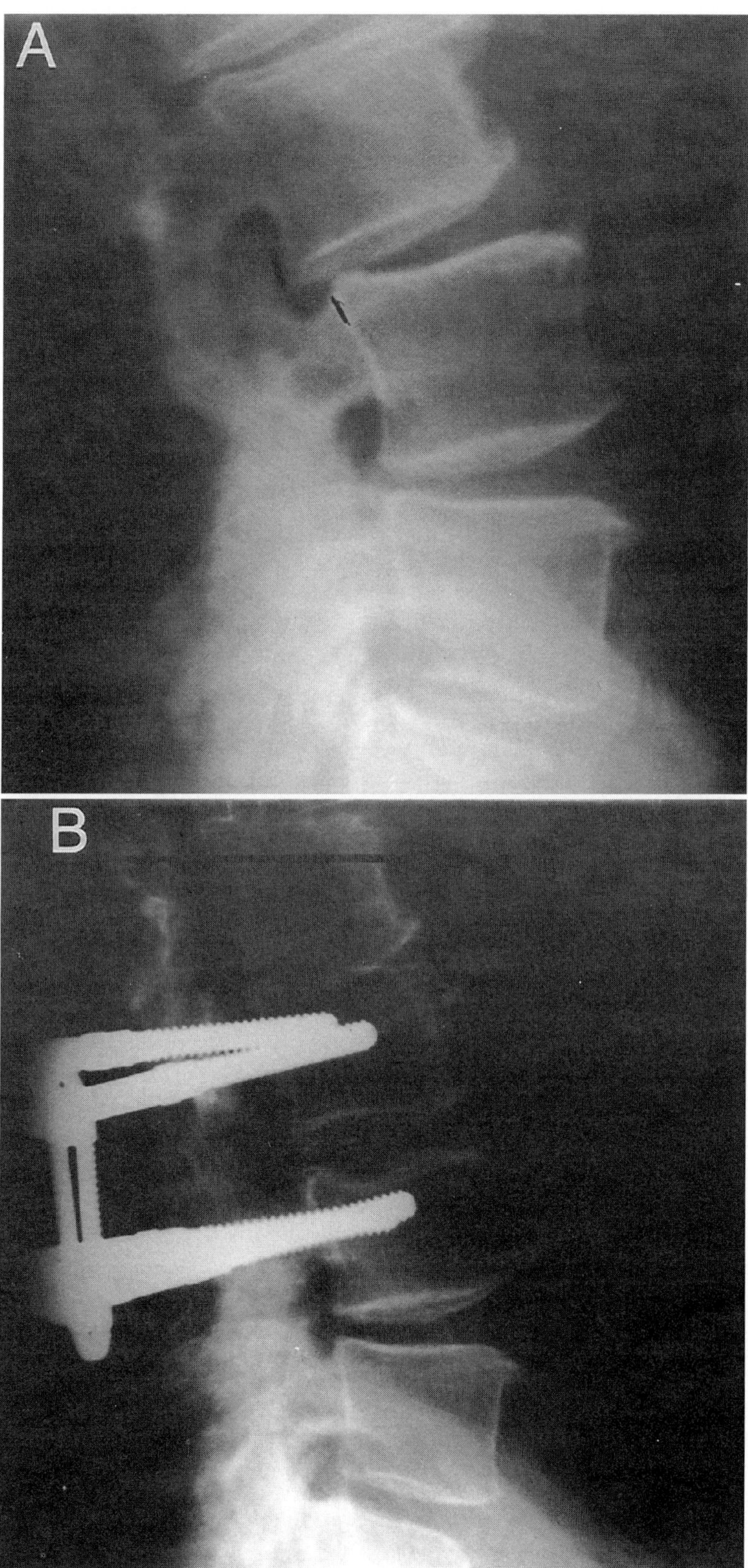
A
B

longitudinal ligament produces tension on well-innervated fibers of the posterior longitudinal ligament and causes pain.[45] The cessation of pain may be related to spontaneous reduction and central migration of these free internal fragments. The pathophysiology of internal disk sequestration is currently subject to clinical, imaging, and anatomic study at The Graduate Hospital's Disk Treatment and Research Center and will be the subject of future publications.

DIAGNOSIS OF LUMBAR INSTABILITY AND ITS TEMPORARY STABILIZATION

In order to ascertain the necessity of lumbar arthrodesis, removable pedicular bolts and subcutaneous plates may be used for temporary fixation of an unstable lumbar motion segment (Fig 16, A and B).

The medullary canals of the pedicles are tapped, probed, and arthroscopically inspected before insertion of the pedicular bolts. The subcutaneous plates are well tolerated and do not usually cause local irritation, and the patients are permitted to become ambulatory after surgery and are kept under observation for a few weeks. If the patient's symptoms are relieved by this subcutaneous stabilization, then the patient is readmitted for arthroscopic lumbar interbody fusion or combined arthroscopic interbody and posterolateral arthrodesis.

BIOPSY OF THE THORACIC AND LUMBAR SPINE

We have used the instruments employed in arthroscopic microdiscectomy to obtain tissue from the intervertebral disks or vertebrae of the thoracic and lumbar spine for the diagnosis of infections and neoplasms.

The vertebral bodies in the mid and upper thoracic spine are accessed through the adjacent intervertebral disks. The access cannula is positioned in the triangular working zone. The entry point is usually about 6 to 8 cm from the midline (see the operative procedure). The annulotomy site is inspected and annular fenestration is accomplished in a routine fashion. Through this fenestration the 5-mm trephine is directed cephalad. The vertebral plate is penetrated, and an adequate quantity of corticocancellous or tumor tissue is removed with the forceps for histologic examination (Fig 17, A and B).

When an intervertebral disk infection is suspected, arthroscopic microdiscectomy instruments inserted through a posterolateral approach may be used for obtaining tissue for culture and performing sensitivity tests and for irrigating and debriding necrotic tissue under arthroscopic visualization. This step is then followed by 6 weeks of intravenous antibiotic therapy.

Arthroscopic inspection of the intervertebral disk invariably provides valuable information concerning the presence or absence of infection. The absence of necrotic or granulation tissue and a normal appearance of the nucleus and annular tissue are commonly associated with a negative culture.

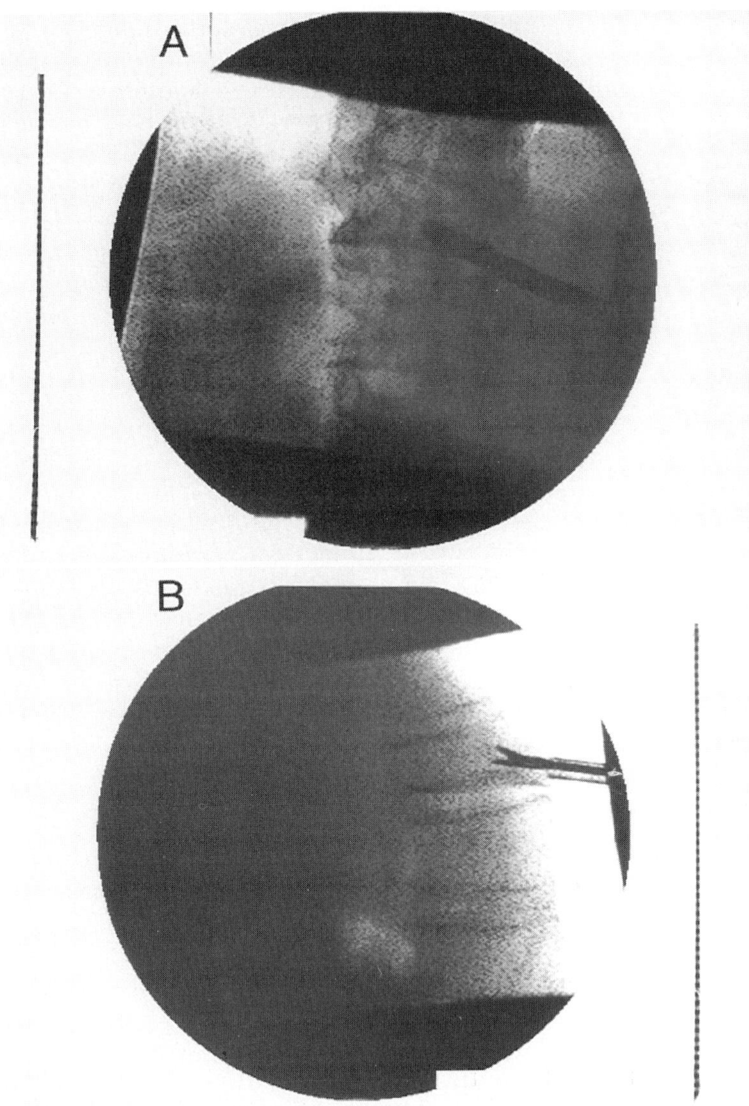

FIGURE 17.
A, antercposterior and lateral intraoperative roentgenographic examination demonstrating the passage of the instruments through the triangular working zone at T7–8 following thorough arthroscopic viewing of the annulotomy site. The access cannula is tilted cephalad, and the vertebral plate is fenestrated. **B,** lateral view demonstrating the introduction of forceps into the vertebral body of T7 to obtain tissue for pathologic examination.

THERAPEUTIC SPINAL ARTHROSCOPY

Herniated disks may be classified into three categories according to the anatomic and arthroscopic appearance of the lumbar intervertebral disk: (1) intra-annular, (2) subligamentous, and (3) extraligamentous herniations.[46, 47] Intra-annular herniations are those in which the nuclear material is still partially supported and contained within the annulus by the remaining intact annular fibers and the posterior longitudinal ligament. Imaging studies show a broad-based bulge or protrusion at the herniation site. Subligamentous herniations result when annular fibers are completely torn but herniated nuclear material is still held under the ventral surface of the posterior longitudinal ligament. Computed tomography and MRI show a pronounced change in the contour of the annulus and obvious compression of neural elements. In extraligamentous herniations, the nuclear fragment has been expelled into the spinal canal or extraforaminal region. In the transverse plane, the herniated nucleus pulposus may be divided into central, paramedial, foraminal, and extraforaminal herniations.[48]

FORAMINAL AND EXTRAFORAMINAL HERNIATIONS

Wiltse et al.[49] have described a paramedial approach for the removal of extraforaminal herniations. These herniations may be accessed and removed with either an intermittent uniportal approach using the videodiscoscope and instruments or by using a working-channel scope. Unilateral biportal access may be used for extraction of extraforaminal herniations. With the aid of cannular jigs, two conversion cannulas may be placed, one anterior to the other, in the triangular working zone. The arthroscope is inserted through one port while the instruments are introduced through the adjacent cannula. The herniation site is visualized and disk material evacuated.

CENTRAL AND PARAMEDIAL HERNIATED NUCLEUS PULPOSUS

Minimally invasive arthroscopic posterolateral disk decompression and fragmentectomy offer important advantages over conventional posteromedial laminotomy techniques. Unavoidable intraoperative injury to the epidural and neural venous system may be associated with venous stasis, neural edema, and perineural and intraneural fibrosis and result in the failed laminotomy syndrome.[45, 50–53]

When laminotomy and annulotomy are performed to extract fragments from an intra-annular or subligamentous herniation, the intact annular fibers are severed. This, in turn, further weakens the posterior containment of the nucleus and increases the incidence of recurrent disk herniation.[22, 23, 54–56] In addition, the incidence of postoperative spondylosis appears to be higher with open laminotomy and discectomy than with arthroscopic microdiscectomy.[57] Postoperative morbidity is reduced since a very small (7-mm) incision is employed, and myoligamentous injury and bleeding are minimized by avoiding the need to detach muscle fibers from the spinal process and lamina. Finally, minimally invasive arthroscopic fragmentectomy is more cost-effective than traditional laminotomy techniques.[58]

Although small central or paramedial herniations are retrievable through a single universal-access cannula or an oval cannula (Fig 18), a large subligamentous or nonmigrated extraligamentous herniation will require the establishment of two portals from the right and left sides to allow for uninterrupted visualization, adequate fluid management, and ex-

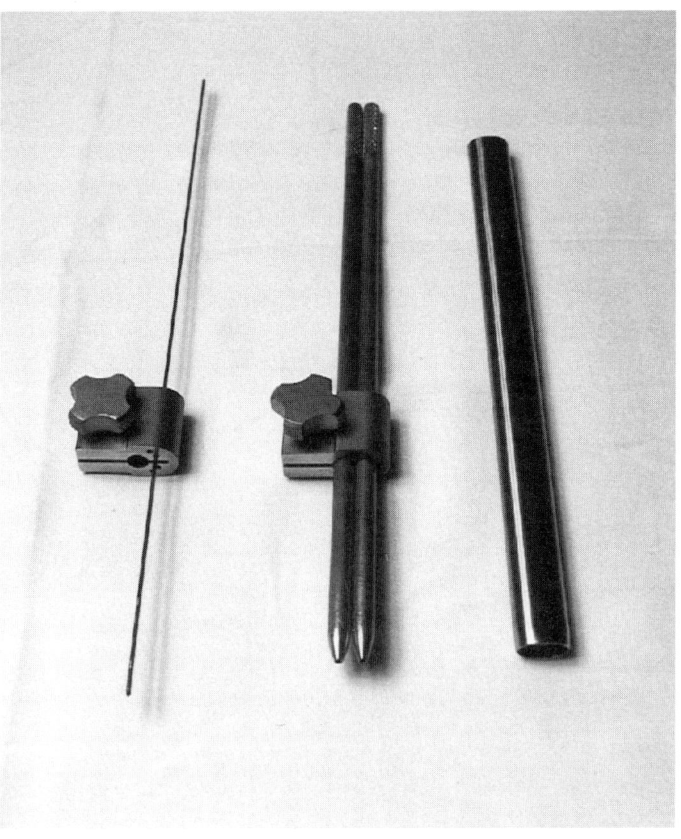

FIGURE 18.

Left to right: jig A—a guide pin is inserted into the bore of jig A in preparation for introduction of a second cannulated obturator anterior to the originally positioned cannulated obturator in the triangular working zone; jig B—two cannulated obturators are passed through the bore of jig B in preparation for insertion of the oval cannula; the oval cannula.

traction of the offending herniated fragments (see Figs 9, 19, and 20).[9, 32, 33, 36, 47, 59] Although extraction of foraminal or paramedial sequestrated fragments through arthroscopic foraminal access is possible, retrieval of a central herniated fragment through this approach is difficult.

In 250 consecutive patients who had signs and symptoms of a herniated nucleus pulposus refractory to nonsurgical modalities and required discectomy through a posterolateral access, we have reported satisfactory outcomes in up to 85% of patients.[32, 36, 56, 60] Our complications have been minimal, and we have not encountered any neurovascular injuries. In a prospective, randomized study comparing the outcome of microscopic discectomy and endoscopic microdiscectomy, Mayer and Brock[61] have reported fewer complications and lower postoperative morbidity following endoscopic access, with a similar outcome in both procedures. Other investigators have also reported satisfactory outcomes in 75% to 80% of properly selected patients following arthroscopic disc surgery.[58, 62–66]

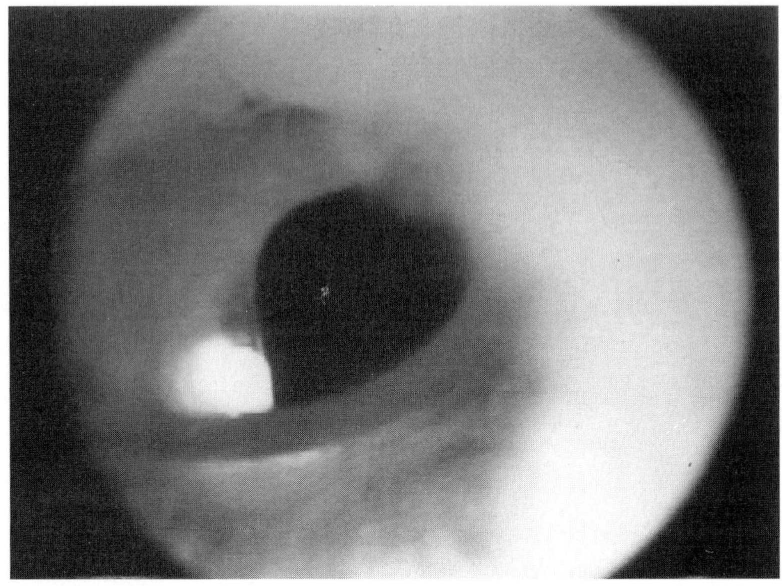

FIGURE 19.
Intraoperative arthroscopic view of the trimmer blade that is used for nuclear resection and creation of a cavity beyond the inner fibers of the posterior of the annulus.

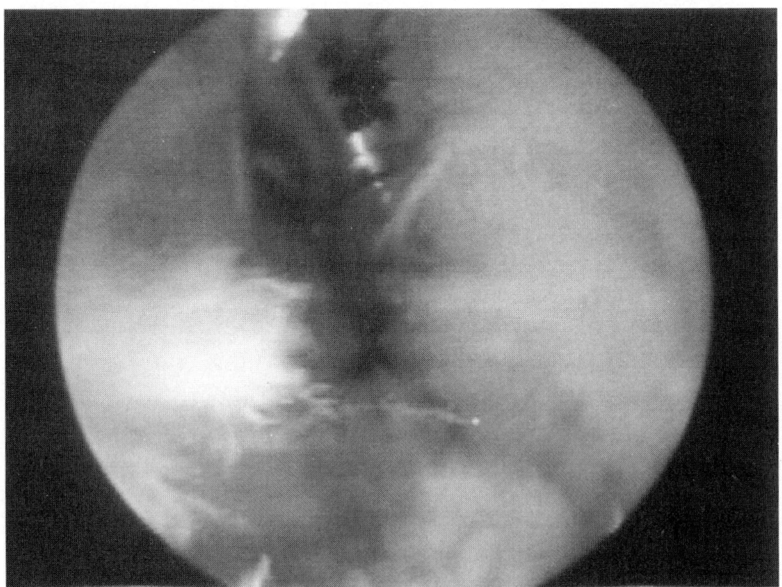

FIGURE 20.
Intraoperative arthroscopic view of biportal access demonstrating the deflecting suction forceps reaching under the posterior longitudinal ligament to grasp and extract a large subligamentous herniation.

ARTHROSCOPIC POSTEROLATERAL INTERBODY FUSION

Interbody fusion is a desirable method of achieving successful stabilization of an unstable lumbar motion segment.[67–71] The availability of compression forces, the broad surface contact of the vertebral bodies, and the good blood supply at the fusion site facilitate the development of rapid arthrodesis. Subsequent improvements, particularly the development of vertebral fixators,[72–79] have contributed to better maintenance of reduction and fusion[80, 81] of the spinal column following either intertransverse or interbody arthrodesis. While interbody fusions have been performed both anteriorly[68, 70] and posteriorly,[67, 69] recent advances in arthroscopic disk surgery and a better understanding of how intervertebral disks can be safely accessed posterolaterally have led to the development of instrumentation for percutaneous interbody fusion and the use of fixators with a minimally invasive surgical technique.

In addition to arthroscopic microdiscectomy instruments, arthroscopic interbody fusion requires the use of an oval access cannula (see Fig 17) in order to provide broader access to the intervertebral disk, thus facilitating ample decortication of the vertebral end plates.

Pedicular bolts are available in a variety of lengths and diameters. These bolts are cannulated to permit their precise positioning in the pedicles at the site of previously inserted guide pins. Straight and offset extension bars in a variety of lengths are available to fasten pedicular bolts to subcutaneous plates and nuts above the deep lumbar fascia. When multiple segments are to be instrumented, the use of offset extension bars facilitates the alignment of pedicular bolts before placement of the subcutaneous plates. These offset extension bars are also useful in preventing convergence of the pedicular bolts when performing an arthrodesis of the L5–S1 segments (Fig 21).

The author's early experience with arthroscopic interbody fusion without the use of pedicular fixators was suboptimal.[82, 83] The availability of instruments that allow decortication of the concave surface of the vertebral plates and the use of autogenous bone and bone protein in conjunction with temporary utilization of subcutaneous fixators[84–89] (see Fig 16) may prove to be an acceptable method of achieving stabilization of lumbar motion segments. Leu and Schreiber also reported a satisfactory rate of stabilization following arthroscopic interbody fusion augmented with external fixators.[90]

Precise positioning of the pedicular bolts in the pedicles is essential. This is achieved by placement of a guide pin in the center of the pedicle under C-arm fluoroscopic control. This step is then followed by insertion of a cannulated obturator and placement of an access cannula with a 10-mm outer diameter. Through this access cannula the pedicle is tapped and examined with the aid of a sonde and arthroscope in preparation for insertion of the pedicular bolts.

At The Graduate Hospital we have used arthroscopic interbody fusion alone or in conjunction with posterolateral intertransverse or facet arthrodesis. At the present time we are augmenting these procedures with pedicular bolt fixation and subcutaneous plating. In 18 patients treated thus far we have not encountered any neurovascular complications, and the outcome has been encouraging.

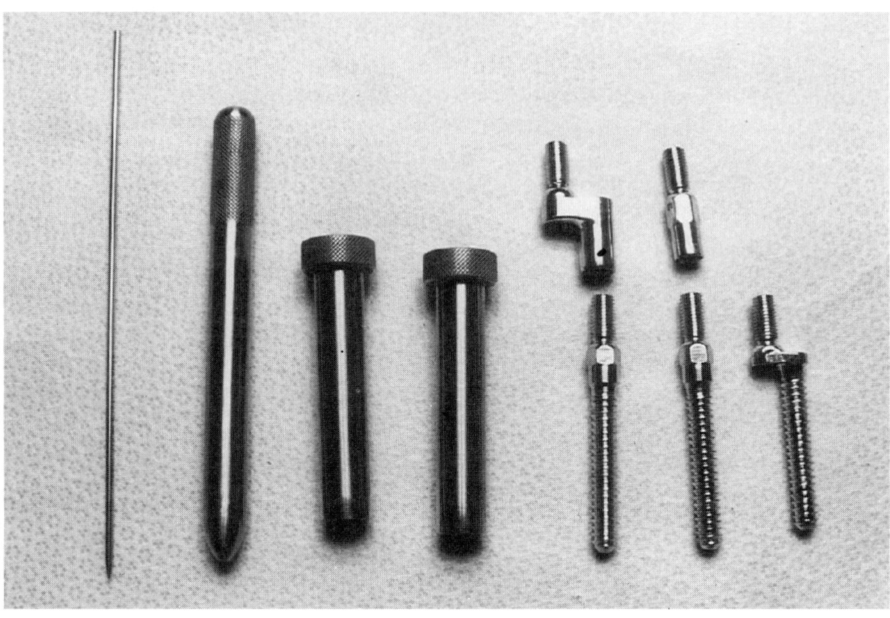

FIGURE 21.
Left to right: pedicular guide pin, cannulator obturator, two pedicular-access cannulas, pedicular bolt with an offset extension bar, pedicular bolt with a straight extension bar, offset pedicular bolt.

DISCUSSION

The field of minimally invasive surgery is expanding rapidly, not only in the area of spine-related disorders but also in gynecologic, gastrointestinal, and thoracic surgery. Minimally invasive spinal surgery performed through a posterolateral approach offers important advantages over conventional procedures.

Nerve root injury and insult to the epidural venous system resulting in chronic neural edema are avoided by establishing portals at a safe distance from the neural elements and by arthroscopic monitoring of the procedure. Postoperative morbidity is reduced since a very small (7-mm) incision is employed, and myoligamentous injury and bleeding are minimized by avoiding the need to detach muscle fibers from the spinal processes and lamina. Thus minimally invasive spinal surgery is more cost-effective than traditional methods because it reduces the hospital stay and permits rapid rehabilitation and early restoration of function. At the present state of the art, the available arthroscopic instruments provide an opportunity for extraction of posteriorly lodged herniated fragments, including nonmigrated extraligamentous herniation, either through a single or biportal access. The working-channel scope is useful for periannular surgery and extraction of extraforaminal and foraminal herniations. A grossly displaced sequestrated fragment is not retrievable with the arthroscopic technique. Our experience with arthroscopic restabilization of lumbar motion segments has been encouraging. This approach reduces soft tissue injuries associated with open operative procedures and promotes early return to a functional level.

Anterior transperitoneal access to the intervertebral disk[91] for discectomy or insertion of cages[92] to achieve arthrodesis may prove to be a useful method of stabilization of the L5–S1 segments. Our expandable cage that may be placed between the vertebral plates through a cannula inserted dorsolaterally provides more rigid stabilization of the anterior column and should enhance the rate of successful lumbar interbody arthrodesis. Technology that provides the capability of extracting posterolateral osteophytes and resecting the stenotic bony elements is currently being developed and implemented (Goldthwait, Reynolds, Pletz, and Kambin, unpublished data).

The development of an expandable disk prosthesis that may be positioned between the vertebral plates through a cannula under arthroscopic control is not unrealistic.

Although posterolateral arthroscopic access has provided surgeons with the opportunity of visualization and diagnosis of certain spine pathologies, further technological advances and clinical trials will certainly broaden our current knowledge in this interesting field.

REFERENCES

1. Dandy WE: Loose cartilage from intervertebral disc simulating tumor of the spinal cord. *Arch Surg* 19:660–672, 1929.
2. Mixter WJ, Barr JS: Rupture of the intervertebral disk with involvement of the spinal canal. *N Engl J Med* 211:205–210, 1934.
3. Paus B, Skalpe IO: Recurrence of pain following operation for herniated lumbar disc: Fresh herniation or extradural scar tissue? *Int Orthop* 3:133–136, 1979.
4. Ramirez LF, Thisted R: Complications and demographic characteristics of patients undergoing lumbar discectomy in community hospitals. *Neurosurgery* 25:226–231, 1989.
5. Shinners BM, Hamby WB: Protruded lumbar intervertebral discs: Results following surgical and nonsurgical therapy. *J Neurosurg* 6:450–458, 1949.
6. Stolke D, Sollman WP, Seifert V: Intra- and postoperative complications in lumbar disc surgery. *Spine* 14:56–59, 1989.
7. Maroon JC, Onik G, Sternau L: Percutaneous automated discectomy: A new approach to lumbar surgery. *Clin Orthop* 238:64–70, 1989.
8. Onik G, Helms C, Ginsburg L, et al: Percutaneous lumbar discectomy using a new aspiration probe. *AJR Am J Roentgenol* 144:1137–1140, 1985.
9. Kambin P: Arthroscopic microdiscectomy: Laser nuclear ablation. *Spine State Art Rev* 7:95–101, 1993.
10. Kambin P: Arthroscopic microdiscectomy laser nucleolysis. *Philadelphia Med* 87:548–549, 1991.
11. Ascher PW, Holzer P, Sutter B, et al: Laser denaturation of the nucleus pulposus of herniated intervertebral disc, in Kambin P (ed): *Arthroscopic Microdiscectomy: Minimal Intervention in Spinal Surgery*. Baltimore, Urban & Schwarzenberg, 1990, pp 137–140.
12. Cummings RS, Progoehl JA, Hermantin FU, et al: Percutaneous laser discectomy using a flexible endoscope: Technical considerations. *Spine State Art Rev* 7:37–40, 1993.
13. Smith L, Gorvin PJ, Gesler RM, et al: Enzyme dissolution of the annulus pulposus. *Nature* 198:1311–1312, 1963.
14. Kahanovitz N, Viola K, Goldstein T, et al: A multicenter analysis of percutaneous discectomy. *Spine* 15:713–715, 1990.

15. Revel M, Payan D, Vallee C, et al: Automated percutaneous lumbar discectomy versus chemonucleolysis in the treatment of sciatica. A randomized multicenter trial. *Spine* 18:1–7, 1993.
16. Epstein NE: Surgically confirmed cauda equina and nerve root injury following percutaneous discectomy at an outside institution: A case report. *J Spinal Disord* 3:380–383, 1990.
17. Rydevik B, Branemark PI, Nordborg C, et al: Effects of chymopapain on nerve tissue: An experimental study on the structure and function of peripheral nerve tissue in rabbits after local application of chymopapain. *Spine* 1:137–147, 1976.
18. Hiroshi E: Transverse myelitis following chemonucleolysis. *J Bone Joint Surg Am* 65:1328–1330, 1983.
19. Jacobson S: Lumbar percutaneous diskectomy. *Bull Hosp Jt Dis* 48:67–74, 1988.
20. Gill K: Retroperitoneal bleeding after automated percutaneous discectomy. A case report. *Spine* 15:1376–1377, 1990.
21. Onik G, Maroon JC, Jackson R: Cauda equina syndrome secondary to an improperly placed nucleotome probe. *Neurosurgery* 30:412–414, 1992.
22. Kambin P, Brager M: Percutaneous posterolateral discectomy: Anatomy and mechanism. *Clin Orthop* 223:145–154, 1987.
23. Kambin P: Research aspect of annular fenestration and discectomy. Presented at the annual symposium of The Graduate Hospital, Philadelphia, Nov 6–7, 1987.
24. Sakamoto T, Tamakawa H, Tajima T, et al: A study of percutaneous lumbar nucleotomy and lumbar intradiscal pressure. Presented at the International Symposium on Percutaneous Lumbar Discectomy, Brussels, March 17, 1989.
25. Stern IJ, Smith L: Dissolution by chymopapain in vitro of tissue from normal or prolapsed intervertebral discs. *Clin Orthop* 50:269–277, 1967.
26. Suguro T, Oegema TR, Bradford DS: The effects of chymopapain on prolapsed human intervertebral disc: A clinical and correlative histochemical study. *Clin Orthop* 213:223–231, 1986.
27. Craig FS: Vertebral-body biopsy. *J Bone Joint Surg Am* 38:93–102, 1956.
28. Kambin P, Gellman H: Percutaneous lateral discectomy of the lumbar spine: A preliminary report. *Clin Orthop* 174:127–132, 1983.
29. Kambin P: Interdepartmental communication, 1973.
30. Kambin P: History of disc surgery, in Kambin P (ed): *Arthroscopic Microdiscectomy: Minimal Intervention in Spinal Surgery*. Baltimore, Urban & Schwarzenberg, 1990, pp 3–8.
31. Kambin P: New surgical procedure aiding herniated spinal disk sufferers. *Image* 6:1–5, 1982.
32. Kambin P: Arthroscopic microdiscectomy. *Arthroscopy* 8:287–295, 1992.
33. Kambin P: Arthroscopic microdiskectomy. *Mt Sinai J Med* 58:159–164, 1991.
34. Kambin P: Percutaneous lumbar discectomy: Current practice. Surg *Rounds Orthop* 31–35, December 1988.
35. Kambin P: Arthroscopic microdiskectomy. *Semin Orthop* 6:97–108, 1991.
36. Schaffer J, Kambin P: Percutaneous posterolateral lumbar discectomy and decompression with a 6.9 millimeter cannula: Analysis of operative failures and complications. *J Bone Joint Surg Am* 73:822–831, 1994.
37. Hijikata S: Percutaneous nucleotomy: A new concept technique and 12 years' experience. *Clin Orthop* 238:93–102, 1989.
38. Hijikata S, Yamagishi M, Nakayama T, et al: Percutaneous diskectomy: A new treatment method for lumbar disk herniation. *J Toden Hosp* 5:5–13, 1975.
39. Schreiber A, Suezawa Y: Transdiscoscopic percutaneous nucleotomy in disk herniation. *Orthop Rev* 15:75–78, 1986.

40. Schreiber A, Suezawa Y, Leu HJ: Does percutaneous nucleotomy with discoscopy replace conventional discectomy? eight years of experience and results in treatment of herniated lumbar disc. *Clin Orthop* 238:35–42, 1989.
41. Castro WH, Halm H, Rondhuis J: The influence of automated percutaneous lumbar discectomy on the biomechanics of the lumbar intervertebral disc. An experimental study. *Acta Orthop Belg* 58:400–405, 1992.
42. Castro WH, Jerosch J, Brinckman P: Changes in the lumbar disc following use of non-automated percutaneous discectomy. A biomechanical study. *Z Orthop Ihre Grenzgeb* 130:473–478, 1992.
43. Kambin P: Posterolateral percutaneous lumbar discectomy and decompression: Arthroscopic microdiscectomy, in Kambin P (ed): *Arthroscopic Microdiscectomy: Minimal Intervention in Spinal Surgery*. Baltimore, Urban & Schwarzenberg, 1991, pp 67–100.
44. Fraser RD, Osti OL, Vernon-Roberts B: Intervertebral disc degeneration. *Eur Spine J* 1:205–213, 1993.
45. Parke WW: Clinical anatomy of the lumbar spine, in Kambin P (ed): *Arthroscopic Microdiscectomy: Minimal Intervention in Spinal Surgery*. Baltimore, Urban & Schwarzenberg, 1990, pp 11–29.
46. Kambin P: Classification of herniated nucleus pulposus based on anatomical and imaging studies. Presented at the International Symposium for Minimal Intervention in Spinal Surgery, The Graduate Hospital, Philadelphia, November 1993.
47. Schaffer J, Kambin P: Minimally invasive spine surgery, in Kelley, Harris, Ruddy, et al (eds): *Textbook of Rheumatology*, update, ed 9. Philadelphia, WB Saunders, 1993, pp 2–12.
48. Bonneville JF: Plaidoyer pour une classification par l'image des hernies discales lombaires: La carte-image. *Rev Imagerie Med* 2:557–560, 1990.
49. Wiltse LL, Bateman JG, Hutchinson RH, et al: The paraspinal sacrospinalis-splitting approach to the lumbar spine. *J Bone Joint Surg Am* 50:919–926, 1968.
50. Olmarker K, Rydevik B, Holm S: Edema formation in spinal nerve roots induced by experimental graded compression. An experimental study in pig cauda equina with special reference to differences in effects between rapid and slow onset of compression. *Spine* 14:569–573, 1989.
51. Park W: The significance of venous return impairment in ischemic radiculopathy and myelopathy. *Orthop Clin North Am* 22:213–222, 1991.
52. Hoyland JA, Freemont AJ, Jayson MIV: Intervertebral foramen venous obstruction: A cause of periradicular pain fibrosis. *Spine* 14:538–568, 1989.
53. Parke WW: The significance of venous return in ischemic radiculopathy and myelopathy. *Clin Orthop* 22:213–220, 1991.
54. Kambin P, Sampson S: Posterolateral percutaneous suction-excision of herniated lumbar intervertebral discs: Report of interim results. *Clin Orthop* 207:37–43, 1986.
55. Kambin P, Schaffer JL: Percutaneous lumbar discectomy: Review of 100 patients and current practice. *Clin Orthop* 238:24–34, 1989.
56. Kambin P, Schaffer J: Percutaneous lumbar discectomy: Prospective review of 100 patients. *Clin Orthop* 238:24–34, 1989.
57. Kambin P, Cohen L, Brooks ML, et al: Comparative incidence of degenerative spondylosis of the lumbar spine following partial discectomy: Laminotomy and discectomy versus posterolateral discectomy: Presented at the North American Spine Society, Boston, July 11, 1992.
58. Hochschuler S, Guyer R: Texas Back Institute experience and results with arthroscopic microdiscectomy. Presented at the International Symposium on Arthroscopic Miscrodiscectomy of the Lumbar Spine sponsored by The

In this review, we highlight some of the recent developments in human glomerular disease. We intentionally confined the discussion to a select group of disorders in which a collective body of information has enhanced the understanding of the basic pathophysiologic mechanisms and/or provided novel therapeutic approaches.

IgA NEPHROPATHY

IgA nephropathy (IgAN), initially described in 1968 by Berger and Hinglais,[1] is the most common form of human glomerulonephritis worldwide, and it accounts for a significant amount of end-stage renal disease (ESRD). The estimated prevalence of glomerular IgA deposits from forensic necropsies is surprisingly common (4–5%) among individuals without prior evidence of renal disease; in contrast, 1.3% of patients with a history of renal disease had IgA deposits at necropsy.[2] IgAN may be idiopathic or associated with one of several systemic illnesses. In this review we will focus primarily on new developments in *primary* IgAN. In particular, after a brief description of the entity, our discussion will largely involve consideration of newer aspects of therapy. The reader is referred to one of many recent reviews for excellent discussions of clinical features and pathogenic mechanisms of this disorder.[3–8]

IgAN is characterized by deposits of IgA and C3 in the mesangium (Fig 1). These deposits are composed primarily of oligomeric IgA1 and co-deposition of IgG and IgM are present in more than 50% of cases.[6] By light microscopy, mesangial expansion with varying degrees of hypercellularity and increased matrix is typical, and the severity of these changes frequently varies among individual glomeruli within the same specimen. Occasionally, crescents are observed; however, crescentic glomerulonephritis is atypical. Electron-dense deposits in the mesangial and paramesangial areas are characteristic; subendothelial deposits may also be present.[8]

Clinically, signs and symptoms vary; i.e., in young patients (<25 yr) macroscopic hematuria associated with low-grade proteinuria (<1 g/day) is common, especially in males, and routine urinalysis screening programs may uncover unsus-

---

FIG 1.

The appearance of glomeruli from patients with IgAN is variable. Among similarly affected glomeruli with purely mesangial lesions, there may be a predominance of cellular proliferation **(A)** or matrix expansion **(C)**, as opposed to a balance between these two elements **(B)**, even within the same patient **(A** vs. **B)**. Similarly, instead of a moderate degree of mesangial change **(A–C)**, equivocal or mild **(D)** or severe **(E)** changes may be evident, again potentially within the same patient **(C** vs. **D)**. In fact, variation even within the same glomerulus (segmental variation) is often recognized (left vs. right halves of glomeruli in **A, C;** 12 and 3 to 4 o'clock vs. remainder of glomerulus in **E)**. Note lucencies in the periodic acid–

(Continued.)

77. Roy-Camille R, Sailant G, Bertezus P, et al: Early treatment of spinal injuries, in MacKibbin B (ed): *Recent Advances in Orthopaedics*. Dublin, Churchill Livingstone, 1979, pp 57–87.
78. Steffee AD, Biscup RS, Sitkowski DJ: Segmental spine plates with pedicle screw fixation: A new internal fixation device for disorders of the lumbar and thoracolumbar spine. *Clin Orthop* 203:45–53, 1986.
79. Kostiuk JP, Errico TJ, Gleason TF: Luque instrumentation in degenerative conditions of the lumbar spine. *Spine* 15:318–321, 1990.
80. Kim SS, Denis F, Lonstein JE, et al: Factors affecting fusion rate in adult spondylolisthesis. *Spine* 15:979–984, 1990.
81. Lorenz M, Zindrick M, Schwaegler P, et al: A comparison of single-level fusions with and without hardware. *Spine* 16(suppl):455–458, 1991.
82. Kambin P: Posterolateral percutaneous lumbar interbody fusion, in Kambin P (ed): *Arthroscopic Microdiscectomy: Minimal Intervention in Spinal Surgery*. Baltimore, Urban & Schwarzenberg, 1991, pp 117–121.
83. Kambin P: Arthroscopic arthrodesis of the lumbar spine. Presented at the International Society for Orthopaedic and Traumatology/International Society for Minimal Intervention in Spinal Surgery (SICOT/ISMISS) Congress, Seoul, Korea, Sept 3, 1993.
84. Kambin P: Posterolateral approach to the lumbar intervertebral discs. From nucleotomy to segmental stabilization. Presented at the International Symposium on Percutaneous Intervertebral Surgery with Discoscopy, Zurich, Switzerland, June 1991.
85. Kambin P: Percutaneous segmental stabilization in situ and with pedicular screws and subcutaneous fixators. Presented at a symposium at The Graduate Hospital, Philadelphia, Nov 1, 1991.
86. Kambin P: Arthroscopic lumbar fusion with pedicular bolts and subcutaneous plates. International Society for Minimal Intervention in Spinal Surgery (ISMISS) Scientific Exhibit, American Academy of Orthopedic Surgeons Meeting, Washington, DC, Feb 20–25, 1992.
87. Kambin P: Arthroscopic lumbar fusion with pedicular bolts and removable subcutaneous plates. International Society for Minimal Intervention in Spinal Surgery (ISMISS) Scientific Exhibit, American Academy of Orthopedic Surgeons Meeting, San Francisco, Feb 18–22, 1993.
88. Kambin P, Schaffer JL: Arthroscopic lumbar fusion augmented with removable pedicular fixators and subcutaneous plates. Presented at an Advanced Course, Scoliosis Research Society/North American Spine Society, Orlando, Fla, May 13–15, 1993.
89. Kambin P, Schreiber A, Shepperd J, et al: Minimal intervention surgical techniques. *Orthop Trans* 17:1132, 1993.
90. Leu HJ, Schreiber A: Percutaneous fusion of the lumbar spine: A promising technique. *Spine State Art Rev* 6:593–604, 1992.
91. Obenchain TG: Laparoscopic lumbar discectomy: Case report. *J Laparoendosc Surg* 1:145–149, 1991.
92. Yuen HA, Zdelblik T, Bagby G, et al: Preliminary report on laparoscopic L5–S1 anterior discectomy and fusion using BAK cage. Presented at the International Society for Orthopaedic and Traumatology/International Society for Minimal Intervention in Spinal Surgery (SICOT/ISMISS) Meeting, Seoul, Korea, Sept 3, 1993.

Fractures of the Spine and Osteoporosis

Michael H. Heggeness, M.D., Ph.D.
Associate Professor, Baylor College of Medicine, St. Luke's Episcopal Hospital Center for Orthopaedic Research and Education, Department of Orthopaedic Surgery, Houston, Texas

Osteoporosis is a clinical condition characterized by decreased skeletal bone mass in which the bone is otherwise normal in its biochemical and histologic characteristics. Osteomalacia is a similar clinical condition in which the bone mass is diminished because of an identifiable metabolic abnormality. The term *osteopenia* may be used to describe any patient with diminished bone mass and patients with either osteomalacia or osteoporosis.

Humans attain peak bone mass during the third decade of life. All individuals lose a small portion of their skeletal bone mass each year thereafter. As a result, elderly patients of both sexes frequently have clinically significant osteoporosis. Female patients rapidly lose skeletal bone mass in the years following menopause. Immediately after oophorectomy or menopause, 5% of cancellous bone mass and 1% to 2% of cortical bone mass are lost each year in the initial 2- to 3-year period. This "postmenopausal" bone loss will gradually diminish over the following 5 years, but the abrupt period of postmenopausal bone loss increases the risk of clinical osteoporosis in female patients significantly.[1–9]

An additional compounding factor is the patient's initial bone mass. Males on average will acquire significant higher peak bone mass during adulthood than will females, and black patients will acquire significantly higher peak bone mass than will Asians or Caucasians.

The incidence of fracture of all bones increases dramatically with age, and it is likely that diminished mineral density is a contributing factor in virtually all fractures sustained in patients over 60 years of age. Fractures particularly associated with lower bone mineral density include fractures of the hip, fractures of the proximal end of the tibia, Colles' fractures of the wrists, and fractures of the thoracic and lumbar spines.

The morbidity of these injuries is staggering. It is estimated that approximately 400,000 hip fractures occur every year in the United States. The cost of acute care of these patients alone is estimated to be in excess of 10 billion dollars per year. Unfortunately, these injuries are also associated with a high incidence of associated mortality, and at least one study has documented a mortality rate of approximately 50% 1 year after a hip fracture.[7, 8]

The morbidity and mortality associated with vertebral fractures is

Advances in Operative Orthopaedics, vol. 3

much harder to estimate because the majority of these injuries go undiagnosed and untreated. Recent estimates indicate a prevalence of up to 27% in the female population older than 65.[3–5, 7–13]

VERTEBRAL FRACTURES

Vertebral fractures associated with osteoporosis are commonly seen in the elderly, although prevalence and incidence rates are extremely difficult to estimate. Precise diagnostic criteria are difficult to establish. Minor degrees of end-plate collapse are often quite difficult to appreciate. In addition, projectional artifact and the low mineral density of the bones themselves contribute to the difficulty.[9]

HEADING AND CLASSIFICATION

The classic epidemiologic work of Drs. Urist, Saville, Riggs, Melton, and others has demonstrated a wide variation in the manifestation and progression of vertebral collapse in osteoporosis.[1–9] Some conclusions can be formed, however. In general, the earliest fracture events are typically seen in the upper thoracic spine. Interestingly, many of these fractures are asymptomatic. Progressive collapse of multiple vertebrae in this area, however, can lead to a significant upper thoracic kyphosis, often unfortunately referred to as a "dowager's hump" (Fig 1).

Adding to the challenge of the physicians, patients are not infre-

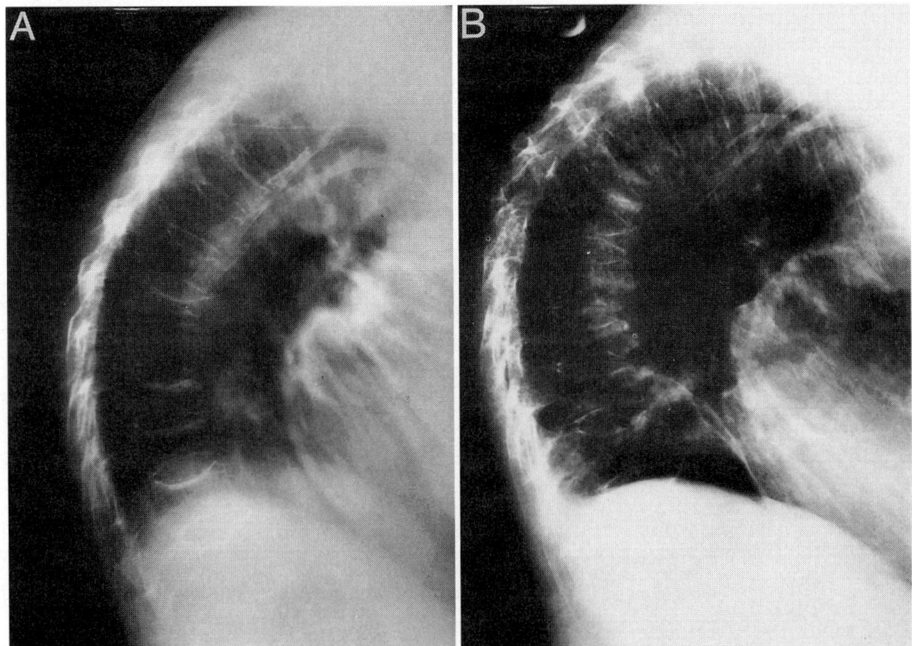

FIGURE 1.

A, lateral x-ray images of an 86-year-old white female with severe idiopathic osteoporosis. **B,** same patient 8 months later documenting the acquisition of multiple new fractures with severe resulting kyphosis.

quently seen for acute back pain with no initial radiographic evidence of fracture. Frequently, images taken days or weeks later will document vertebral collapse.

This phenomenon illustrates an important point about osteoporotic compression fractures: the fractured vertebra frequently demonstrates insidious progressive collapse over weeks or months to a degree not seen in younger patients. The majority of osteoporotic vertebral fractures are the result of failure under axial compression.[14, 15] These injuries are commonly referred to as compression fractures, although they are known to quite frequently involve the posterior cortex of the vertebral body. Many such fractures are therefore technically true burst fractures. Because very few of these fractures can be imaged by computed tomography (CT) or magnetic resonance imaging (MRI) technology, the true incidence of middle column injury is not known. Classic anatomic studies by Schmorl and Junghans and by Jaffe have shown, however, that this is a very frequent feature of these fractures.[16, 17]

Most attempts to classify these injuries have been based on plain radiographic criteria, and the classification system of Eastell et al.[18] has proved useful. Vertebral fractures are often referred to by their gross morphology as "biconcave" or "codfish" fractures, "wedge" fractures, or "crush" fractures. A crush fracture represents gross failure of the anterior and middle columns. It is not known what percentage of biconcave or wedge fractures also have some posterior cortex (or middle column) involvement. Indeed, as mentioned earlier, it is frequently observed that what appears to be an isolated fracture may undergo progressive collapse to a wedge and subsequently a crush fracture appearance over days and weeks of observation. On rare occasion, this sequence of events can lead to devastating late neurologic dysfunction.[19–24] Management of a patient with an osteoporosis-related compression fracture includes careful patient evaluation, diagnostic studies to include an investigation of other possible causes of pathologic fractures, and in the vast majority of cases, nonoperative care. The patient's history should include specific reference to risk factors for osteoporosis such as a smoking history, excessive alcohol intake, and a detailed surgical and medical history. The possibility of multiple myeloma must specifically be kept in mind. A history of weight loss may be particularly suggestive of malignancy. Radiographs should be carefully examined for fracture morphology. A history of previous fractures can be very useful.

A laboratory screen should be routinely performed and should include a complete blood count, sedimentation rate, serum protein electrophoresis, urinalysis, and thyroid function tests. In an elderly Caucasian female without evidence of other contributing history, a tentative diagnosis of idiopathic osteoporosis may be entertained if this workup is negative. Male patients with osteoporosis or young female patients may require additional workup and endocrinologic consultation.

A careful neurologic examination is mandatory, particularly of the lower extremities. A general physical examination to include a breast examination and palpation of the thyroid is encouraged. The presence of objective neurologic dysfunction presents a strong indication for CT or MRI.

The patient's education should be part of the initial phase of management. It is very useful for the patient to understand this diagnosis and its implication. The possibility of future fracture events should be discussed with the patient, although it is important to stress to the patient that vertebral fractures do heal successfully in the overwhelming majority of cases and that spontaneous resolution of pain may be expected in 2 to 10 weeks regardless of treatment. Patients are counseled to seek prompt re-evaluation should neurologic signs or symptoms develop.

Pain management is a critical concern in these patients. When pain is inadequately addressed, many such patients become limited to bed rest, which places them at risk for venous thrombosis and a worsening of their osteoporosis on the basis of inactivity. The exact effect of prolonged bed rest on the mineral density of osteoporotic patients has not been studied. Bed rest studies on younger patients, however, have indicated that bone loss of up to 1% per week can be expected.[25] On this basis, this author strongly discourages bed rest as treatment and defines patient mobilization as a critical component of care. A short course of oral narcotics is often indicated in these situations to allow the patient a reasonable level of activity.

The use of braces for acute fracture events is controversial. It is certainly true that many elderly patients, despite their pain, are unable to tolerate brace wear. Attempts to brace fractures in the upper thoracic spine are particularly difficult and too rarely successful for pain management. On the other hand, simple braces such as canvas corsets can be extremely useful for lumbar fractures and often afford a dramatic level of pain relief. Bracing of thoracolumbar and midthoracic fractures is more difficult because a lumbosacral corset often does not provide adequate support to this region. Many patients with such thoracolumbar fractures find significant relief with the use of custom-molded soft foam braces.

There is also ongoing controversy about brace use for these problems because of the theoretical possibility of stress shielding of the spine through brace use. It is argued that stress shielding from brace use may exacerbate osteoporosis. It is the author's experience that osteoporotic patients will use the brace only as long as it is useful for severe pain management and that the benefits of keeping the patient ambulatory may significantly outweigh the potential risks afforded by the stress shielding. Unfortunately, no scientific data exist on which to form a firm conclusion on this issue.

A minority of patients will experience such severe pain and physical limitation from fractures that hospitalization is required for supportive care and parenteral pain medication. Mobilization of these patients, even when hospitalized, is encouraged.

Parenteral calcitonin use is gaining popularity in the acute management of vertebral compression fractures. This polypeptide hormone functions naturally to downregulate osteoclast function and has been approved for the treatment of osteoporosis on this basis. For unknown reasons, in many patients who have sustained vertebral compression fractures, dramatic analgesia also results from the use of calcitonin. Although the basis of this phenomenon may lie in the documented central nervous system receptors for this hormone, its precise mode of action in analgesia remains unknown. Parenteral doses of calcitonin of approximately 100 IU/day are extremely effective in pain relief for some patients. Hypersensitivity reactions have been described, however, and most patients do experience transient gastrointestinal symptoms of nausea and vomiting during the initial days of therapy. Because of this, small doses are usually given initially (5 to 20 IU), and the dosage is slowly increased over a matter of 3 to 5 days into the therapeutic range. Symptomatic treatment of associated nausea is often helpful during this interval. Calcitonin treatment and external bracing can usually be discontinued within 4 to 10 weeks of the fracture event.

Because progressive bone loss is inevitable for all of us, some patients unfortunately experience the relentless occurrence of multiple vertebral fractures through their sixth, seventh, and eighth decades. Dramatic kyphotic deformity and severe postural problems often result. Chronic back pain with associated degenerative disease and kyphosis can be an extremely frustrating problem.

Progression of the kyphosis will usually stop when the lower ribs begin to impinge on the iliac wings. Unfortunately, this is frequently associated with local pain caused by irritation of the soft tissues and costal nerves in this area. In rare cases, severe intractable pain may be managed by costal nerve blocks. Spinal osteotomy, rib resection, and multiple-level spinal fusions are strongly contraindicated.

SPINE FRACTURE WITH NEUROLOGIC DEFICIT

The literature suggests that although the incidence of vertebral fractures in the aging population is high, neurologic dysfunction results from these fractures only in extremely rare cases. Reports of such cases are appearing with much greater frequency in recent years, however, and it is likely that this phenomenon is more common than has been previously appreciated.[19–24] All of these reports describe the clinical manifestation of these injuries as quite distinct from fracture events in younger patients. In nearly every case, the fractures occurred either spontaneously or after minor trauma, and the initial complaint was for back pain only. These patients subsequently experienced progressive insidious collapse of the fractured vertebra and acquired radicular pain and neurologic deficits weeks or months after the index fracture event. It is this author's observation that radicular pain always precedes the development of motor deficits.

Shikata et al.,[22] Kaneda et al.,[23] and others have advocated aggressive surgical management of these injuries with decompression and operative stabilization. This author has found that conservative management consisting of aggressive bracing, analgesics, and physical therapy can also lead to excellent results in patients with relatively minor deficits. In patients with major neurologic deficits and dramatic motor dysfunction, there is general agreement that operative management, although difficult, is usually indicated. These patients are frequently elderly and often have medical problems associated with smoking, alcohol, or other complicating conditions. Surgical techniques for dealing with these injuries must be individualized to the specific patient in question.

In general, operative intervention consists of an anterior approach to the spine, corpectomy, and reconstruction. This author favors anterior instrumentation, although simultaneous or staged posterior stabilization may also be appropriate, depending on the surgeon's preference and the individual clinical situation. Iliac crest autograft struts as well as allograft

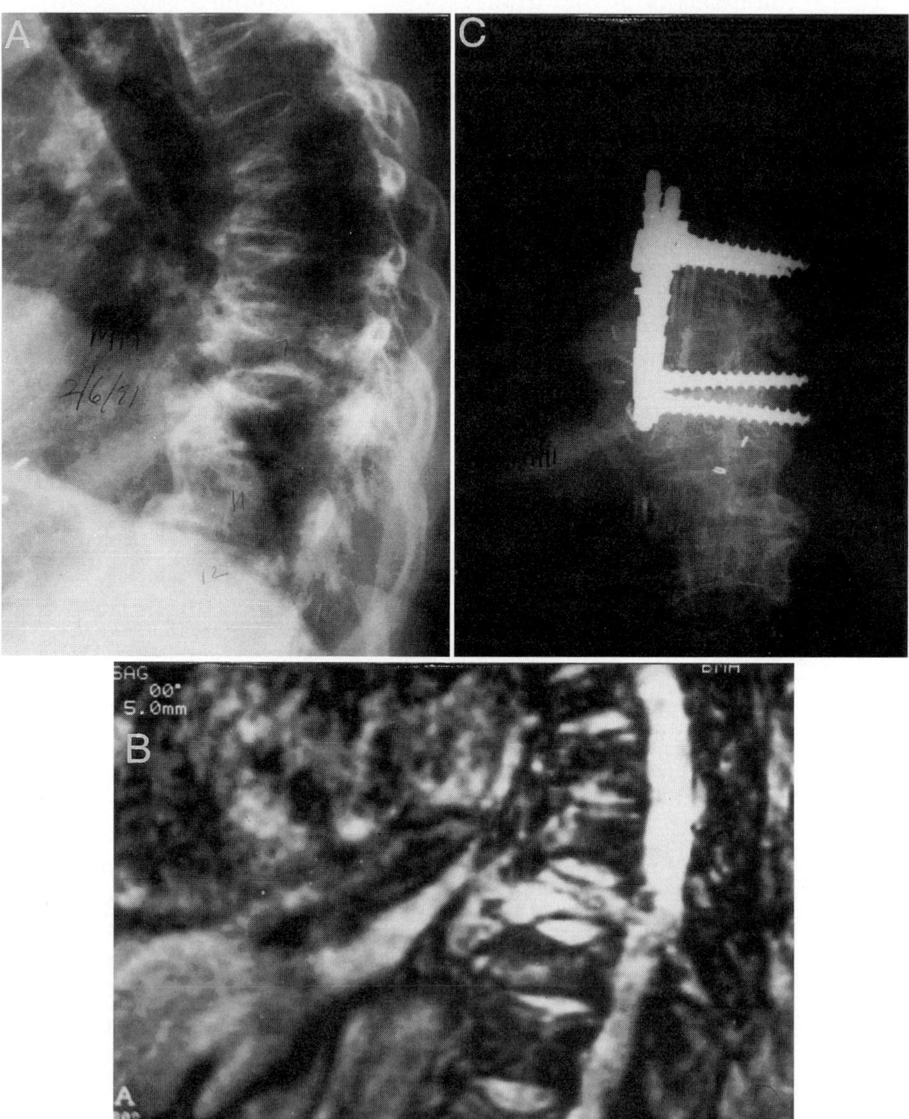

FIGURE 2.

A, lateral radiograph of a 73-year-old female documenting a spontaneous fracture of T9. Six weeks after her original injury, dense paraparesis developed. **B,** a magnetic resonance image of the injured area confirms collapse of the ninth thoracic vertebra and documents extrusion of bony material into the canal. **C,** anteroposterior view of this patient's thoracic spine after anterior decompression (corpectomy) and reconstruction with an iliac crest bone graft and Kostuik-Harrington instrumentation.

and ceramic spacers may all have a role in the surgical treatment of this injury.

Instrumentation of the anterior spine in badly osteopenic patients requires meticulous technique and the creation of a construct with load sharing between unfractured posterior elements, the strut graft itself, and the instrumentation system.

This author personally favors the Kostuik-Harrington device[26] for instrumentation of these fractures because the screw thread design allows excellent purchase in the vertebral bodies (Fig 2). Extended biomechanical studies have not addressed the question of the relative advantage of different screw designs; however, large cancellous threads would seem to offer some advantage in this situation. Bicortical technique is also advised because this does add substantially to the biomechanical stability of such screws.[27]

Biomechanical studies of posterior instrumentation techniques have suggested that hook constructs may offer some advantage over pedicle screw constructs in osteoporotic individuals,[28] although specific techniques such as rigid cross-linking and hook screw constructs leave many options for the surgeon in individualizing treatment.

The author's experience suggests that the clinical phenomenon of neurologic deficit associated with osteoporosis-related spinal fracture is probably a good deal more common than is generally appreciated and that the insidious manifestation of the neurologic deficits frequently leads to a missed or delayed diagnosis. Increased awareness of this injury may lead to more prompt and accurate diagnosis and, it is hoped, more appropriate treatment.

Late follow-up of conservatively treated patients who have resolved their neurologic deficit reveals progressive resorption and remodeling of the offending bone fragments within the canal, although the resorption occurs much more slowly than the clinically observed neurologic recovery.

PREVENTION OF FRACTURE

Treatment of spinal osteoporosis and fractures can be very frustrating for the physician and patient alike. It is likely that the best solution for this problem may result not from its cure but from its prevention. Lifestyle modification, including increased exercise throughout life, postmenopausal estrogen supplementation, and adequate calcium and vitamin D intake, may together significantly decrease the magnitude of this problem in the future. To be effective, however, this approach must rely on identification, education, and treatment of patients in their early and middle adult years.

For a patient with established osteoporosis, acute treatment of fractures can significantly decrease patient suffering. Home safety and fall prevention, however, may assist patients in avoiding these problems entirely. Activities and situations where falls are likely should be approached with great caution. An obstacle-strewn living environment (with exposed lamp cords and throw rugs), icy sidewalks, and dimly lit stairways represent preventable causes of fracture. A discussion of these issues should be part of the treatment of any patient with osteoporosis.

REFERENCES

1. Urist MR, Gurvey MS, Fareed DO: Long term observations on aged women with pathologic osteoporosis, in Barzel US (ed): *Osteoporosis*. New York, Grune & Stratton, 1970, pp 3–37.
2. Saville PD: Observations on 80 women with osteoporotic spine fractures, in Barzel US (ed): *Osteoporosis*, New York, Grune & Stratton, 1970, pp 38–46.
3. Kanis JA, Pitt FA: Epidemiology of osteoporosis. *Bone* 13(suppl):7–15, 1992.
4. Iskrant AP, Smith RW: Osteoporosis in women 45 years and over related to subsequent fractures. *Public Health Rep* 84:33–38, 1969.
5. Melton LJ III, Kan SH, Frye MA, et al: Epidemiology of vertebral fractures during 30 years. *Am J Epidemiol* 129:1000–1011, 1989.
6. Bengner U, Johnell O, Redlund-Johnell I: Changes in incidence and prevalence of vertebral fractures during 30 years. *Calcif Tissue Int* 42:293–296, 1988.
7. Avioli LV: Significance of osteoporosis: A growing international health problem. *Calcif Tissue Int* 49:55–57, 1991.
8. Leidig G, Minne HW, Sauer P, et al: A study of complaints and their relation to vertebral destruction in patients with osteoporosis. *Bone Miner* 8:217–229, 1990.
9. Cooper C, Atkinson E, O'Falcon M, et al: Incidence of clinically diagnosed vertebral fractures: A population-based study in Rochester, Minnesota, 1985–1989. *J Bone Miner Res* 7:221–229, 1990.
10. White BL, Fisher WD, Laurin CA: Rate of mortality for elderly patients after fracture of the hip in the 1980's. *J Bone Joint Surg Am* 69:1335–1340, 1987.
11. Miller CW: Survival and ambulation following hip fracture. *J Bone Joint Surg Am* 60:930–934, 1978.
12. Kleerekoper M, Nelson DA: Vertebral fracture or vertebral deformity? *Calcif Tissue Int* 50:5–6, 1992.
13. Lane JM, Cornell CN, Healey JH: Orthopaedic consequences of osteoporosis, in *Osteoporosis: Etiology, Diagnosis and Management*. New York, Raven Press, 1988, pp 433–455.
14. Denis R: The three column spine and its significance in the classification of acute thoracolumbar spinal injuries. *Spine* 8:817–831, 1983.
15. Holdsworth FW: Fractures, dislocations and fracture dislocations of the spine. *J Bone Joint Surg Am* 52:1534–1551, 1970.
16. Schmorl G, Junghans H: *The Human Spine in Health and Disease*. New York, Grune & Stratton, 1971.
17. Jaffe HL: *Metabolic Degenerative and Inflammatory Diseases of Bone and Joints*. Philadelphia, Lea & Febiger, 1972.
18. Eastell R, Cedel SL, Wahner HW, et al: Classification of vertebral fractures. *J Bone Miner Res* 6:207–215, 1991.
19. Arciero RA, Leung KYK, Pierce JH: Spontaneous unstable burst fracture of the thoracolumbar spine in osteoporosis: A report of two cases. *Spine* 14:114–117, 1989.
20. Salomon C, Chopin D, Benoist M: Spinal cord compression: An exceptional complication of spinal osteoporosis. *Spine* 13:222–224, 1988.
21. Tan SB, Kozak JA, Mawad ME: The limitations of magnetic resonance imaging in the diagnosis of pathologic vertebral fractures. *Spine* 16:919–923, 1991.

22. Shikata J, Yamamuro T, Iida H, et al: Surgical treatment of paraplegia resulting from vertebral fractures in senile osteoporosis. *Spine* 15:485–489, 1990.
23. Kaneda K, Asano S, Hashimoto T, et al: Treatment of osteoporotic-posttraumatic vertebral collapse using the Kaneda device and a bioactive ceramic vertebral prosthesis. *Spine* 17(suppl):295–303, 1992.
24. Heggeness MH: Spine fracture with neurological deficit in osteoporosis. *Osteopor Int* 3:215–221, 1993.
25. LeBlanc AD, Schneider VS, Evans HJ, et al: Bone mineral loss and recovery after 17 weeks of reduction. *J Bone Miner Res* 5:843–850, 1990.
26. Kostuik JP: Anterior fixation for burst fractures of the thoracic and lumbar spine with or without neurological involvement. *Spine* 13:286–293, 1988.
27. Breeze S, Alexander J, Noble PS, et al: A biomechanical study of thoracolumbar screw fixation. Presented at the North American Spine Society, Minneapolis, 1994.
28. Coe JD, Warden KE, Herzig MA, et al: Influence of bone mineral density on the fixation of thoracolumbar implants. *Spine* 15:902–907, 1988.

The Use of Technetium Scintigraphy in the Assessment of Musculoskeletal Trauma

Scott F. Dye, M.D.
Department of Orthopaedic Surgery, University of California, San Francisco, School of Medicine, San Francisco, California

Living human musculoskeletal tissues are among the most complex systems known. Over the 400 million years of vertebrate existence, musculoskeletal components have evolved developmental, homeostatic, and reparative mechanisms designed to generate and transmit great loads, often on the order of multiples of body weight.[1, 2] The response of such tissues to trauma, either direct or indirect, acute or chronic, is of great interest to the orthopedic surgeon whose *raison d'etre* is the restoration of musculoskeletal function.

The development of orthopaedic concepts of musculoskeletal trauma and tissue response to trauma has been profoundly influenced by the preponderance of *structural* information gained from surgery (including arthroscopy) and most imaging modalities. Radiographs, arthrography, computed tomography (CT), ultrasound, and magnetic resonance imaging (MRI) provide primarily structural and pathoanatomic data rather than a direct assessment of physiologic parameters of perturbed musculoskeletal tissues.[3]

The current lexicon reflecting orthopaedic conceptualization of musculoskeletal trauma is therefore replete with "structurally loaded" terminology. Fractured tibia, ruptured anterior cruciate ligament (ACL), torn meniscus, sprained ankle, etc.—the very language of orthopaedic trauma—reflect gross structural failure rather than the physiologic properties of those tissues.[4–6] The limitation of our conceptualization of orthopaedic trauma to only structural characteristics restricts one's understanding of the process of musculoskeletal injury, healing, and ultimately our ability to explain, predict, and control the long-term clinical result. For example, it has recently been shown that early degenerative changes may still develop in patients even when seemingly normal structural and biomechanical properties have been restored following ACL reconstruction.[7, 8] The addition of *physiologic* parameters of such perturbed systems can help clarify this apparent paradox.

Of all of the imaging modalities readily available to the practicing or-

Advances in Operative Orthopaedics, vol. 3

thopaedist, only scintigraphy *absolutely requires* a living, metabolically functioning system in order to be performed. Interestingly, MRI using current sequences cannot readily distinguish between living and nonliving musculoskeletal tissues up to 72 hours postmortem in a porcine model.[9] Technetium 99m methylene diphosphonate (MDP) scintigraphy is an inexpensive, safe, and mature technology that provides a sensitive manifestation of the metabolic activity of living osseous tissues. No current, easily available imaging technology is capable of manifesting similar metabolic characteristics of soft tissues.[11]

Long used to detect possible occult osseous processes such as stress fractures, bone contusions, osteolysis, and reflex sympathetic dystrophy, technetium scintigraphy has, in newer applications, revealed unexpected findings. Over the past decade, the systematic use of this modality in clinical conditions previously thought to encompass only structural failure of soft tissue (e.g., torn meniscus, ACL failure, chondromalacia, etc.) has manifested a heretofore unknown and unappreciated process of associated increased osseous metabolic activity (Fig 1, A and B). The results of many independent research efforts in North America and Europe have convincingly demonstrated that there commonly exists an underlying periarticular increased osseous remodeling phenomenon in association with soft tissue damage of the knee, the persistence of which is predictive of eventual radiographically identifiable degenerative changes.

The purpose of this chapter is to delineate and summarize the latest

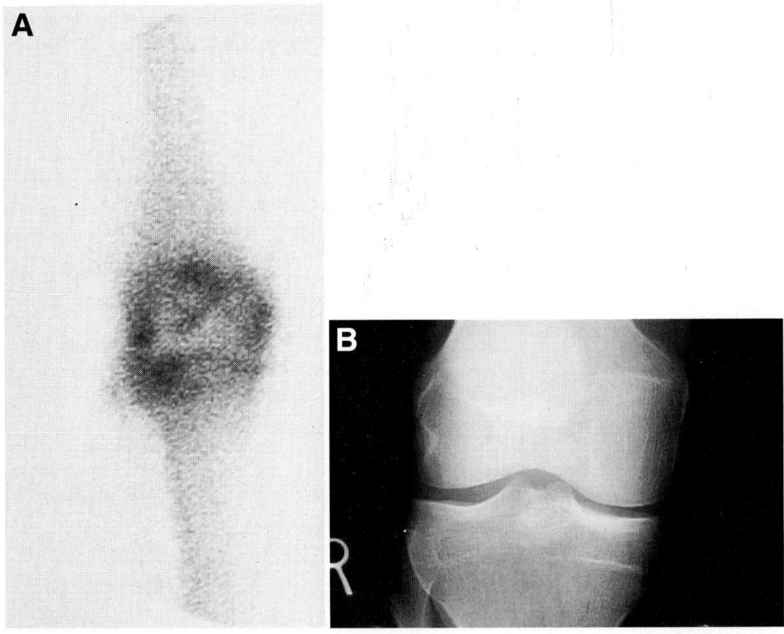

FIGURE 1.

A, technetium scintiscan of a patient with chronic anterior cruciate ligament deficiency of the right knee manifested as increased uptake in all three compartments. **B,** radiograph of the same anterior cruciate ligament–deficient patient manifesting *normal* findings in the face of widespread abnormal scintigraphic activity.

research regarding periarticular bone scintigraphy in the setting of sports-related musculoskeletal trauma and to interpret the clinical significance of these findings for the practicing orthopaedist. This research strongly suggests that our current concepts of musculoskeletal trauma and response of tissues to injury need to be expanded to include these previously unrecognized, physiologic phenomenon. Our treatment goals should likewise be expanded to include restoration of homeostasis of musculoskeletal tissues, if possible, rather than mere restoration of gross structural characteristics.

BIOPHYSICS OF TRACER ACCUMULATION

In order to understand and properly interpret the results of ^{99m}Tc-MDP scintigraphy, one should be familiar with the physiology and biophysics of tracer accumulation in metabolically active tissues. Technetium 99m (m for metastable) is a short (6-hour) half-life emitter of high-energy (140-kEv) γ-ray photons. This radioactive elemental species is produced in a generator by transmutation from molybdenum 99.[12] The high energy of the γ-ray photons enables easy penetration of tissues and radiolucent structures and allows them to be detected by a gamma camera (Fig 2). Such a camera is composed of a large disk-shaped sodium iodide crystal and a set of photomultiplier tubes. The sodium iodide crystal captures the high-energy γ-ray photon and then immediately scintillates a lower-energy photon of visible wavelength. A set of photomultiplier tubes positioned next to the sodium iodide crystal increases the gain of the signal, which with appropriate computer enhancement then generates a visual depiction of the frequency distribution of the technetium tracer accumulation in tissues. Different collimators positioned between the patient and the sodium iodide crystal are available to modify the image. For

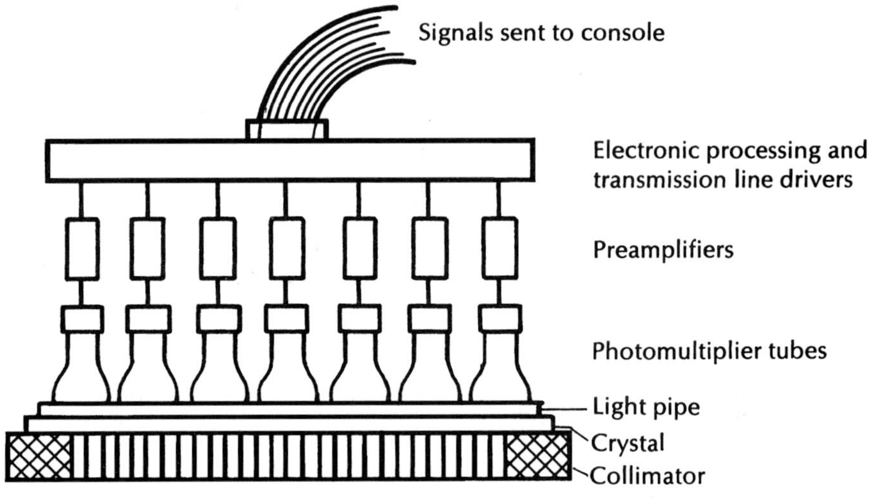

FIGURE 2.
Schematic representation of the components of a gamma camera. (From Rollo F (ed): *Nuclear Medicine, Physics, Instrumentation, and Agents.* St Louis, Mosby, 1977. Used by permission.)

most imaging of the musculoskeletal system, we currently use a low-energy, all-purpose (LEAP) collimator. On occasion, a pinhole collimator can be helpful in defining uptake in small osseous structures such as the carpal bones. Most current systems (at our institution we use a Siemens 750 S-ZLC gamma camera, Erlangen, Germany) depict the distribution of tracer activity as black dots on a clear background.

Until recently it was believed that the MDP moiety, with the technetium 99m attached, became incorporated together into the hydration shell surrounding living osseous cells.[13] Recent research, however, indicates that the technetium 99m and the MDP moiety may become dissociated in the osseous tissues with the technetium 99m component preferentially taken up by the organic phase of bone whereas the phosphorus of the MDP moiety is preferentially taken up in the inorganic phase of bone.[14] Tracer accumulation is a function of both the metabolic activity of living bone and blood flow to osseous tissues—the two factors being, of necessity, linked phenomena.[15] The whole-body radiation exposure resulting from a standard study using 20 mEq of ^{99m}Tc-MDP is about equal to that of a lumbosacral spine radiographic series. (Whole-body vs. spot imaging of musculoskeletal structures does not affect tissue radiation exposure in that the only variable is time near the gamma camera.)

Images of the musculoskeletal components captured immediately after the ^{99m}Tc-MPD aliquot is injected reflect the arterial supply of the examined region; this is termed the *blood flow*, or the first phase of a three-phase study. Images captured a few minutes later are believed to depict the relative vascularity of the examined region and are termed the *blood pool*, or the second phase.[13] The study used most frequently in assessing musculoskeletal trauma is termed the third phase and consists of *delayed static images* captured 2 to 3 hours after intravenous injection of the aliquot to allow for soft tissue clearance of the agent. These images primarily reflect the osseous metabolic activity of the musculoskeletal region of interest. However, soft tissue uptake of the ^{99m}Tc-MDP is possible on occasion in strained or damaged muscle and other inflamed tissues.[16, 17]

Single-photon emission computed tomography (SPECT) is a technique that allows greater specification of tracer accumulation by providing tomographic images that reflect tracer distribution.[18] Although this technique has many advocates,[19–22] I believe that it is most useful for imaging deep structures such as the spine[23] or pelvis rather than more peripheral musculoskeletal structures such as the knee,[24] wrist,[25] or ankle, where multiple high-resolution planar views are most often adequate in accurately depicting tracer distribution.

STANDARD USES OF TECHNETIUM SCINTIGRAPHY IN MUSCULOSKELETAL TRAUMA

The use of technetium scintigraphy to assess the possibility of osseous trauma and the subsequent response of damaged tissues has been recognized and accepted by the orthopedic and nuclear medicine communities for over two decades.[12, 13, 26–31] The majority of articles discussing stress fractures, for example, have used scintigraphic criteria (e.g., increased uptake on a technetium bone scan) as the method of detection rather than radiographic criteria.[29, 32–44] It is now well documented that the earliest stages of the spectrum of increased osseous remodeling termed a "stress fracture" are associated with normal radiographic findings. In the early phase of this phenomenon it is presumed that the repetitive submaximal loads placed across the involved osseous component induce greater osteoclastic than osteoblastic activity, thus resulting in increased bone turnover favoring bone loss. A significant amount of bone can be resorbed by such osteoclastic activity without detection by standard radiographs. Bone scans are capable of detecting this process *at least* 2 to 3 weeks before radiographic changes occur.[45] Only after extensive bone resorption has occurred will the structural integrity of the osseous components be sufficiently compromised to predispose toward overt fracture. This phenomenon has been documented histologically in an animal model[46] and in humans.[47]

Such an osseous stress reaction phenomenon, documented by increased scintigraphic uptake, is not rare and can occur in virtually any osseous structure under the appropriate excessive loading conditions. The classic stress fracture secondary to repetitive supraphysiologic loads of the lower extremities has been well documented in military recruits participating in sudden increases in physical activity. The most common sites tend to be the tibia, femur, and the metatarsals. This same phenomenon has been demonstrated in competitive athletes, particularly distance runners, whose patterns of uptake are similar to that documented in the military population[29, 32, 45, 48] (Fig 3). Detection of the early stages of a stress fracture is of clinical significance in order to alter the biomechanical environment and thus avert the development of an overt fracture. An early stress fracture, especially in the region of the femoral neck, that is allowed to evolve to an overt fracture and displacement can have serious clinical consequences.

In the foot, stress fractures secondary to overuse are most commonly found in the distal diaphysis of the second metatarsal. This fracture was so commonly seen in new military recruits secondary to forced ambulation that it has been termed a "march fracture." Any repetitive supraphysiologic loading activities sufficient to induce increased osseous remodeling can trigger the process.[44]

Stress fractures have also been documented in the fourth and fifth metatarsals. Other osseous components of the foot have been documented to manifest osseous stress phenomena, including the tarsal navicular, cuneiform, sesamoids, calcaneus, and talus.[44, 49–51] Healed stress fractures in bones with high cancellous bone content such as the calcaneus often ultimately manifest radiographically increased radiodensity (typically a sclerotic band).

In the ankle, stress fractures of the medial malleolus at the junction of the tibial plafond have been reported by Schils et al.,[52] primarily in patients participating in running and jumping activities. These authors emphasize a high index of suspicion and recommend obtaining a technetium bone scan in patients with persistent malleolar pain who have been involved in repetitive excessive loading activities. Stress fractures of the fibula are less common, with a recent report in the literature associated with the distal tibiofibular synostosis.[53]

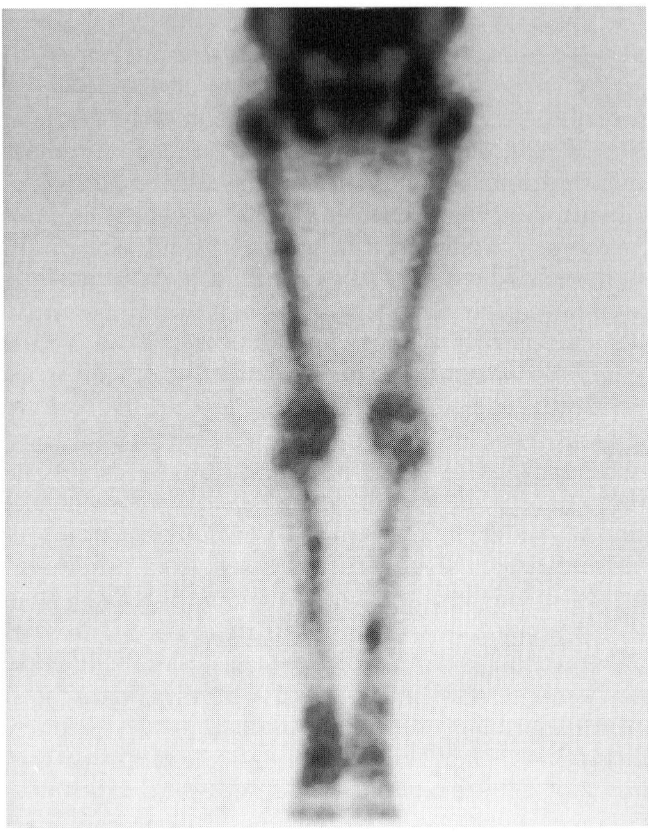

FIGURE 3.
Technetium scintiscan of a long-distance runner with multiple stress fractures of the tibiae and femora detected by increased tracer uptake.

Urman et al.[54] have emphasized the value of technetium scintigraphy in the evaluation of patients with chronic ankle pain for the possibility of occult talar dome fractures. In their series of 122 patients with ankle pain they found the bone scan to have a sensitivity of 0.96 and were able to establish the presence and location of occult osseous lesions of the talus. These authors recommend follow-up with a CT study in patients with a positive bone scan of the talar dome. If a negative bone scan is obtained, they interpret this finding as indicative of no active bony process, which obviates the need for further osseous imaging studies. They found a high number of patients (41%) with positive talar dome scans who also demonstrated multiple related sites of increased scintigraphic uptake such as the os trigonum, and distal end of the tibia, etc. This finding along with our knee research, to be presented later in this chapter, emphasizes the *mosaic* nature of musculoskeletal trauma. It is quite common that many different zones within a symptomatic joint may become metabolically active. The technetium bone scan sensitively manifests the increased osseous metabolic "tiles" of that mosaic.

The tibia has been reported to be the bone most commonly documented to manifest stress fracture phenomena. In one of the most extensive surveys of stress fractures of athletes, Matheson et al. report in a study of 320 bone scan–positive cases that the tibia was by far the most common site of involvement at 49% (157/320).[55] They note that the technetium bone scan is the "single most useful diagnostic aid in making the diagnosis of a stress fracture." In a similar study documenting the location of stress fractures in athletes, Ha et al. note that the tibia was involved more than twice as frequently as the second most involved bone, the femur.[38] The most common sites of involvement in the tibia are the medial midshaft area and the medial proximal portion of the metaphysis. Clement reports that in his experience middle-distance runners were the most commonly involved group manifesting tibial stress phenomena.[56]

About the knee, the inferior pole of the patella has been frequently documented to manifest overt stress fractures.[39, 42, 57, 58] This anatomic region is subjected to the highest loads of any component in the knee,[2] which may account for its predisposition to scintigraphically detectable osseous symptoms.

Stress fractures of the femur are common phenomena, especially in runners.[33, 37, 40, 59] The diaphysis is the anatomic area most often involved,[60] followed by the lesser trochanter, intertrochanteric region, and femoral neck. Early detection of the process leading to impending structural failure of the femoral neck is imperative. Fullerton and Snowdy emphasize the high likelihood of progression to structural failure of a tension side (superior neck) stress fracture of the femoral neck.[37]

Stress fractures have been documented in and about the pelvis and involving the anterior iliac crest,[61] iliac apophysis,[34] and the ischium.[62] Technetium scintigraphy is also well suited for the early detection of osteitis pubis in athletes.[63] Single-photon emission CT has successfully demonstrated stress fractures of the pars interarticularis of the lumbar vertebrae.[25, 64]

Technetium scintigraphy is also well accepted in the detection of occult osseous trauma in the upper extremity, particularly in the region of the hand and wrist[24, 65–69] (Fig 4). High-resolution planar technetium bone scans can sensitively manifest occult fractures of all of the osseous structures, including the scaphoid,[70–73] pisiform, and metacarpals,[74] as well as lunate avascular necrosis[65] and precise localization of regions of active degenerative joint disease.[24] The combination of a screening scintigraphic study followed by high-resolution CT in cases with a positive bone scan has been reported as a highly effective diagnostic algorithm in assessing a painful wrist.[69, 73]

Other traditional uses for technetium scintigraphy in the setting of musculoskeletal trauma involve the diagnosis of Osgood-Schlatter disease,[75] osteochondral fractures,[76] osteolysis,[75] and osteonecrosis.[77]

REFLEX SYMPATHETIC DYSTROPHY

In some individuals the normal osseous homeostatic control mechanisms are so significantly altered that intense osteoclastic activity is stimulated

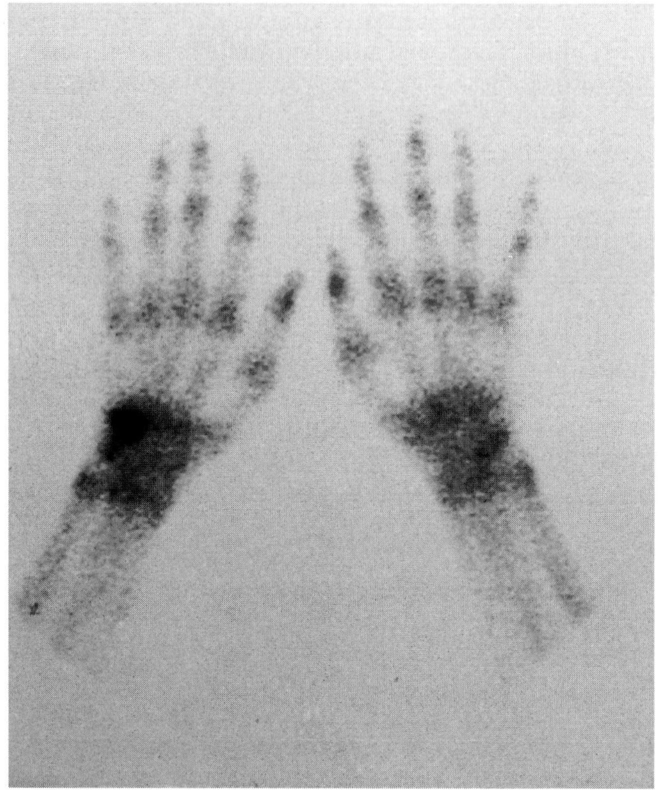

FIGURE 4.
Technetium scintiscan of a patient with occult osseous injury to the hamate of the left carpus.

without an effective compensatory osteoblastic response. In a small subset of susceptible patients, persistent nociceptive factors combine to induce a spectrum of intense osteoclastic activity that when unchecked, is manifested radiographically as Sudeck's atrophy and clinically as reflex sympathetic dystrophy. The technetium bone scan patterns in these patients typically manifest intense periarticular uptake in all three phases[68, 78, 79] (Fig 5). At present there is poor understanding of the factors that initiate, sustain, and resolve the intense osteoclastic remodeling seen in patients with reflex sympathetic dystrophy. Some patients with more localized intense periarticular scintigraphic activity following slight trauma may well represent a milder variant of reflex sympathetic dystrophy—a so-called mini–reflex sympathetic dystrophy.[3]

SOFT TISSUE UPTAKE

The uptake of ^{99m}Tc-MDP is not always exclusively in living osseous tissues; it has also occasionally been documented in physiologically overstressed or inflamed soft tissues, notably muscle and synovium.[17, 80–83] For example, leg muscles of long-distance runners have manifested increased uptake on technetium scintigraphy.[16] Teres major uptake has

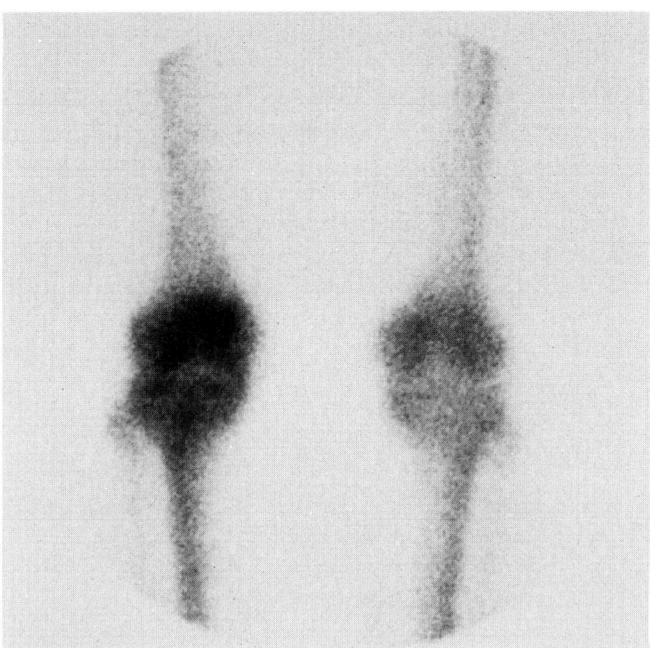

FIGURE 5.
Technetium scintiscan of a patient with active reflex sympathetic dystrophy and intense three-compartment uptake in the right knee.

been shown as well in a weight lifter.[19] We have documented increased uptake in the synovium of patients with chronic inflammation of the knee joint, although many patients with active synovitis do not demonstrate abnormal uptake in the synovial soft tissues. We have also seen increased uptake in contusion of soft tissues about the knee (Fig 6).

Patients with "shin splints," that is, lower leg pain associated with muscle tearing and periosteal inflammation rather than a primary bone process, may also demonstrate soft tissue uptake in a fusiform pattern, particularly in the posteromedial region of the tibia.[28, 84, 85] So-called arm splints have also been documented scintigraphically in a volleyball player.[86]

The phenomenon of soft tissue technetium uptake is but a limited manifestation of the fact that alterations in the metabolic activity of soft tissue are common phenomena in musculoskeletal trauma. In the future the process of soft tissue damage and repair may be more accurately documented for research and possible treatment purposes. Perhaps the best candidate for such a modality is positron emission tomography,[87, 88] another advanced scintigraphic technology that has not yet been used widely in orthopaedic research. It is clear that there are differential rates of injury and repair of the myriad musculoskeletal tissues involved in sports-type trauma. It is the summation of all of these processes plus other factors (e.g., restoration of cerebellar-proprioceptive mechanisms) that determines the ultimate functional capacity of perturbed musculoskeletal systems.

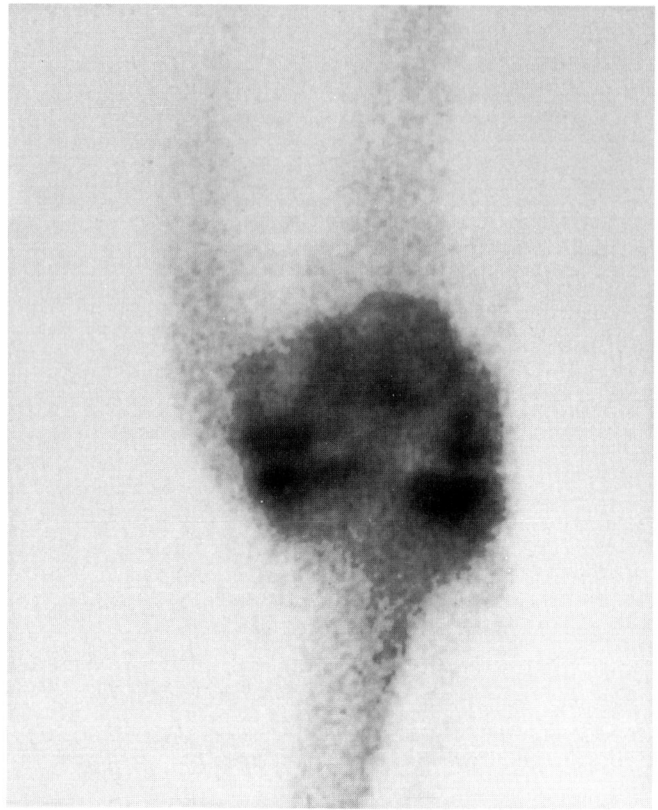

FIGURE 6.
Technetium scintiscan of a patient with medial soft tissue injury of the left knee and distal portion of the thigh manifested as increased medial soft tissue uptake. This patient also has increased medial and lateral compartment uptake associated with meniscal tears.

NONTRADITIONAL USES OF BONE SCINTIGRAPHY

ANTERIOR KNEE PAIN

The first nontraditional clinical area in which standard scintigraphic techniques were used was in the assessment of patients with anterior knee pain. This large subset of patients remains a significant clinical challenge to the orthopaedic community, in large part because there is often a lack of objectively identifiable structural pathology to account for the presence and persistence of symptoms. In an earlier era, chondromalacia was thought to be so commonly associated with complaints of anterior knee pain that it was the accepted clinical diagnostic term to describe such patients.[89–91] It is now well documented that many patients with anterior knee pain have grossly normal articular cartilage.[3, 90, 92, 93] I have also seen patients with extensive chondromalacia of the patella without anterior knee symptoms. During this past decade varying degrees of "malalignment" have been considered to be of prime etiologic significance in the genesis of most anterior knee pain.[94–102] The experience of our clinical research group at Letterman Army Medical Center in San Francisco led us to a different conclusion regarding the significance of objectively identifiable malalignment in the genesis of anterior knee pain in the majority of patients seen for the first time. In a study performed in the early 1980s our group examined and compared a large number of patients with anterior knee symptoms with a large group of controls.[103] Several objectively identifiable factors of malalignment, including many radiologic parameters obtained from views described by both Merchant[104] and Laurin[104a] and their colleagues, were documented in this study. All patients received a ^{99m}Tc-MDP bone scan in addition to the standard history, physical examination, and radiographic assessment. Patients were excluded if they had evidence of fracture, osteophytes, osteopenia, or a history of prior knee surgery. We found no statistical difference in the presence of objective malalignment characteristics between our control and symptomatic population, including Q angle, Insall-Salvati index, patellar facet sclerosis, congruence angle, and the measurements from Laurin views.[104a] However, 49% of the patients with symptomatic anterior knee pain had abnormal scintigraphic uptake in the patella as compared with only 4% of our controls ($P < .001$) (Fig 7). We also developed a sensitive quantitative method of assessing patellar scintigraphic activity that confirmed our qualitative evaluations.[105] At that time, a significant report in the literature indicated that technetium bone scans are most often normal in patients with anterior knee pain, except in the presence of radiographic changes (e.g., fracture, osteophytes, or osteopenia).[106] Our data indicated just the opposite—that increased patellar scintigraphic findings are common in patients with anterior knee pain even in the pres-

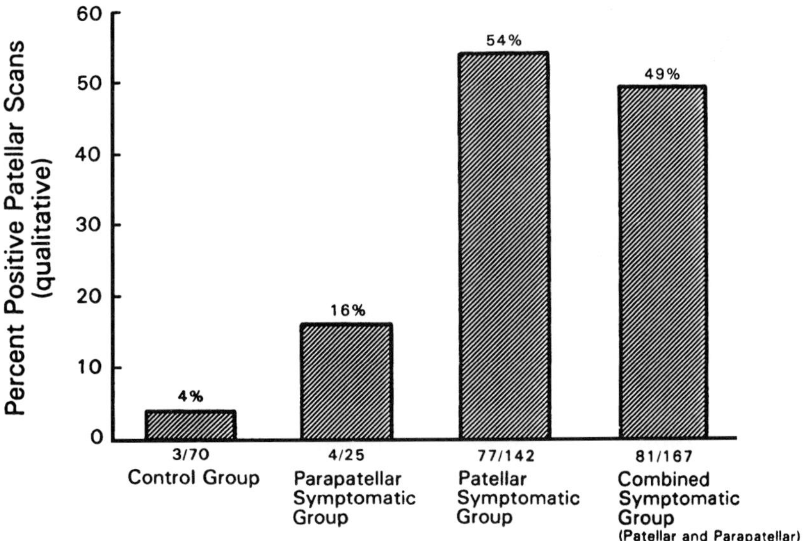

FIGURE 7.

Bar graph depicting the percentage of qualitatively positive patellar bone scan in patients with anterior knee pain by clinical group. Forty-nine percent of the symptomatic patients manifested abnormal patellar uptake vs. only 4% of the controls. (From Dye SF, Boll DA: *Orthop Clin North Am* 17:255, 1986. Used by permission.)

ence of *normal* radiographic findings. Similar scintigraphic findings have now been documented by other researchers with an interest in the patellofemoral joint.[107–111] The results of our initial study profoundly changed my conceptualization of the knee (and other joints). I came to view human joints not as mere collections of macrostructures, but as assemblages of billions of living cells with unseen mechanisms of homeostasis. Technetium scintigraphy thus provided a sensitive "window" to view the underlying physiologic characteristics of living bone.

After documenting that nearly half of a large number of patients with anterior knee pain and normal radiographs manifested increased scintigraphic uptake in the patella, we were curious as to the clinical outcomes after treatment. Therapy included restricting any excessive loading activities, muscle strengthening, hamstring stretching, daily icing, and anti-inflammatory medication. The fates of these patients on follow-up scans within 18 months revealed essentially five scintigraphic patterns. Those patients with initially normal uptake had the highest percentage of subjective recovery with conservative treatment. There were two positive bone scan patterns that were associated with resolution of symptoms and scan activity: diffuse patellar activity (Fig 8, A and B) and focal patellar activity excluding the inferior pole (Fig 9, A and B).[112] We also identified two positive bone scan patterns of the patella with poor clinical outcomes that predicted persistence of symptoms and scan activity: trochlear and patellar activity and focal inferior pole patellar activity[113] (Fig 9, C and D). It was subsequently noted that patients with persistent inferior patellar pole activity responded well to early surgical intervention, i.e., drilling the inferior pole. Based on this and subsequent work, I now believe that the majority of patients with anterior knee pain do not initially manifest overt malalignment and that the genesis of pain is a function of repetitive supraphysiologic loading of the often anatomically normal patellofemoral components.[114] Vastus medialis obliquus atrophy, when present, may well represent a secondary phenomenon caused by the persistence of pain. The reports of high percentages of malalignment factors in the literature may be due in part to evaluation of highly selected and therefore statistically skewed populations of patients who failed treatment.

Having discovered that a large number of patients with anterior knee pain had increased uptake on technetium scintigraphy in the face of normal radiographs, we were interested in discovering the actual osseous process manifested by these abnormal scans. The concept was widely held at the time that a technetium bone scan was so nonspecific as to be essentially useless (except in the standard cases covered earlier in this chapter) because multiple stimuli are capable of triggering remodeling of bone, including infection[115] and tumors.[116] We therefore decided to de-

FIGURE 8.

A, technetium scintiscan of a patient with anterior knee pain showing diffuse patellar uptake. **B,** a technetium scintiscan of the same patient 4 months later following resolution of symptoms with a conservative treatment program shows complete resolution of abnormal patellar activity.

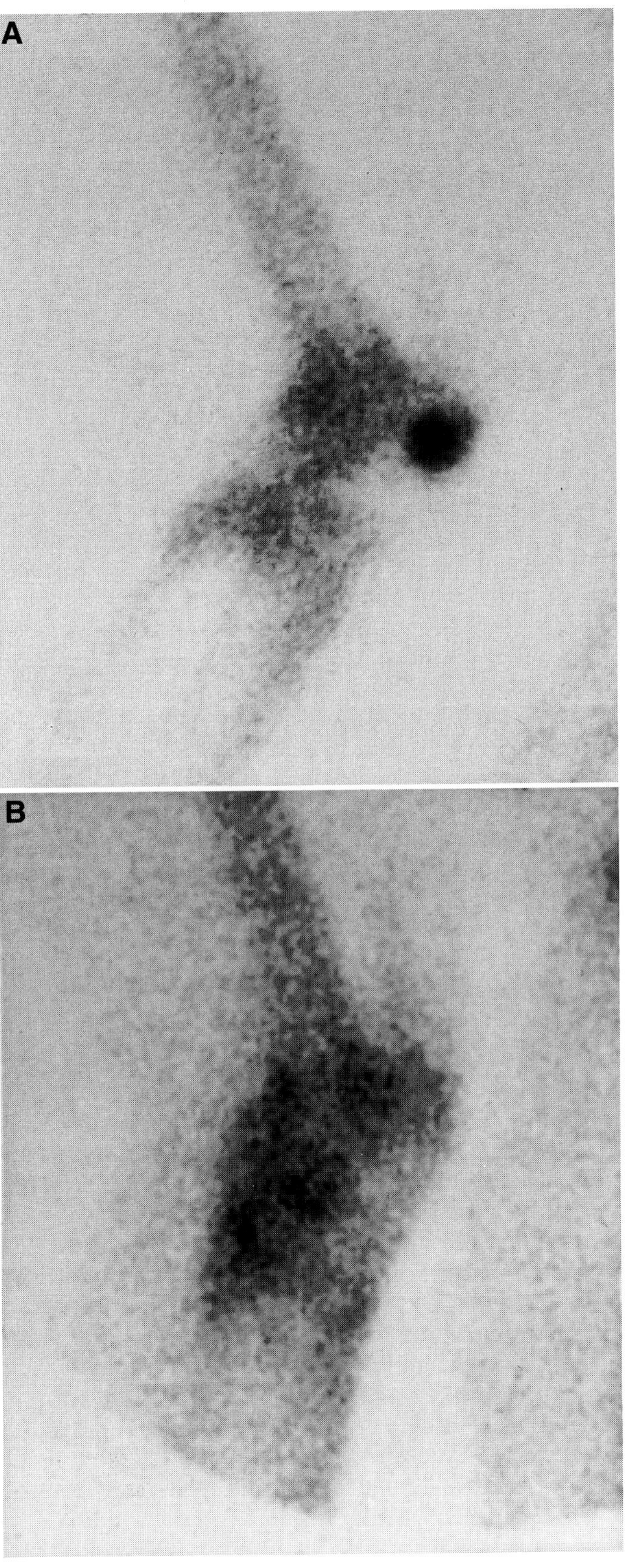
A
B

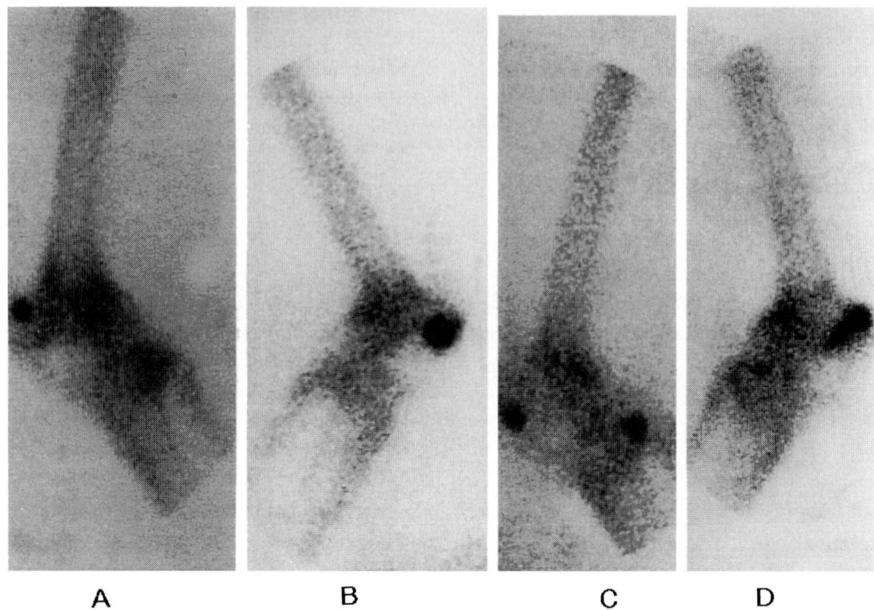

FIGURE 9.
Technetium scintiscans of increased patellar activity. **A,** the focal pattern, which is associated with likely resolution of symptoms. **B,** the diffuse pattern, which is associated with likely resolution of symptoms. **C,** the focal inferior pole pattern, which is associated with persistence of symptoms. **D,** the trochlear-patellar pattern, which is associated with persistence of symptoms. (From Dye SF, Chew MH: *J Bone Joint Surg Am* 75:1400, 1993. Used by permission.)

lineate the actual osseous pathology manifested in our patients with anterior knee pain and a positive bone scan.[117] We obtained small patellar core biopsy specimens with the patient's permission (and clearance through the research committee) in 17 cases. These results were compared with those of age-matched control cadaver patellas. No control patellas manifested regions of identifiable active osteoclastic or active osteoblastic activity. We found only normal-appearing, rather thin interior trabeculae and normal tide mark zones in the subchondral region (Fig 10, A). In all of the patellar biopsy specimens from regions of increased scintigraphic uptake in the patients with anterior knee pain we found regions of increased bone turnover (vs. controls), with increased numbers of reversal lines on polarized light and thickened trabeculae in some areas (Fig 10, B) and active osteoclastic activity (Fig 10, C) and regions of primitive woven bone in others. We did not find evidence of infection or tumor in any of the 17 cases. In none of the patients was there an abnormal white blood cell count or increased sedimentation rate. We therefore concluded that a positive bone scan in these patients denoted a spectrum of increased osseous metabolic activity without infection or tumor. The persistence of recurrent patterns of subchondral activity in patients with anterior knee pain and in most patients with meniscal and ACL pathology allows one to easily recognize patterns that are different, such as the intensive pancondylar periarticular activity associated with reflex sympathetic dystrophy, infection, or tumor.

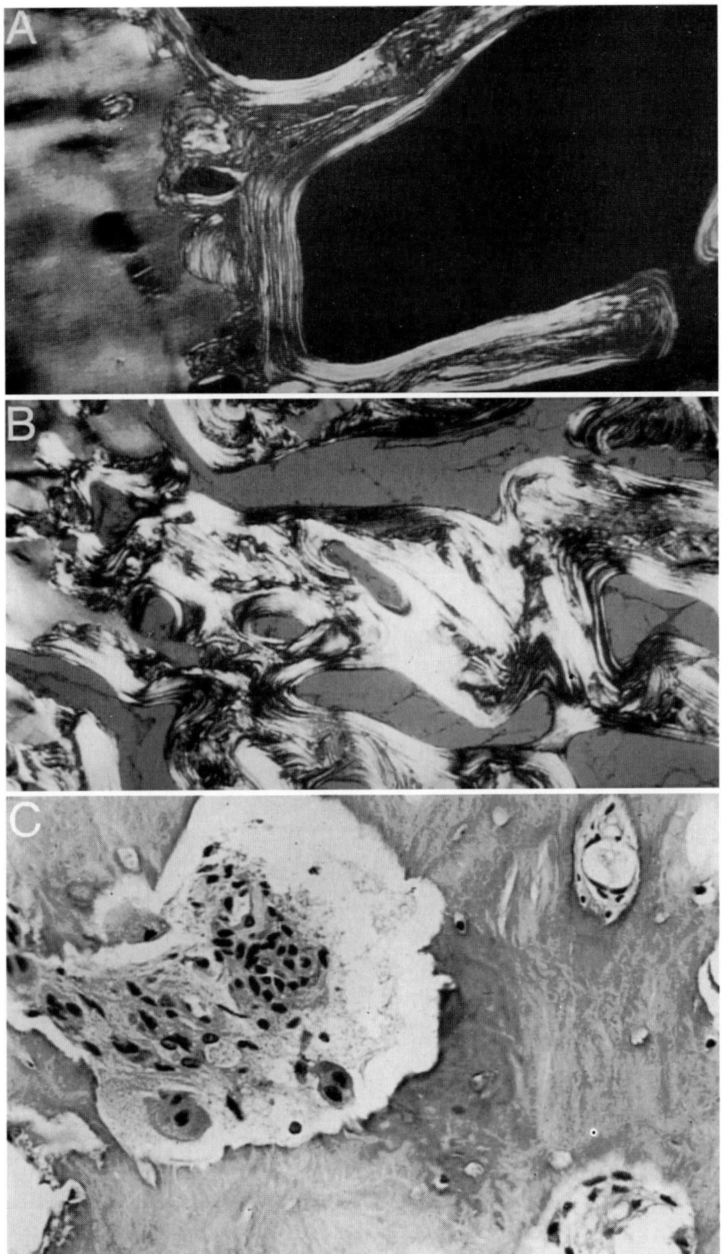

FIGURE 10.

Histologic section of the subchondral region of a normal patella showing trabeculae and regular lamellations with polarized light (hematoxylin-eosin, ×250). **B,** histologic section of the subchondral region of a symptomatic patella with increased scintigraphic activity, thickened trabeculae, an increased number of reversal lines, and a whorled lamellar pattern on polarized light (hematoxylin-eosin, ×250). **C,** histologic section of a symptomatic patella with increased scintigraphic activity and a Howship lacuna (hematoxylin-eosin, ×350). (**A** and **B,** from Dye SF: Radionuclide imaging of the knee, in Aichroth P, Cannon WD (eds): *Knee Surgery, Current Practice*. London, Martin Dunitz, 1992, p 41; **C,** from Dye SF, Chew MH: *J Bone Joint Surg Am* 75:1395, 1993. All used by permission.)

ETIOLOGY OF INCREASED OSSEOUS METABOLIC ACTIVITY

Having established that patients with anterior knee pain and a positive bone scan manifest histologic evidence of increased bone remodeling and turnover, we were interested in determining the factors that are significant in the genesis of this process. There are three clinical areas well understood by both orthopaedists and nuclear medicine physicians that we believe are of importance.

Mechanical Bone Overload

Mechanical bone overload, either through a single event such as an acute fracture or through repetitive supraphysiologic loading, as is manifested in the early phases of a stress fracture, can induce increased remodeling detectable scintigraphically. Many patients with anterior knee pain reported high levels of supraphysiologic loading of the type that could induce increased bone remodeling. We also believe that the pathokinematics associated with soft tissue disruptions, such as a meniscus tear or ACL insufficiency, can also induce supraphysiologic loading of osseous tissues sufficient to induce increased osseous metabolic activity. McBride et al.[118] in an animal model has shown that scintigraphically detectable increased periarticular osseous turnover is induced following section of the ACL long before radiographic changes of post-traumatic degenerative arthritis occur.

Neurovascular Factors

Neurovascular disturbances of bone can also induce increased remodeling as exemplified by the often intense osteoclastic activity associated with reflex sympathetic dystrophy.[68, 98, 119, 146] The factors that control the neurovascular component of osseous homeostasis are not understood, but it is my belief that some of our patients with anterior knee pain and associated intense remodeling of the patella following a mild or moderate retinacular strain represent a process mentioned previously, namely, a localized "mini–reflex sympathetic dystrophy" process.[3]

Humoral Factors

Systemic or local humoral factors have also been known to be capable of inducing scintigraphically detectable increased osseous metabolic activity.[120–124] High circulating levels of parathyroid hormone, for example, are quite capable of inducing osteoclastic activity throughout the skeleton.[125,126] Increased osseous metabolic activity was diagnosed in such an individual with high circulating parathyroid hormone levels only after an overt fracture of the inferior pole of the patella during sports activity.[57] It is clear that regions of high bone stresses, such as found at the inferior pole of the patella, are sites where increased levels of certain hormones and cytokines can be first manifested as a result of the combined effect of the local humoral and biomechanical environment.

Klein and Raisz have documented that prostaglandin E is a potent stimulator of osteoclastic activation and bone resorption.[127] It is likely that the powerful action of cytokines produced secondary to either soft tissue or osseous injury is a process common to most factors inducing increased bone remodeling.[128] Prostaglandins and other cytokines released from soft tissue or osteocyte injury can thus induce a biological cascade resulting in increased osseous remodeling.

THEORETICAL MODEL OF OSSEOUS HOMEOSTASIS

Synthesizing all available data, Chew and I have developed a theoretical model of osseous homeostasis (Fig 11) that takes into account multiple potential triggers of increased osseous metabolic activity as well as possible remodeling effects.[23] If the induced increased bone remodeling results in equal turnover and the process eventually returns to homeostasis, there will be no net change of bone morphology in the involved osseous structure. However, if there is a net increase in bone resorption secondary to the induced increased osteoclastic activity such as seen with reflex sympathetic dystrophy (e.g., Sudeck's atrophy) and osteolysis, the process may still come to eventual homeostasis, with stable osteopenia manifested radiographically. If net bone formation is triggered, as manifested by active osteophyte production or osteosclerosis, the region may also come to homeostasis ultimately identifiable by a normal bone scan, but the region would retain the structural change, e.g., a dormant osteophyte. Living osseous tissues are complex physiologic systems, and regions of net bone resorption, formation, and equal turnover can exist within different zones of a symptomatic joint. We believe that this theoretical model of osseous homeostasis explains the variety of scintigraphic and radiographic findings in patients with musculoskeletal trauma.

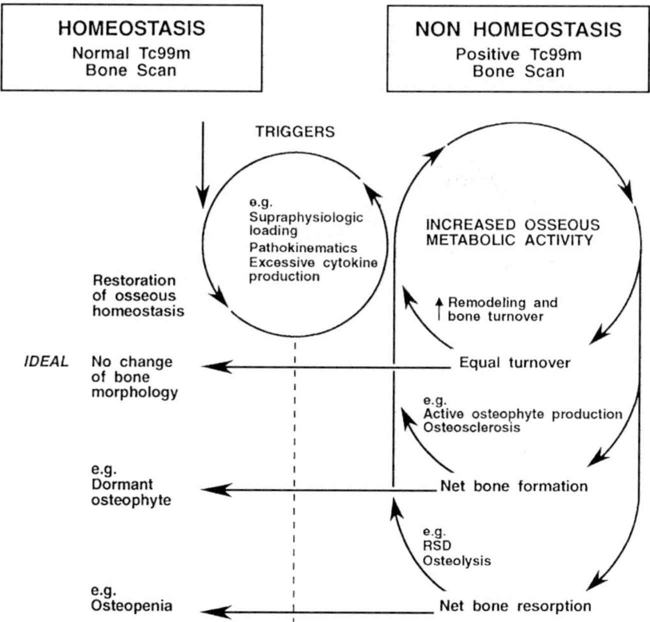

FIGURE 11.

Theoretical model of osseous homeostasis with multiple triggers inducing increased remodeling activity detectable by technetium scintigraphy. The increased osseous metabolic activity can continue for an indefinite period because of the effects of recurrent triggers. If bone turnover is equal, no change in bone morphology occurs; if osteoclastic activity predominates, osteopenia can develop; and if osteoblastic activity predominates, osteosclerosis and osteophytes can develop. Restoration of osseous homeostasis, documentable by normal findings on a technetium scan, is possible with or without osseous morphologic changes. *RSD* = reflex sympathetic dystrophy. (From Dye SF, Chew MH: *J Bone Joint Surg Am* 75:1398, 1993. Used by permission.)

NONTRADITIONAL USES OF SCINTIGRAPHY: MENISCUS TEARS

Many traumatic conditions previously thought to be limited to structural failure of soft tissue are frequently associated with increased osseous metabolic activity of periarticular bone. One of the most common diagnoses of injuries about the knee—a torn meniscus—has now been well documented to have an associated increased metabolic activity of subchondral tibial and femoral osseous tissues. As early as 1983, Marymont et al.[129] noted the common finding of a positive bone scan of the involved knee compartment with a proven symptomatic meniscal tear. Our research group[23, 130–132] along with Bauer et al.,[133] Mooar et al.,[134] Lohmann et al.,[135] and Rockett[136] have also shown that metabolically activated perimeniscal bone is the *expected norm* in patients with symptomatic torn menisci, even though the radiographic appearance of the knee is found to be normal. This increased osseous metabolic activity of periarticular bone in patients with meniscal tears can and frequently does occur even in the presence of a normal osseous signal on MRI. Research performed by our group in San Francisco[137] comparing MRI osseous signal changes with technetium bone scan findings in patients with a variety of types of structural failure of soft tissue about the knee documented that MRI as currently used is *insensitive* in detecting the process of increased osseous metabolic activity of bone. (Soft tissue diagnoses are those including meniscal tears, chondromalacia, and ACL tears.) In this group of 53 patients, MRI indicated bony change of any type in only 22% as compared with 86% with technetium bone scintigraphy. Meyers and Wintch have reported similar findings of insensitivity of MRI in the detection of osseous processes.[138]

This work starkly proves the principle that MRI, contrary to popular belief, is not an omniscient or pathognomonic technique but is, in fact, rather insensitive to the process of metabolically active bone remodeling.

Regions of metabolically activated bone manifested by technetium scintigraphy in patients with meniscal tears are not necessarily exclusive to the involved compartment and are often abnormal in areas of the knee without overt structural failure of soft tissue. The often widespread abnormal osseous metabolic activity in such patients reflects, in my opinion, the resultant pathokinematic and pathophysiologic factors secondary to the torn meniscus (Fig 12, A). One of the most interesting phenomena regarding the use of scintigraphy in patients with meniscal tears is the dynamic character of the increased osseous metabolic activity in these patients following surgical treatment. Our research team has demonstrated that in a group of 34 patients with documented meniscal pathology, 82% (28/34) manifested abnormal increased activity before surgery.[137] On follow-up examination within 18 months, 62% (21/34)

FIGURE 12.

A, technetium scintiscan of a patient with a large bucket-handle tear of the lateral meniscus. Note the three-compartment uptake despite normal structural findings of the medial and patellofemoral compartments. **B,** technetium scintiscan of the same patient 23 months following arthroscopic repair of the lateral meniscus tear. Resolution of abnormal scintigraphic activity is nearly complete. (From Dye SF, Chew MH: *J Bone Joint Surg Am* 75:1391, 1993. Used by permission.)

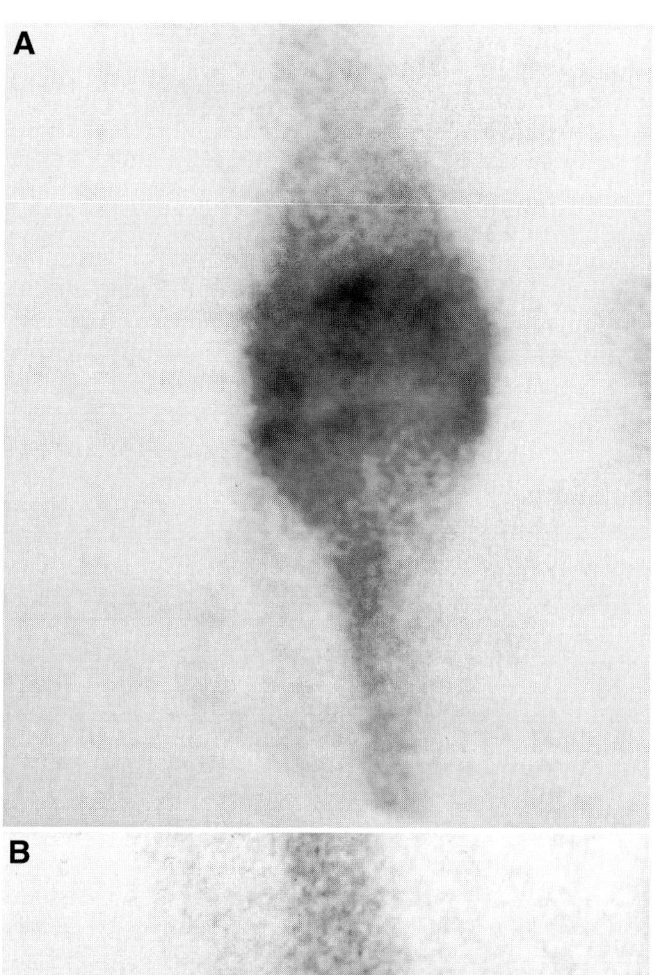
A

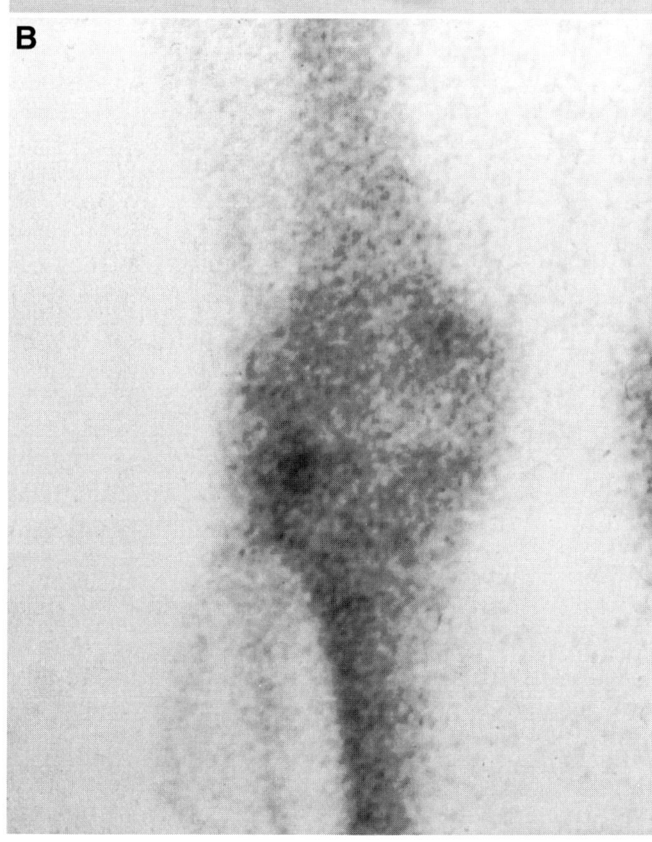
B

showed resolution or significant improvement of abnormal scintigraphic activity, with radiographically identifiable degenerative Fairbank[139] changes occurring in only 5% (1/20) of these patients (Fig 12, B).

Of the 14 patients whose postoperative bone scans remained positive or worsened, early Fairbank changes developed in 42% (6/14) (Fig 13, A to D). Thus, the persistence of increased osseous metabolic activity documented by a continued positive postoperative bone scan was predictive of early overt radiographically identifiable degenerative changes. This compelling finding has been supported by the independent work of Dieppe et al., who concluded that a positive technetium bone scan was a "powerful predictor" of progression of radiographically identifiable degenerative changes in patients with established early osteoarthritis.[140–142] Thomas et al.[143] and Egund et al.[144] indicate that scintigraphy is a sensitive method of detecting early degenerative joint disease. Thus,

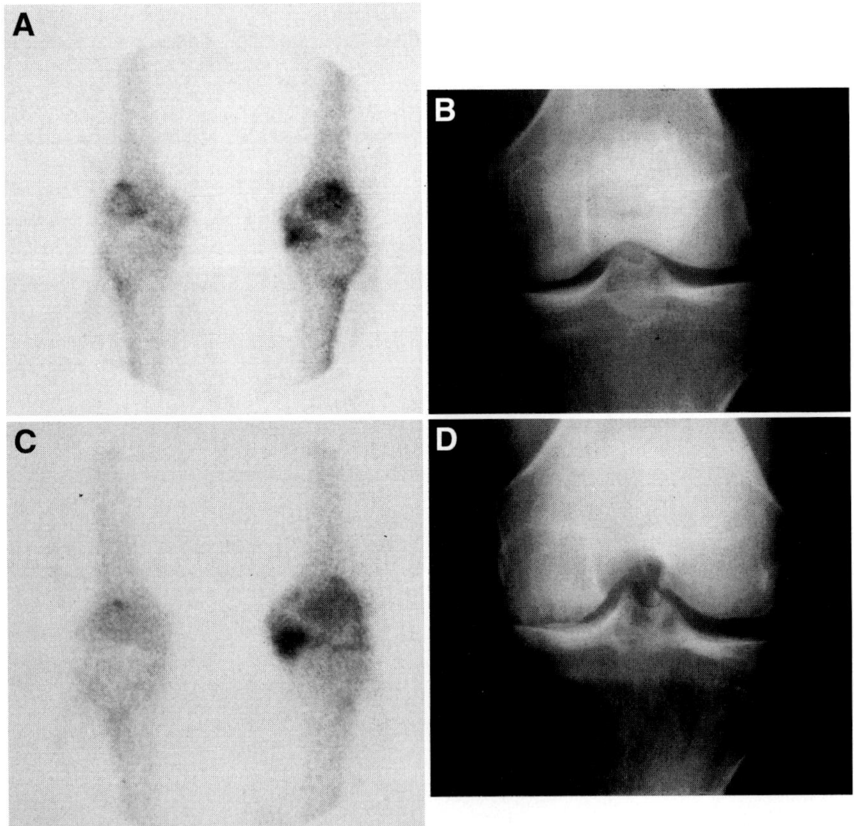

FIGURE 13.

A, scintiscan of a heavyset patient with an extensive tear of the left medial meniscus and significantly increased medial compartment uptake of the left knee. **B,** radiograph of the left knee of the same patient before surgery showing no degenerative changes at a time when the medial compartment manifested significantly increased activity. **C,** technetium scintiscan of the patient 15 months after arthroscopic partial meniscectomy with increasing abnormal uptake of the left medial compartment. **D,** radiograph of the left knee of the patient 15 months postsurgery showing structural Fairbank changes of the medial compartment.

scintigraphy has the capability of identifying that subset of knee patients who are "at risk" of early degenerative changes at a time when the radiographic findings are still normal, as well as those patients whose established degenerative changes will progress. The micro-osseous events that lead to overt degenerative structural changes, e.g., osteophytes, osteosclerosis, etc., can be manifested by scintigraphy at a time when that process may still be reversible to homeostasis. This evidence tends to strongly support the concept of Radin regarding the importance of osseous events in the etiology of early degenerative arthrosis of joints.[145–147]

SCINTIGRAPHIC FINDINGS IN ANTERIOR CRUCIATE LIGAMENT–DEFICIENT KNEES

Scintigraphic findings similar to those patients with meniscal tears have now been well documented in ACL-deficient knees. In 1987 we documented that the majority (46/61) of a group of patients with symptomatic chronic ACL-deficient knees manifested increased osseous metabolic activity.[131] Similar scintigraphic findings have also been documented in ACL-deficient patients by Dorchak et al.[141] I believe that these regions of dynamic bone stress in the *chronic ACL-deficient* population reflect the persistent pathokinematics of the involved regions of the knee. The patterns of increased uptake in chronically ACL-deficient patients show a higher percentage in the medial compartment as compared with the lateral compartment. This finding contrasts to the work of Vellet et al., who found a higher percentage of lateral compartment activity by MRI and bone scan evaluation in *acute* ACL injuries.[76] I believe that the reason for these differences is that the initial osseous injury (bone infraction/contusion/edema) shown on MRI and easily manifested as well scintigraphically[148] (Fig 14, A and B) is an area of acute bone overload of the lateral compartment secondary to sudden, dramatic, and ephemeral anterolateral subluxation of the acute injury. Such contusion zones frequently heal given time. Whereas the increased frequency of medial compartment scintigraphic uptake in *chronically* ACL-deficient patients reflects the inability of this more normally constrained region of the knee to accept pathologic increases in translation as compared with the lateral compartment, the higher rate of medial meniscal tears vs. lateral tears in chronically ACL-deficient patients also reflects this underlying pathokinematic reality. By contrast, the lateral compartment is designed for greater mobility and can therefore more easily absorb subtle residual pathologic increases in motion secondary to chronic ACL deficiency with less tendency to activate abnormal osseous metabolic activity.

In landmark studies directed by Daniel (developer of the KT-1000 laxity tester), surgically reconstructed ACL-deficient patients were shown by radiography and technetium scintigraphy to be at risk of postoperative degenerative changes developing even if static laxity parameters were restored to normal limits.[7, 8] The current standard of ACL reconstructive surgery—laxity equal to the uninjured knee—may not represent the singular ideal method of determining success. Some patients, as shown in Daniel's work, manifest active progression of degenerative changes despite restoration of normal laxity parameters. Therefore, restoration of

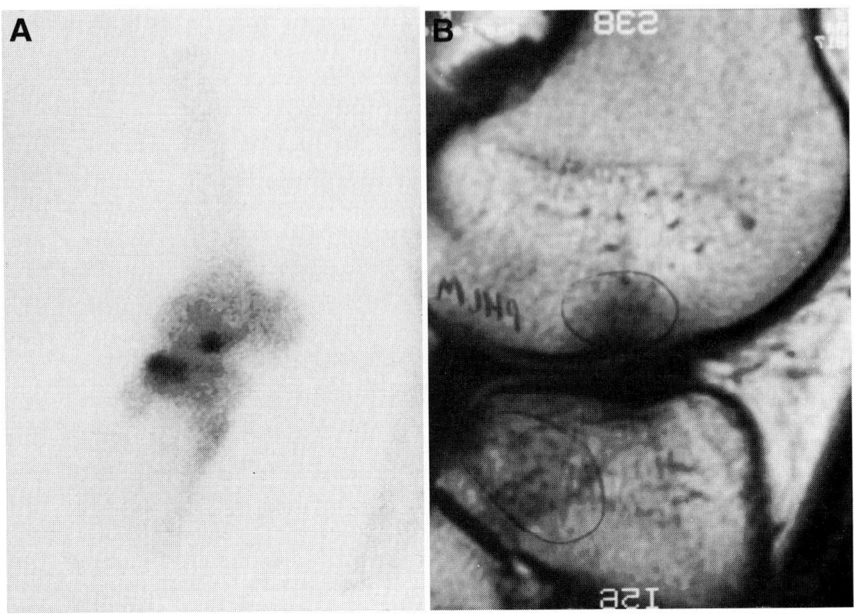

FIGURE 14.
A, technetium scintiscan of a patient with an acute anterior cruciate ligament rupture demonstrating increased uptake of the lateral femoral condyle and the posterior lateral tibial plateau. **B,** MRI of the patient with an acute anterior cruciate ligament rupture showing bone contusions matching the sites detected in the scintiscan.

normal measurable biomechanical properties does not necessarily prove that the functional *load acceptance capacity* of the knee has been fully restored. Currently, technetium scintigraphy provides the most sensitive view of the overall physiologic status of the knee as a complex living biomechanical transmission system.[23] I believe that our goals of treatment should be not only restoration of normal laxity parameters but also restoration of homeostasis. We have shown that restoration of osseous homeostasis is possible following ACL reconstructive surgery[131] (Fig 15). Main et al. have also documented significant improvement in postoperative scintigraphic activity in ACL-reconstructed patients.[149] Kaplan and Clancy[150] and Bergfeld (personal communication, 1992) have discovered persistent abnormal scintigraphic patterns in patients with chronic posterior cruciate ligament instability in the face of normal radiographs.

SCINTIGRAPHY OF JOINTS OTHER THAN THE KNEE

We have now noted that increased post-traumatic periarticular osseous metabolic activity is also commonly associated with joints other than the knee in the face of normal radiographic findings. For example, we currently have a series of 21 patients with normal radiographs and persistent ankle pain in all of whom "ankle sprains" have been diagnosed. *All* of these patients have manifested increased periarticular scintigraphic uptake on technetium scintiscans. These patients' symptoms and abnormal scan results are slow to resolve, taking an average of 8 to 9 months. This

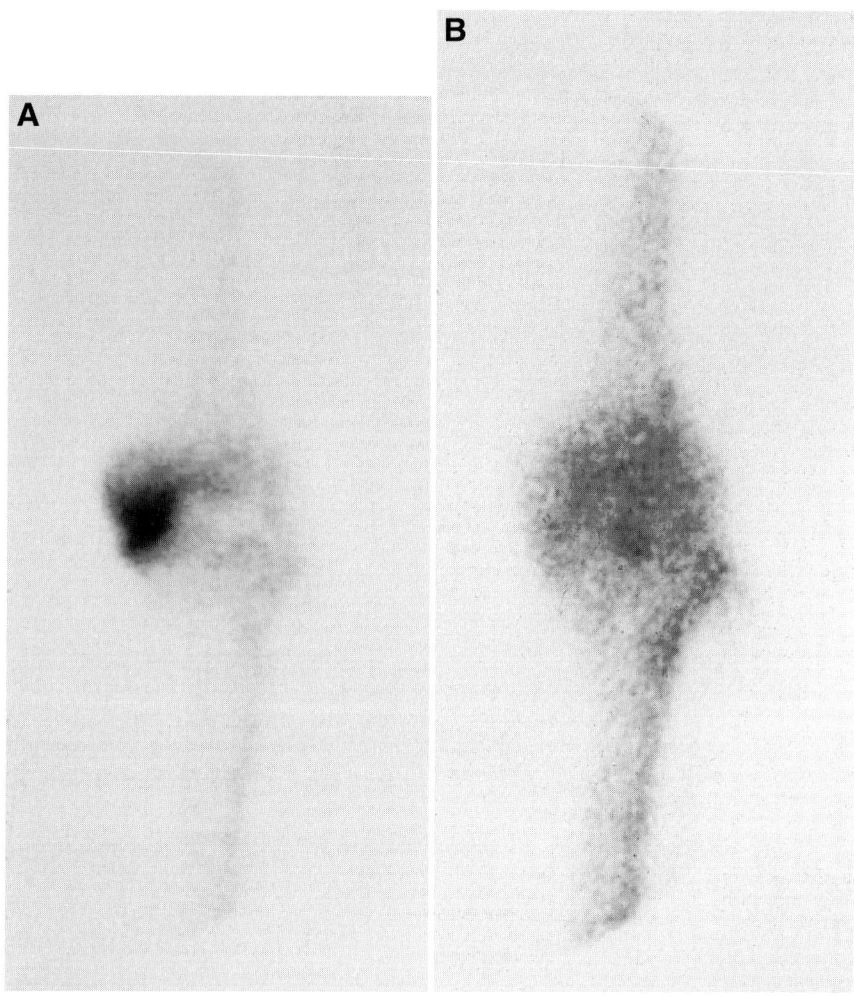

FIGURE 15.

A, technetium scintiscan of a patient with chronic anterior cruciate ligament deficiency of the left knee showing medial compartment uptake. **B,** a technetium scintiscan of the anterior cruciate ligament–deficient patient 21 months after anterior cruciate ligament reconstruction using the central third of the patellar tendon demonstrates essential restoration of osseous homeostasis. (From Dye SF: *Am J Sports Med* 21:748–750, 1993. Used by permission.)

finding is similar to our experience with patients with patellofemoral pain. The occult osseous involvement in patients with chronic ankle symptoms manifested by scintigraphic methods also once again indicates the *mosaic* nature of periarticular musculoskeletal trauma (Fig 16). Perhaps those with an interest in orthopedic foot and ankle research should consider the addition of scintigraphic data in future clinical reports. I believe that the same micro-osseous processes are common to all mammalian joint systems and proven restoration of osseous homeostasis would be a commendable treatment goal for all joints.

The acromioclavicular joint has now also been documented to manifest increased osseous metabolic activity in symptomatic patients with

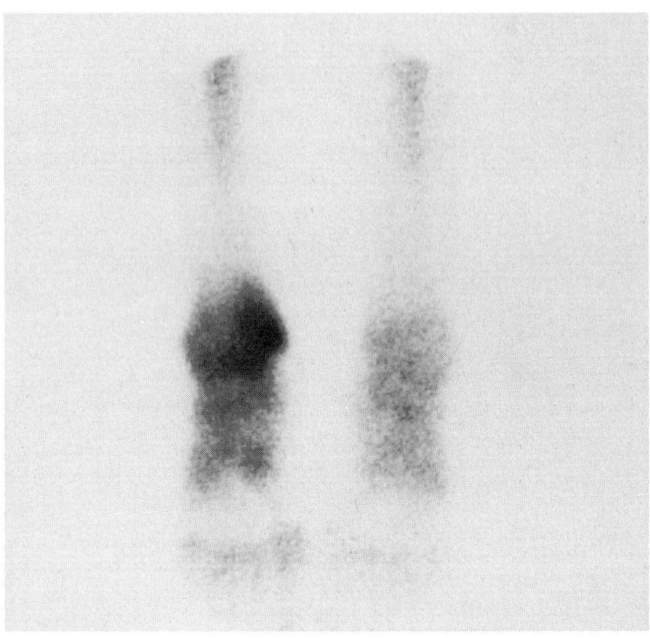

FIGURE 16.
A technetium scintiscan of a symptomatic patient with a diagnosis of an "ankle sprain" following sports activity 7 months before this study shows increased activity of the right distal tibia and talus. This patient has normal radiographic findings.

normal radiographic findings.[151, 152] Johnson[152] uses scintigraphic criteria to determine which symptomatic patients with acromioclavicular pain should have an arthroscopic excision.

The periarticular scintigraphic findings summarized earlier from the orthopaedic literature have been independently confirmed in the temporomandibular joint.[153, 154] Scintigraphic activity of this joint identifies those patients who are metabolically active, and these data are used in treatment decisions (Kaban L, personal communication, 1991).

CLINICAL RECOMMENDATIONS

The use of technetium scintigraphy can sensitively manifest regions of radiographically occult increased osseous metabolic activity in patients who have sustained musculoskeletal injury. The addition of such physiologic information can be a valuable adjunct in the diagnosis of musculoskeletal symptoms, as well as in the assessment of therapy.

DIAGNOSIS OF MUSCULOSKELETAL SYMPTOMS

A technetium bone scan is indicated in cases of persistent unexplained musculoskeletal pain or where the source and significance of symptoms remain in doubt. The discovery of bone scan patterns consistent with nascent stress fractures and other osseous stress-related phenomena can quickly lead to an appropriate diagnosis and early rational therapeutic intervention. No other imaging modality, including MRI or CT, has this capability.

The newer applications of scintigraphy in the assessment of patients with possible periarticular soft tissue damage can often help clarify an otherwise confusing clinical situation. For example, vague knee pain developed in a patient following increased athletic activity involving running and stair climbing. An orthopaedist obtained an MRI scan whose only abnormal finding was a grade II signal of the posterior horn of the meniscus, and the patient was told that surgery was indicated. This patient came to our office with an MRI in hand and requested a second opinion. Following a history and physical examination plus review of the MRI, I thought that this patient was most likely experiencing supraphysiologic overload of the patellofemoral components rather than structural failure of meniscal fibrocartilage. A bone scan obtained in this patient revealed intense diffuse patellar uptake with nearly normal activity of the medial compartment, thus confirming my impression that the MRI-detected meniscus "lesion" was clinically and physiologically silent. Based on this physiologic insight, I strongly recommended that the patient modify his activity and participate in an appropriate anti-inflammatory therapeutic regimen (outlined later in this chapter). The bone scan image was unequivocal; it helped the patient understand his problem and led him to fully cooperate in the appropriate nonsurgical therapeutic approach. This patient was symptom free within 4 weeks and has remained so 2 years after this incident by participating in loading activities within the *envelope of load acceptance* for his knee.[155]

A bone scan in a similar patient with vague symptoms and MRI evidence of medial meniscal failure manifested the presence of increased osseous metabolic activity in the involved compartment, thus independently confirming the clinical significance of the possible structural pathology. Such a patient is a much stronger candidate for arthroscopic inspection. To date, in cases in which both MRI and the bone scan indicate pathology in a symptomatic patient, surgical findings have always been present.

On one occasion we have seen a symptomatic patient in whom both MRI and the bone scan were normal, yet structure pathology was found at surgery, e.g., trochlear cartilage chondromalacia.

ASSESSMENT OF THERAPY

Many patients have persistent residual symptoms following periarticular surgery such as partial meniscectomy or ACL reconstruction. We recommend a technetium scan 12 to 24 months following such surgery to determine whether osseous homeostasis has been achieved. If the study indicates a significant loss of osseous homeostasis, the physician should caution the patient that the joint is being supraphysiologically loaded and may be at risk of early degenerative changes.

THERAPEUTIC RECOMMENDATIONS

A positive periarticular bone scan manifests loss of osseous homeostasis that should be addressed therapeutically in three areas: correction of pathomechanics, anti-inflammatory therapy, and rehabilitation.

Pathomechanics

Any persisting pathomechanical factors must be sought and corrected as the clinical circumstances permit. These factors may be external supraphysiologic loading secondary to high-impact sports activities (e.g., basketball, racquetball) or aggravating activities of daily living (e.g., excessive stair climbing). Such activities can trigger increased osseous remodeling and should be at least temporarily restricted. Patients must decrease their loading to within the joint's *envelope of load acceptance*. Loading activities that do not produce symptoms are more likely to be within this "envelope." Malalignment such as significant varus or patellar subluxation should be considered for surgical correction.

Extant internal pathomechanical factors such as structurally damaged cartilage or ligaments should also be assessed for possible surgical treatment. A correlative abnormal technetium study supports consideration of surgical intervention.

Anti-Inflammatory Therapy

I believe that regions of persistently increased osseous metabolic activity manifested by a positive bone scan are associated with excessive local cytokine production (see the section on humoral factors). A program of chronic anti-inflammatory therapy is therefore indicated in patients with a significantly abnormal technetium study. I recommend an appropriate daily low-dose oral anti-inflammatory agent of the physician's choice along with icing of the involved area two to three times per day for 15 to 20 minutes. Such a program should be continued at least until resolution of symptoms. We have shown that increased periarticular osseous metabolic activity can be temporarily suppressed at least 80% with a 20-minute episode of icing.

Rehabilitation

The maintenance of free range of motion, muscle tone, strength, and coordination[156–158] is an appropriate concurrent therapeutic goal in patients with positive bone scans, as long as the actual exercise program is within the patient's envelope of load acceptance. Even patients with significantly abnormal scintigraphic values can participate in exercises such as a gentle swimming program and stretching, progressing as symptoms allow.

CONCLUSIONS

It is now well documented that regions of metabolically active bone manifested scintigraphically are common phenomena in patients with sports and related musculoskeletal trauma. No imaging method other than scintigraphy—including MRI—is capable of reliably manifesting these regions of increased osseous metabolic activity. Orthopaedists need to expand their conceptualization of musculoskeletal trauma to include these previously unrecognized osseous phenomena. This is especially true in patients with periarticular soft tissue structural damage such as meniscal tears and ACL ruptures. The persistence of increased osseous metabolic activity reflects the pathophysiologic effect of such soft tissue damage on the osseous component of joints even in the presence of normal radiographs and MRI osseous assessments.

The persistence of such abnormal periarticular scintigraphic activity identifies patients who may be at risk of early degenerative changes because the same micro-osseous events leading to radiographically identifiable changes can be detected by technetium scintigraphy at a time when the process is still reversible. An analogy of this concept that I often use with patients is that a bone scan is similar to the use of an infrared camera in assessing cams in an engine. All of the cams may look structurally normal (analogous to normal radiographs of femoral condyles), but if three of the cams are cool and one is hot by infrared assessment, this identifies which component is being excessively stressed and therefore at risk of ultimate overt failure.

The addition of osseous physiologic data provides an enhanced understanding of the dynamic osseous adaptations to musculoskeletal injury for both the physician and patient. I have found that because of their simplicity and starkness, technetium images are comprehensible to patients and often lead them to a more profound understanding of their condition and heightened cooperation in a rational therapeutic program to regain musculoskeletal function, including appropriate surgical intervention when indicated.

The achievement of homeostasis is a well-established principle in the field of medicine.[159] It should be no less a goal for orthopaedists who have long sought restoration of biomechanical parameters as the prime criteria of therapeutic success.[155] The recent work on manifesting early degenerative changes following ACL reconstructive surgery proves the limitations of a purely biomechanical and structural conceptual paradigm.

Perturbed musculoskeletal tissues are ultracomplex metabolically activated systems, the parameters of which we are just now beginning to discover. The physiologic insight provided by scintigraphic methods, including positron emission tomography and other advanced techniques, will allow a more precise understanding of tissue response to injury that will continue to refine our conceptualization and therapeutic approaches well into the future.

REFERENCES

1. Dye SF: An evolutionary perspective of the knee. *J Bone Joint Surg Am* 69:976–983, 1987.
2. Dye SF: Functional anatomy and biomechanics of the patellofemoral joint, in Scott WN (ed): *The Knee*. St Louis, Mosby, 1994, pp 381–389.
3. Dye SF, Boll DA: Radionuclide imaging of the patellofemoral joint in young adults with anterior knee pain. *Orthop Clin North Am* 17:249–262, 1986.
4. Hutchins WC: Miscellaneous affections of joints, in Edmonson AS, Crenshaw AK (eds): *Campbell's Operative Orthopedics*, ed 6. St Louis, Mosby, 1971, pp 1004–1029.
5. Rockwood CA Jr, Green DP (eds): *Fractures in Adults*, ed 2. Philadelphia, JB Lippincott, 1984, p 17.
6. Thomas CL (ed): *Taber's Cyclopedic Medical Dictionary*, ed 16. Philadelphia, FA Davis, 1989.
7. Daniel DM, Stone ML, Dobson BE, et al: Fate of the ACL-injured patient, a prospective outcome study. *Am J Sports Med* 22:632–644, 1994.
8. Fritschy D, Daniel DM, Rossman D, et al: Bone imaging after acute knee hemarthrosis. *Knee Surg Sports Traumat Arthrosc* 1:20–27, 1993.

9. Lang P, Jergesen HE, Genant HK, et al: Magnetic resonance imaging of the ischemic femoral head in pigs. Dependency of signal intensities and relaxation times on elapsed time. *Clin Orthop* 244:272–280, 1989.
10. Deleted in proofs.
11. Dye SF, Bessolo R, Chew MH, et al: Comparison of magnetic resonance imaging and technetium scintigraphy in the detection of increased osseous metabolic activity about the knee. *Orthop Trans* 17:1060–1061, 1993.
12. Rollo FD (ed): *Nuclear Medicine Physics, Instrumentation, and Agents.* St Louis, Mosby, 1977, pp 398–399.
13. Holder LE: Radionuclide bone-imaging in the evaluation of bone pain. *J Bone Joint Surg Am* 64:1391–1396, 1982.
14. Schwartz Z, Shani J, Soskolne A, et al: Uptake and biodistribution of technetium-99m-MD^{32}P during rat tibial bone repair. *J Nucl Med* 34:104–108, 1993.
15. Siegel BA, Donovan RL, Alderson P, et al: Skeletal uptake of ^{99m}Tc-diphosphonate in relation to local bone blood flow. *Radiology* 120:121–123, 1976.
16. Delpassand ES, Dhekne RD, Barron BJ, et al: Evaluation of soft tissue injury by Tc-99m bone agent scintigraphy. *Clin Nucl Med* 16:309–314, 1991.
17. Morris E, Seeherman HJ, O'Callaghan MW, et al: Scintigraphic identification of skeletal muscle damage in horses 24 hours after strenuous exercise. *Equine Vet J* 23:347–352, 1991.
18. Collier BD, Johnson RP, Carrera GF, et al: Chronic knee pain assessed by SPECT: Comparison with other modalities. *Radiology* 157:795–802, 1985.
19. Grevitt MP, Taylor M, Churchill M, et al: SPECT imaging in the diagnosis of meniscal tears. *J R Soc Med* 86:639–641, 1993.
20. Murray IP: The role of SPECT in evaluation of skeletal trauma. *Ann Nucl Med* 7:1–9, 1993.
21. Murray IP, Dixon J, Kohan L: SPECT for acute knee pain. *Clin Nucl Med* 15:828–840, 1990.
22. Ryan PJ, Taylor M, Grevitt M, et al: Bone single-photon emission tomography in recent meniscal tears: An assessment of diagnostic criteria. *Eur J Nucl Med* 20:703–707, 1993.
23. Traughber PD, Havlina JM Jr: Bilateral pedicle stress fractures: SPECT and CT features. *J Comput Assist Tomogr* 15:338–340, 1991.
24. Dye SF, Chew MH: The use of scintigraphty to detect increased osseous metabolic activity about the knee. *J Bone Joint Surg Am* 75:1388–1406, 1993.
25. Patel N, Collier BD, Carrera GF, et al: High-resolution bone scintigraphy of the adult wrist. *Clin Nucl Med* 17:449–453, 1992.
26. Brill DR: Sports nuclear medicine. Bone imaging for lower extremity pain in athletes. *Clin Nucl Med* 8:101–116, 1983.
27. Holder LE: Bone scintigraphy in skeletal trauma. *Radiol Clin North Am* 31:739–781, 1993.
28. Holder LE, Methews LS: The nuclear physician and sports medicine, in Freeman LM, Weissman HS (eds): *Nuclear Medical Annual 1984.* New York, Raven Press, 1984, pp 81–140.
29. Marymont JV, Bergfeld JA: Nuclear scintigraphy in the diagnosis of sports-related injuries. *Mediguide Orthop* 10:1–5, 1991.
30. Matin P: Bone-scanning of trauma and benign conditions, in Freeman LM, Weissman HS (eds): *Nuclear Medicine Annual 1982.* New York, Raven Press, 1982, pp 81–118.
31. Rupani HD, Holder LE, Espinola DA, et al: Three phase radionuclide bone imaging in sports medicine. *Radiology* 156:187–196, 1985.

32. Blatz DJ: Bilateral femoral and tibial shaft stress fractures in a runner. *Am J Sports Med* 9:322–325, 1981.
33. Butler JE, Brown SL, McConnell BG: Subtrochanteric stress fractures in runners. *Am J Sports Med* 10:228–232, 1982.
34. Clancy WG, Foltz AS: Iliac apophysitis and stress fractures in adolescent runners. *Am J Sports Med* 4:214–218, 1976.
35. Daffner RH: Stress fracture: Current concepts. *Skeletal Radiol* 2:221–229, 1978.
36. Englaro EE, Gelfand MJ, Paltiel HJ: Bone scintigraphy in preschool children with lower extremity pain of unknown origin. *J Nucl Med* 33:351–354, 1992.
37. Fullerton LR Jr, Snowdy HA: Femoral neck stress fractures. *Am J Sports Med* 16:365–377, 1988.
38. Ha KI, Hahn SH, Chung MY, et al: A clinical study of stress fractures in sports activities. *Orthopedics* 14:1089–1095, 1991.
39. Jerosch JG, Castro WHM, Jantea C: Stress fracture of the patella. *Am J Sports Med* 17:579–580, 1989.
40. Lombardo SJ, Benson DW: Stress fractures of the femur in runners. *Am J Sports Med* 10:219–226, 1982.
41. McBryde AM Jr: Stress fractures in athletes. *J Sports Med* 3:212–217, 1975.
42. Rockett JF, Freeman BL III: Stress fracture of the patella confirmation by triple-phase bone imaging. *Clin Nucl Med* 15:873–875, 1990.
43. Rosenthall L, Hill RO, Chuang S: Observation on the use of ^{99m}Tc-phosphate imaging in peripheral bone trauma. *Radiology* 119:637–641, 1976.
44. Santi M, Sartoris DJ: Diagnostic imaging approach to stress fractures of the foot. *J Foot Surg* 30:85–97, 1991.
45. Hulkko A, Orava S: Stress fractures in athletes. *Int J Sports Med* 8:221–226, 1987.
46. Li G, Zhang S, Chen G, et al: Radiographic and histologic analysis of stress fracture in rabbit tibias. *Am J Sports Med* 13:285–294, 1985.
47. Johnson LC, Stradford Capt HT, et al: Histogenesis of stress fractures. *J Bone Joint Surg Am* 45:1542, 1963.
48. Courtenay BG, Bowers DM: Stress fractures: Clinical features and investigation. *Med J Aust* 153:155–156, 1990.
49. Pavlov H: Imaging of the foot and ankle. *Radiol Clin North Am* 28:991–1018, 1990.
50. Pavlov H, Torg JS, Freiberger RH: Tarsal navicular stress fractures: Radiographic evaluation. *Radiology* 148:641–645, 1983.
51. Prather JL, Nusynowitz ML, Snowdy HA, et al: Scintigraphic findings in stress fractures. *J Bone Joint Surg Am* 59:869–874, 1977.
52. Schils JP, Andrish JT, Paraino DW, et al: Medial malleolar stress fractures in seven patients: Review of the clinical and imaging features. *Radiology* 185:219–221, 1992.
53. Kottmeier SA, Hangs GA, Kalenak A: Fibular stress fracture associated with distal tibiofibular synostosis in an athlete. *Clin Orthop* 281:195–198, 1992.
54. Urman M, Ammann W, Sisler J, et al: The role of bone scintigraphy in the evaluation of talar dome fractures. *J Nucl Med* 32:2241–2244, 1991.
55. Matheson GO, Clement DB, McKenzie DC, et al: Stress fractures in athletes, a study of 320 cases. *Am J Sports Med* 15:46–58, 1987.
56. Clement DB: Tibial stress syndrome in athletes. *J Sports Med* 2:81–85, 1974.
57. Maddox PA, Garth WP Jr: Tendinitis of the patellar ligament and quadriceps (jumper's knee) as an initial presentation of hyperparathyroidism. *J Bone Joint Surg Am* 68:288–292, 1986.
58. Tibone JE, Lombardo SJ: Bilateral fractures of the inferior poles of the patellae in a basketball player. *Am J Sports Med* 9:215–216, 1981.

59. Clement DB, Ammann W, Taunton JE, et al: Exercise-induced stress injuries to the femur. *Int J Sports Med* 14:347–352, 1993.
60. Masters S, Fricker P, Purdam C: Stress fractures of the femoral shaft—four case studies. *Br J Sports Med* 20:14–16, 1986.
61. Rockett JF: Three-phase radionuclide bone imaging in stress injury of the anterior iliac crest. *J Nucl Med* 31:1554–1556, 1990.
62. Metzmaker JN, Pappas AM: Avulsion fractures of the pelvis. *Am J Sports Med* 13:349–358, 1985.
63. Briggs RC, Kolbjornsen PH, Southall RC: Osteitis pubis, Tc-99m MDP, and professional hockey players. *Clin Nucl Med* 17:861–863, 1992.
64. Glazer M, Sagar VV, Welch K: Radiograph of the month. Acute stress fracture of the pars interarticularis of the right half of L2 vertebral body. *Del Med J* 66:91–92, 1994.
65. Hawkes DJ, Robinson L, Crossman JE, et al: Registration and display of the combined bone scan and radiograph in the diagnosis and management of wrist injuries. *Eur J Nucl Med* 18:752–756, 1991.
66. Linn MR, Mann FA, Gilula LA: Imaging the symptomatic wrist. *Orthop Clin North Am* 21:515–541, 1990.
67. Maurer AH: Nuclear medicine in evaluation of the hand and wrist. *Hand Clin* 7:183–201, 1991.
68. Shewring DJ, Savage R, Thomas G: Experience of the early use of technetium 99 bone scintigraphy in wrist injury. *J Hand Surg [Br]* 19:114–117, 1994.
69. Tiel-van Buul MM, van Beek EJ, Dijkstra PF, et al: Significance of a hot spot on the bone scan after carpal injury—evaluation by computed tomography. *Eur J Nucl Med* 20:159–164, 1993.
70. Engel A, Feldner-Busztin H: Bilateral stress fracture of the scaphoid. A case report. *Arch Orthop Trauma Surg* 110:314–315, 1991.
71. Tiel-van Buul MM, van Beek EJ, van Dongen A, et al: The reliability of the 3-phase bone scan in suspected scaphoid fracture: An inter- and intraobserver variability analysis. *Eur J Nucl Med* 19:848–852, 1992.
72. Tiel-van Buul MM, van Beek EJ, Broekhuizen AH, et al: Radiography and scintigraphy of suspected scaphoid fracture. A long-term study in 160 patients. *J Bone Joint Surg Br* 75:61–65, 1993.
73. Tiel-van Buul MM, van Beek EJ, Borm JJ, et al: The value of radiographs and bone scintigraphy in suspected scaphoid fracture. A statistical analysis. *J Hand Surg Br* 18:403–406, 1993.
74. Howard RS II, Conrad GR: Ice cream scooper's hand. Report of an occupationally related stress fracture of the hand. *Clin Nucl Med* 17:721–723, 1992.
75. Rosenberg ZS, Kawelblum M, Cheung YY, et al: Osgood-Schlatter lesion: Fracture or tendinitis? Scintigraphic, CT, and MR imaging features. *Radiology* 185:853–858, 1992.
76. Vellet AD, Marks PH, Fowler PJ, et al: Occult posttraumatic osteochondral lesions of the knee: Prevalence, classification, and short-term sequelae evaluated with MR imaging. *Radiology* 178:271–276, 1991.
77. Lotke PA, Ecker ML: Osteonecrosis of the knee. *Orthop Clin North Am* 16:797–808, 1985.
78. Kozin F, Ryan LM, Carrera GF, et al: The reflex sympathetic dystrophy syndrome (RSDS). III: Scintigraphic studies, further evidence of therapeutic efficacy with systemic corticosteroids, and proposed diagnostic criteria. *Am J Med* 70:23–30, 1981.
79. Simon H, Carlson DH: The use of bone scanning in the diagnosis of reflex sympathetic dystrophy. *Clin Nucl Med* 5:116–121, 1980.

80. Malki AA, Elgazzar A, Ashqar T, et al: New technique for assessing muscle damage after trauma. *J R Coll Surg Edinb* 37:131–133, 1992.
81. Mochizuki T, Tauxe WN, Perper JA: Technetium-99m MDP scintigraphy of rhabdomyolysis induced by exertional heat stroke: A case report. *Ann Nucl Med* 4:111–113, 1990.
82. Peller PJ, Ho VB, Kransdorf MJ: Extraosseous Tc-99m MDP uptake: A pathophysiologic approach. *Radiographics* 13:715–734, 1993.
83. Rockett JF, Freeman BL: 3D scintigraphy demonstration of pectineus muscle avulsion injury. *Clin Nucl Med* 15:800–803, 1990.
84. Holder LE, Michael RH: The specific scintigraphic pattern of "shin splints in the lower leg": Concise communication. *J Nucl Med* 25:865–869, 1984.
85. Nielsen MB, Hansen K, Holmer P, et al: Tibial periosteal reactions in soldiers. *Acta Orthop Scand* 62:531–534, 1991.
86. Roach PJ, Cooper RA, Watson AS: Arm splints on bone scan in a volleyball player. *Clin Nucl Med* 18:900–901, 1993.
87. Muehllehner G, Karp JS: A positron camera using positron-sensitive detectors: PENN-PET. *J Nucl Med* 27:90–98, 1986.
88. Muehllehner G, Karp JS: Positron emission tomography imaging. *Semin Nucl Med* 16:35–50, 1986.
89. Bentley G: Chondromalacia patellae. *J Bone Joint Surg Am* 52:221–232, 1970.
90. Bentley G, Dowd G: Current concepts of etiology and treatment of chondromalacia patellae. *Clin Orthop* 189:209–228, 1984.
91. Insall J, Falvo KA, Wise DW: Chondromalacia patellae. A prospective study. *J Bone Joint Surg Am* 58:1–8, 1976.
92. DeHaven KE, Collins HR: Diagnosis of internal derangements of the knee. The role of arthroscopy. *J Bone Joint Surg Am* 57:802–810, 1975.
93. McGinty JB, McCarthy JC: Endoscopic lateral retinacular release: A preliminary report. *Clin Orthop* 158:120–125, 1981.
94. Aglietti P, Insall JN, Cerulli G: Patellar pain and incongruence. I: Measures of incongruence. *Clin Orthop* 176:217–224, 1983.
95. Carson WG Jr, James SL, Larson RL, et al: Patellofemoral disorders: Physical and radiographic evaluation. Part I: Physical examination. *Clin Orthop* 185:165–177, 1984.
96. Carson WG Jr, James SL, Larson RL, et al: Patellofemoral disorders: Physical and radiographic evaluation. Part II: Radiographic examination. *Clin Orthop* 185:178–186, 1984.
97. Ficat P, Hungerford DS: *Disorders of the Patellofemoral Joint*. Baltimore, Williams & Wilkins, 1977.
98. Fulkerson JP: The etiology of patellofemoral pain in young, active patients: A prospective study. *Clin Orthop* 179:129–133, 1983.
99. Hughston JC, Walsh WM, Pudda G: *Patellar Subluxation and Dislocation*. Philadelphia, WB Saunders, 1984.
100. Hughston JC: Subluxation of the patella. *J Bone Joint Surg Am* 50:1003–1026, 1968.
101. Insall J: "Chondromalacia patellae": Patellar malalignment syndrome. *Orthop Clin North Am* 10:117–127, 1979.
102. Insall J, Aglietti P, Tria AJ: Patellar pain and incongruence. II: Clinical application. *Clin Orthop* 176:225–232, 1983.
103. Dye SF, Boll DA: An analysis of objective measurements including radionuclide imaging in young patients with patellofemoral pain. *Am J Sports Med* 13:432, 1985.
104. Merchant AC, Mercer RL, Jacobsen RH, et al: Roentgenographic analysis of patellofemoral congruence. *J Bone Joint Surg Am* 56:1391–1396, 1974.

104a. Laurin CA, Dussault R, Leveque HP: The tangential x-ray investigation of the patellofemoral joint: X-ray technique, diagnostic criteria and their interpretation. *Clin Orthop* 144:16–26, 1979.
105. Dye SF, Boll DH, Westin GH, et al: Assessing patellar scintigraphic activity; a new quantitative method. *Orthop Trans* 9:459, 1985.
106. Insall J: Current concepts review—Patellar pain. *J Bone Joint Surg Am* 64:147–152, 1982.
107. Butler-Manuel PA, Guy RL, Heatley FW, et al: Scintigraphy in the assessment of anterior knee pain. *Acta Orthop Scand* 61:438–442, 1990.
108. Hejgaard N, Diemer H: Bone scan in the patellofemoral pain syndrome. *Int Orthop* 11:29–33, 1987.
109. Kahn D, Wilson MA: Bone scintigraphic findings in patellar tendonitis. *J Nucl Med* 28:1768–1770, 1987.
110. Kipper MS, Alazraki NP, Fieglin DH: The "hot" patella. *Clin Nucl Med* 7:28–32, 1982.
111. Kohn HS, Guten GN, Collier BD, et al: Chondromalacia of the patella. Bone imaging correlated with arthroscopic findings. *Clin Nucl Med* 13:96–98, 1988.
112. Dye SF, Chew MH: Restoration of osseous homeostasis after anterior cruciate ligament reconstruction. *Am J Sports Med* 21:748–750, 1993.
113. Dye SF, Peartree PK: Sequential radionuclide imaging of the patellofemoral joint in symptomatic young adults (abstract). *Am J Sports Med* 17:727, 1989.
114. Dye SF: The pathophysiology of patellofemoral pain. *Sports Med Arthrosc Rev* 2:203–210, 1994.
115. Handmaker H, Leonards R: The bone scan in inflammatory disease. *Semin Nucl Med* 6:95–015, 1976.
116. McNeil BJ: Value of bone scanning in neoplastic disease. *Semin Nucl Med* 14:277–286, 1984.
117. Dye SF, Daniel JA, Fry MF, et al: The correlation of increased scintigraphic activity and patellar osseous pathology in young patients with patellofemoral pain. *Orthop Trans* 10:480, 1986.
118. McBride JT, Rodkey WG, Brooks DE, et al: Early detection of osteoarthritis using technetium 99m MDP imaging, radiographs, histology, and gross pathology in an experimental rabbit model. *Orthop Trans* 15:348–349, 1991.
119. MacKinnon SE, Holder LE: The use of three-phase radionuclide bone scanning in the diagnosis of reflex sympathetic dystrophy. *J Hand Surg* 9:556–563, 1984.
120. Bertolini DR, Nedwin GE, Bringman TS, et al: Stimulation of bone resorption and inhibition of bone formation in vitro by human tumour necrosis factors. *Nature* 318:516–518, 1986.
121. Evans DB, Bunning RA, Russell RG: The effects of recombinant human granulocyte-macrophage colony-stimulating factor (rhGM-CSF) on human osteoblast-like cells. *Biochem Biophys Res Commun* 160:588–595, 1989.
122. Gowen M, Mundy GR: Actions of recombinant interleukin-1, interleukin-2, and interferon-gamma on bone resorption in vitro. *J Immunol* 136:2478–2482, 1986.
123. Mundy GR: Cytokines and local factors which affect osteoclast function. *Int J Cell Cloning* 10:215–222, 1992.
124. Sato K, Fujii Y, Kasono K, et al: Stimulation of prostaglandin E_2 and bone resorption by recombinant human interleukin 1 alpha in fetal mouse bones. *Biochem Biophys Res Commun* 138:618–624, 1986.
125. Krishnamurthy G, Brickman AS, Blahd W: Technetium-99m-Sn-pyrophosphate pharmacokinetics and bone image changes in parathyroid disease. *J Nucl Med* 18:236–242, 1977.

126. Sy W: Bone scan in primary hyperparathyroidism. *J Nucl Med* 15:1089–1091, 1974.
127. Klein DC, Raisz LG: Prostaglandins: Stimulation of bone resorption in tissue culture. *Endocrinology* 86:1436–1440, 1970.
128. Lorenzo J: Cytokines and bone metabolism: Resorption and formation, in Kimball S (ed): *Cytokines and Inflammation*. Boca Raton, Fla, CRC Press, 1991, pp 145–168.
129. Marymont JV, Lynch MA, Henning CE: Evaluation of meniscus tears of the knee by radionuclide imaging. *Am J Sports Med* 11:432–435, 1983.
130. Dye SF: Radionuclide imaging of the knee, in Aichroth P, Cannon WD (eds): *Knee Surgery, Current Practice*. London, Martin Dunitz, 1992, pp 38–44.
131. Dye SF, Andersen CT, Stowell MT: Unrecognized abnormal osseous metabolic activity about the knee of patients with symptomatic anterior cruciate ligament deficiency. *Orthop Trans* 11:492, 1987.
132. Dye SF, McBride JT, Chew MH, et al: Unrecognized abnormal osseous metabolic activity in patients with documented meniscal pathology (abstract). *Am J Sports Med* 17:723–724, 1989.
133. Bauer HC, Persson PE, Nilsson OS: Tears of the medial meniscus associated with increased radionuclide activity of the proximal tibia. Report of three cases. *Int Orthop* 13:153–155, 1989.
134. Mooar P, Gregg J, Jacobstein J: Radionuclide imaging in internal derangements of the knee. *Am J Sports Med* 15:132–136, 1987.
135. Lohmann M, Kanstrup IL, Gerfvary I, et al: Bone scintigraphy in patients suspected of having meniscus tears. *Scand J Med Sci Sports* 1:123–127, 1991.
136. Rockett JH: Demonstration of medial meniscus tear by three-phase bone imaging. *Clin Nucl Med* 16:47–48, 1991.
137. Dye SF, Chew MH, McBride JT, et al: Restoration of osseous homeostasis of the knee following meniscal surgery. *Orthop Trans* 16:725, 1992.
138. Meyers A, Wintch KM: Positive bone images in patients with normal or equivocal MRI studies: Two case reports. *J Nucl Med Tech* 21:24–26, 1993.
139. Fairbank TJ: Knee joint changes after meniscectomy. *J Bone Joint Surg Br* 30:664–670, 1948.
140. Dieppe P, Cushnaghan J, Young P, et al: Prediction of the progression of joint space narrowing in osteoarthritis of the knee by bone scintigraphy. *Ann Rheum Dis* 52:557–563, 1993.
141. Dorchak JD, Barrack RL, Alexander AH, et al: Radionuclide imaging of the knee with chronic anterior cruciate ligament tear. *Orthop Rev* 22:1233–1241, 1993.
142. Dieppe P, Cushnaghan J, Young P, et al: Bone scintigraphy predicts progression of knee osteoarthritis. *J Musculoskeletal Med* 10:7–8, 1993.
143. Thomas RH, Resnick D, Alazraki NP, et al: Compartmental evaluation of osteoarthritis on the knee. A comparative study of available diagnostic modalities. *Radiology* 116:585–594, 1975.
144. Egund N, Frost S, Brismar J, et al: Radiography and scintigraphy in the assessment of early gonarthrosis. *Acta Radiol* 29:451–455, 1988.
145. Radin EL: Aetiology of osteoarthrosis. *Clin Rheum Dis* 2:509–522, 1976.
146. Radin EL: The relationship between biological and mechanical factors in the aetiology of osteoarthritis. *J Rheumatol Suppl* 9:20–21, 1983.
147. Radin EL, Rose RM: Role of subchondral bone in the initiation and progression of cartilage damage. *Clin Orthop* 213:34–40, 1986.
148. Marks PH, Goldenberg JA, Vezina WC, et al: Subchondral bone infractions in acute ligamentous knee injuries demonstrated on bone scintigraphy and magnetic resonance imaging. *J Nucl Med* 33:516–520, 1992.

149. Main JD, Alexander AH, Barrack RL, et al: Radionuclide imaging of the ACL reconstructed knee. *Orthop Trans* 17:572, 1993.
150. Kaplan MJ, Clancy WG Jr: Alabama sports medicine experience with isolated and combined posterior cruciate ligament injuries. *Clin Sports Med* 13:545–552, 1994.
151. Grimm ES, Bekerman C: The bench press mark. *Clin Nucl Med* 17:56–57, 1992.
152. Johnson LL: *Diagnostic and Surgical Arthroscopy of the Shoulder*. St Louis, Mosby, 1993, pp 406–408.
153. Blankestijn J, Panders AK, Vermey A, et al: Synovial chondromatosis of the temporo-mandibular joint. Report of three cases and a review of the literature. *Cancer* 55:479–485, 1985.
154. Epstein DH, Graves RW, Higgins WL: Clinical significance of increased temporomandibular joint uptake by planar isotope bone scan. *Clin Nucl Med* 12:705–707, 1987.
155. Dye SF: Knee as biologic transmission/envelope of load acceptance: A rational paradigm of function. *Clin Orthop* 1993, in press.
156. Marr D: A theory of cerebellar cortex. *J Physiol* 202:437–470, 1969.
157. Sanes JS: A theory of cerebellar function. *Math Biosci* 10:25–51, 1971.
158. Schmahmann JD: An emerging concept. The cerebellar contribution to higher function. *Arch Neurol* 48:1178–1187, 1991.
159. Guyton AC (ed): *Textbook of Medical Physiology*, ed 7. Philadelphia, WB Saunders, 1986, p 3.

Current Concepts in Shoulder Instability

Jon J.P. Warner, M.D.
Director, Shoulder Service Center for Sports Medicine, Department of Orthopaedic Surgery, University of Pittsburgh, Pittsburgh, Pennsylvania

Kary R. Schulte, M.D.
Shoulder Service Center for Sports Medicine, Department of Orthopaedic Surgery, University of Pittsburgh, Pittsburgh, Pennsylvania

Andreas B. Imhoff, M.D.
Shoulder Service Center for Sports Medicine, Department of Orthopaedic Surgery, University of Pittsburgh, Pittsburgh, Pennsylvania

ANATOMY AND BIOMECHANICS: RISK FACTORS

The shoulder is the most mobile joint in the body, and unlike the other large ball-in-socket joint, the hip, it has little inherent stability from articular and bony anatomy. In fact, this minimally constrained arrangement is an anatomic configuration necessary for the large range of motion in this joint. The surrounding soft tissue envelope of the capsule, ligaments, and rotator cuff muscles functions as the primary stabilizer of this joint. Furthermore, in order to allow for multiplanar motion in this joint, the capsule and ligaments are relatively lax but become passive static restraints to excessive translation and rotation of the humeral head on the glenoid at the end ranges of rotation. The rotator cuff and long head of the biceps brachii function during active shoulder motion to stabilize the humeral head in the glenoid through the entire range of rotation. Balancing the mobility and stability of this joint is a unique challenge of this anatomic region, and this arrangement explains why this joint is at risk for clinical instability.

Historically, most of our insight into the normal and abnormal function of the shoulder has been based on clinical intuition and anecdotal observations of pathology. However, over the past 20 years, specific experimental and clinical studies have greatly clarified our understanding of the factors that contribute to stability of this joint. This first section of this chapter will outline some of these factors and give examples of various pathologic lesions that may contribute to glenohumeral instability. However, before consideration can be given to these stability factors, it is necessary to define the term *instability* and distinguish it from the term

Advances in Operative Orthopaedics, vol. 3

TABLE 1.
Factors Influencing Stability of the Glenohumeral Joint

Factors Influencing Stability of the Glenohumeral Joint
Static factors
Articular components
Glenoid labrum
Capsule and ligaments
Negative intra-articular pressure
Adhesion/cohesion
Dynamic factors
Rotator cuff
Biceps tendon

laxity. Instability is defined as excessive, symptomatic translation of the humeral head on the glenoid during active shoulder motion. Laxity is defined as the amount of passive, asymptomatic translation of the humeral head on the glenoid as determined by clinical examination. It is extremely important to distinguish between these two terms when examining a patient with suspected instability because a relatively lax shoulder in an asymptomatic young athlete may be physiologically normal whereas a less lax ("tighter") shoulder in an individual with a known prior shoulder dislocation may be abnormal. Laxity is a necessary feature of normal shoulder capsuloligamentous anatomy.

The factors responsible for stability of the glenohumeral joint may be divided into static and dynamic anatomic constraints (Table 1). Disruption of one or more of these restraint mechanisms can lead to glenohumeral instability. Each of these factors, along with relevant lesions, is briefly considered in the following text and outlined in Table 2.

STATIC CONSTRAINTS

ARTICULAR COMPONENTS (HUMERUS/GLENOID)

The glenoid face offers a nearly "pear-shaped" surface, being narrow superiorly and wide inferiorly, with average anteroposterior and superoinferior dimensions of 25 mm and 35 mm, respectively. By contrast, the respective humeral head dimensions measure 45 and 48 mm.[1] Soslowsky et al.[2] measured the radii of the humeral head and glenoid fossa by stereophotogrammetry. They found radii measuring 25.2 ± 1.6 and 27.0 ± 1.7 mm, respectively. Therefore, in any position of rotation there is a surface area mismatch so that only 25% to 30% of the humeral head is in contact with the glenoid surface.[3–7] Saha[5,6] described this relationship as the glenohumeral index, which is a ratio of the maximum glenoid diameter to the maximum humeral head diameter. This ratio has been determined to be approximately 0.6 in the transverse plane and 0.75 in the sagittal plane.[5,6,8]

Examinations of the congruency of the articular surface of this joint have revealed the radii of curvature of the humeral head and glenoid to

TABLE 2.
Glenohumeral Stability

Stability Factor	Stability Function	Pathology
Articular surface congruity	Concavity-compression effect	Dysplasia Fracture Hill-Sachs lesion Reverse Hill-Sachs lesion
Glenoid labrum	Increased socket depth and surface area Acts like a "chock block" anchor for ligaments	Bankart lesion
Negative pressure	Vacuum effect for stability	Capsular rupture "Rotator interval" defect Capsular laxity
CHL/SGHL*	Limits: ER and inferior translation in adduction Posterior translation in FF	Capsular injury or laxity "Rotator interval" lesion
MGHL	Limits: ER and inferior translation in adduction Anterior translation in midabduction	Bankart lesion
IGHLC	Limits: Anterior, posterior, and inferior translation in abduction	Bankart lesion
Rotator cuff	Dynamic joint compression "Steering effect"	Overuse injury (fatigue) Rupture with/without dislocation
Biceps (long head)	Dynamic restraint to superior and anterior translation	SLAP lesion Rupture
Posterior capsule	Restraint to posterior translation in the flexed, adducted, internally rotated shoulder	Posterior capsular laxity

*CHL = coracohumeral ligament; SGHL = superior glenohumeral ligament; ER = external rotation; FF = forward flexion; MGHL = middle glenohumeral ligament; IGHLC = inferior glenohumeral ligament complex; SLAP = superior labral detachment anterior and posterior.

be 23 and 24.5 mm, respectively.[2] Soslowsky et al.[2] have shown the anatomic relationship between the two articular surfaces by stereophotogrammetry and determined that the glenoid cartilage was thicker peripherally than centrally whereas the humeral cartilage was thicker centrally than peripherally. Consequently, the articular surfaces are closely congruent and nearly spherical even though the underlying bone of the glenoid may appear to be flat (Fig 1). Therefore the tendency for instability is not due to a mismatch in articular congruity but rather to an oversized humeral head in a smaller glenoid.

A normal proximal end of the humerus has a neck shaft angle of 130 to 150 degrees and is retroverted about 20 to 30 degrees in relation to the transverse epicondylar axis of the elbow. The degree of normal glenoid

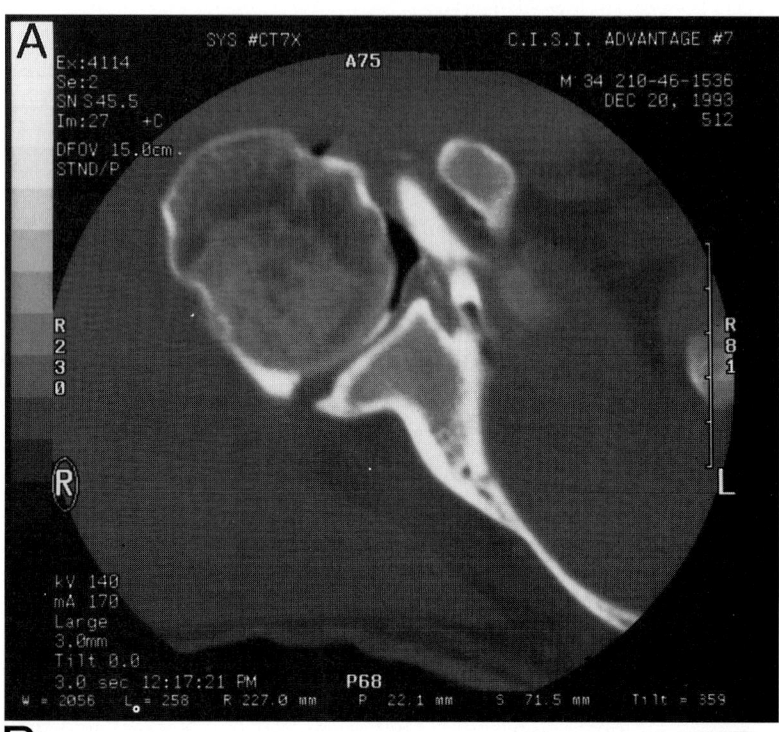

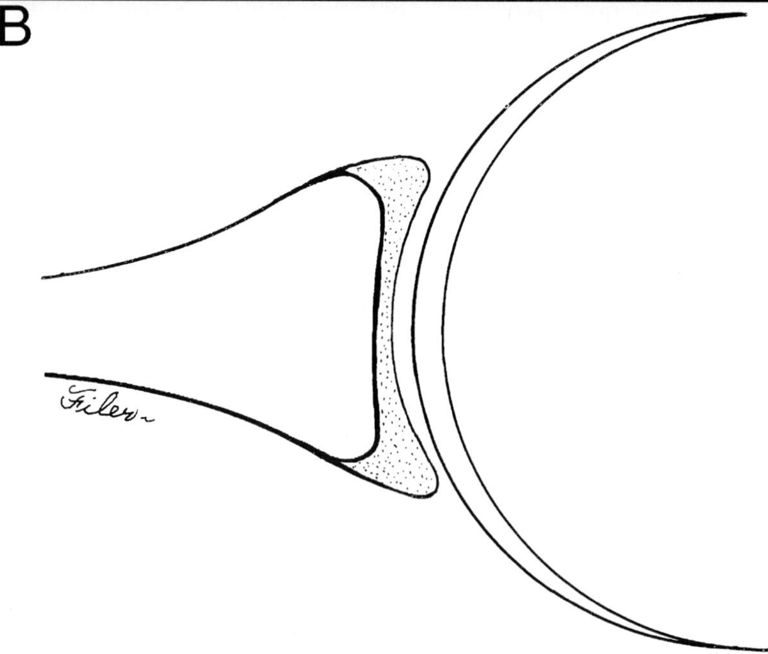

FIGURE 1.

A, computed tomographic arthrogram showing matched articular congruity of the glenohumeral joint. **B,** drawing demonstrating that the glenoid cartilage is thicker peripherally whereas the humeral head cartilage is thicker centrally. This creates articular congruence.

version may vary greatly, whereas 75% of individuals have a glenoid that is retroverted an average of 7.4 degrees in relation to the plane of the scapula, the remaining 25% can have 2 to 10 degrees of anteversion.[5, 6, 9] Therefore the glenohumeral joint articular surfaces average a combined retroversion of 20 to 40 degrees.[3, 5, 6, 10–17] It has been suggested that this relationship is important in maintaining stability of the joint and that excessive anteversion or retroversion may contribute to instability in either an anterior or posterior direction, respectively.[12, 17–26] However, this concept remains a subject of debate, and clinical experience has shown that the need for corrective osteotomy of either the glenoid or the humeral component of this joint is rare.

Additional bony lesions that may disrupt the normal anatomic articular relationship of this joint and thus contribute to instability are glenoid fracture, glenoid dysplasia, and a large Hill-Sachs or reverse Hill-Sachs lesion (Figs 2 and 3). These last two lesions are impression fractures of the posterolateral and anterolateral margins of the humeral head, respectively. They are created when the humeral head dislocates over the anterior or posterior glenoid rim.[27–31] In the case of anterior instability, this lesion is present in over 80% of anterior dislocations and 25% of anterior subluxations,[27, 29] and it is larger with dislocations of longer duration, with recurrent dislocations, and in cases with inferior displacement of the humeral head.[28, 32–34] In most instances this lesion is relatively small, and therefore it plays little role in ongoing shoulder instability[30, 35, 36] and anterior capsular repair is all that is necessary to correct the instability. However, when the Hill-Sachs lesion involves more than 30% of the humeral articular surface, it may contribute to anterior instability even if an adequate anterior capsular repair is performed.[31, 35] In these relatively rare situations, external rotation allows the posterior humeral head defect to come into contact with the anterior glenoid rim, thus allowing the humeral head to fall out of the glenoid cavity (Fig 3). Therefore some surgeons perform surgical procedures that either eliminate the humeral head defect (i.e., infraspinatus tendon transfer or allograft reconstruction)[31, 32, 37] (Gerber, personal communication, 1993) or rotate it out of contact with the glenoid by a proximal humeral osteotomy.[25, 26] In the senior author's experience (J.P.W.), surgical treatment of a Hill-Sachs or reverse Hill-Sachs lesion is only necessary in those rare cases in which it is greater than 30% of the articular surface. In older individuals the humeral head is usually replaced with a prosthesis; however, in younger individuals, reconstruction with a bone graft or allograft has been successful in a few rare cases (Fig 3).

GLENOID LABRUM

The perimeter of the glenoid fossa is lined by a fibrocartilaginous ring that acts as a transition to the glenohumeral ligaments and the tendon of the long head of the biceps brachii. This anatomic structure is the glenoid labrum, and it contributes to stability of the glenohumeral joint through three mechanisms: (1) it increases the depth and surface area of the glenoid socket, thus increasing the conforming fit of the humeral head

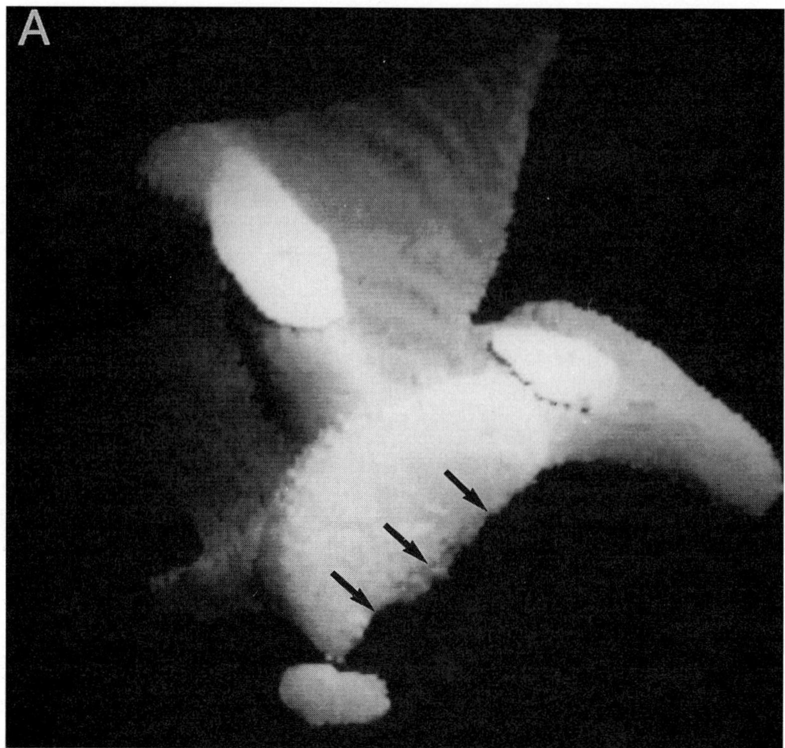

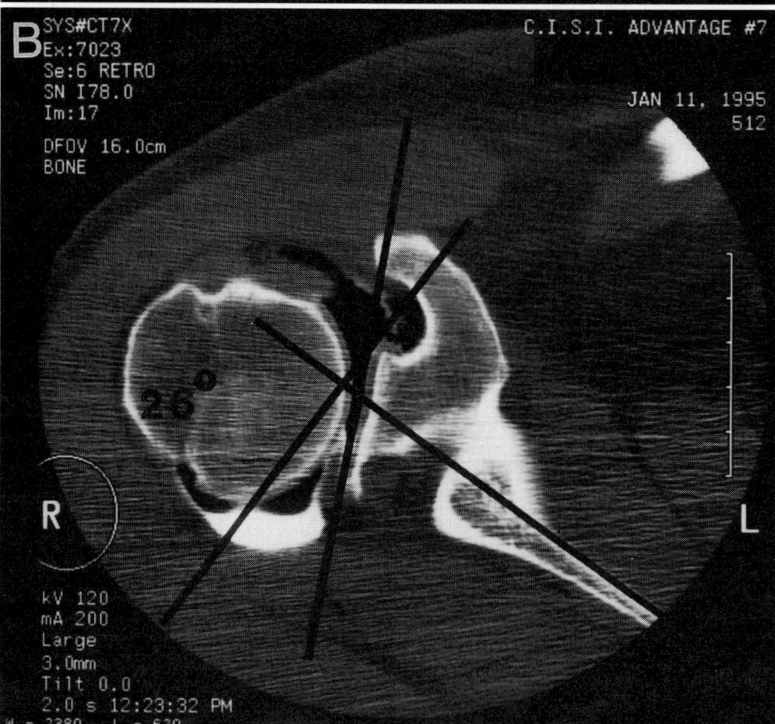

FIGURE 2.

A, three-dimensional computed tomographic reconstruction in a patient with a glenoid fracture (right shoulder) showing loss of the anterior third of the glenoid fossa (*arrows*). **B,** computed tomographic arthrogram showing 26 degrees of glenoid retroversion secondary to a posterior glenoid osteochondral fracture. This patient had pain caused by posterior humeral subluxation.

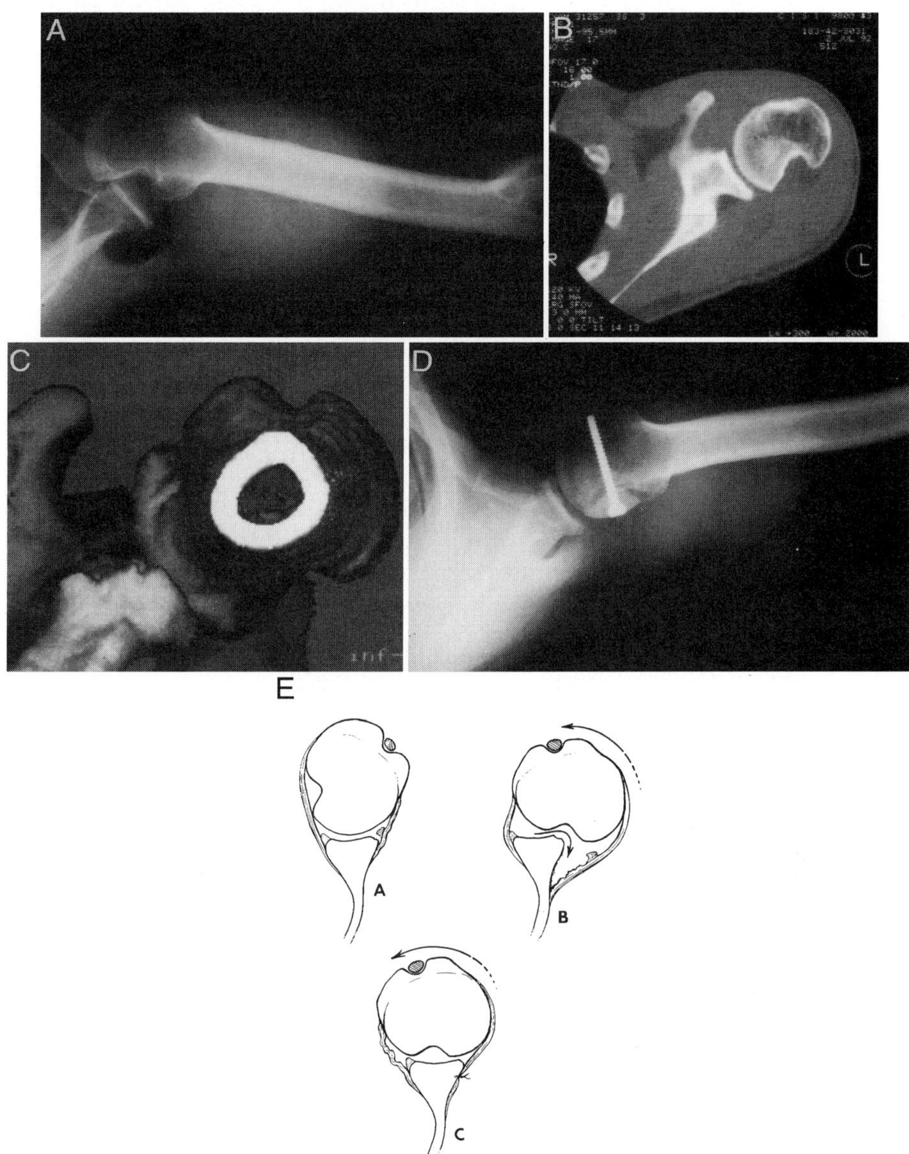

FIGURE 3.

A, anterior dislocation in a patient with a large Hill-Sachs lesion (>30% of the humeral head). **B,** computed tomographic scan in the same patient. **C,** three-dimensional computed tomographic reconstruction also shows a large Bankart lesion in addition to the large Hill-Sachs lesion. **D,** this was treated with a Bankart repair and osteochondral allograft reconstruction of the humeral head. **E,** role of the Hill-Sachs lesion in anterior shoulder instability: *A,* with the arm in internal rotation, the Hill-Sachs lesion is not in contact with the glenoid. *B,* with external rotation, the humeral head translates anteriorly because of the incompetent anterior capsular mechanism. This allows the humeral head to dislocate through the Hill-Sachs lesion. *C,* an adequate Bankart repair keeps the Hill-Sachs lesion contained on the glenoid, unless it is greater than 30% of the humeral articular surface.

in the glenoid[38, 39] (Fig 4); (2) it acts as a "chock block" to translation of the humeral head out of the glenoid[38]; (3) it forms the anchoring point for the glenohumeral ligaments and long head of the biceps brachii.[1, 40]

The "Bankart lesion" represents a detachment of the glenoid labrum from the glenoid rim, and historically this lesion has been implicated as the primary injury occurring with a traumatic anterior dislocation (Fig 5).[30, 31, 35, 36, 41–43] However, there is often confusion about what this lesion actually is. Cooper et al.[40] have shown that the labrum has significant anatomic variability around the periphery of the glenoid. Above the equator of the glenoid the labrum is frequently quite loosely attached and may therefore function more as a mobile extension of the glenoid surface rather than a rigid "chock block." Below the equator of the glenoid the labrum is consistently tightly attached to the glenoid articular cartilage. Therefore, labral detachments below the equator of the glenoid are more likely to represent a true Bankart lesion in association with instability, whereas a loosely attached labrum above the level of the equator most likely represents a normal variant of anatomy.

The consequences of a Bankart lesion (detachment of the glenoid labrum) are a decrease in the depth of the socket by 50% and detachment of the inferior glenohumeral ligament.

CAPSULOLIGAMENTOUS STRUCTURES

It is necessary to clearly understand the range of normal glenohumeral capsuloligamentous anatomy in order to rationally treat shoulder instability (Fig 6). Historically, these ligaments were first described as thickenings in the capsule of the shoulder joint. Recent arthroscopic observations and experimental biomechanical studies of these structures have contributed to a more quantitative appreciation of their functional anatomy. The function of each glenohumeral ligament is considered briefly in the following text and is also outlined in Table 2.

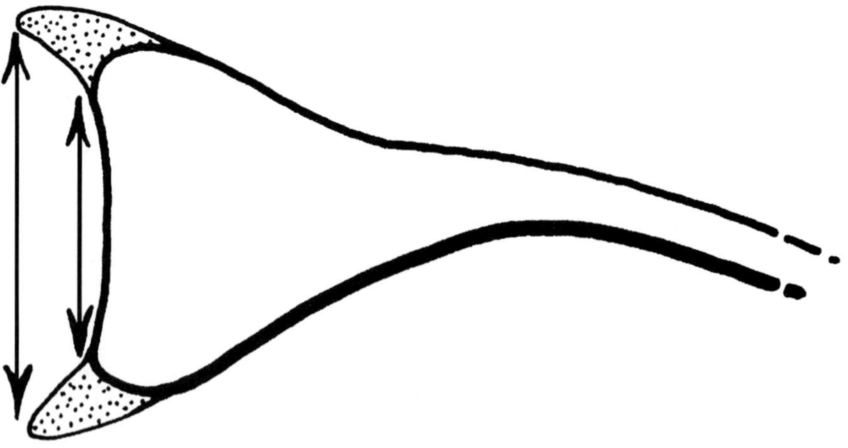

FIGURE 4.
The glenoid labrum broadens and deepens the glenoid fossa, thus enhancing stability by increasing the surface area and concavity for a conforming fit of the humeral head.

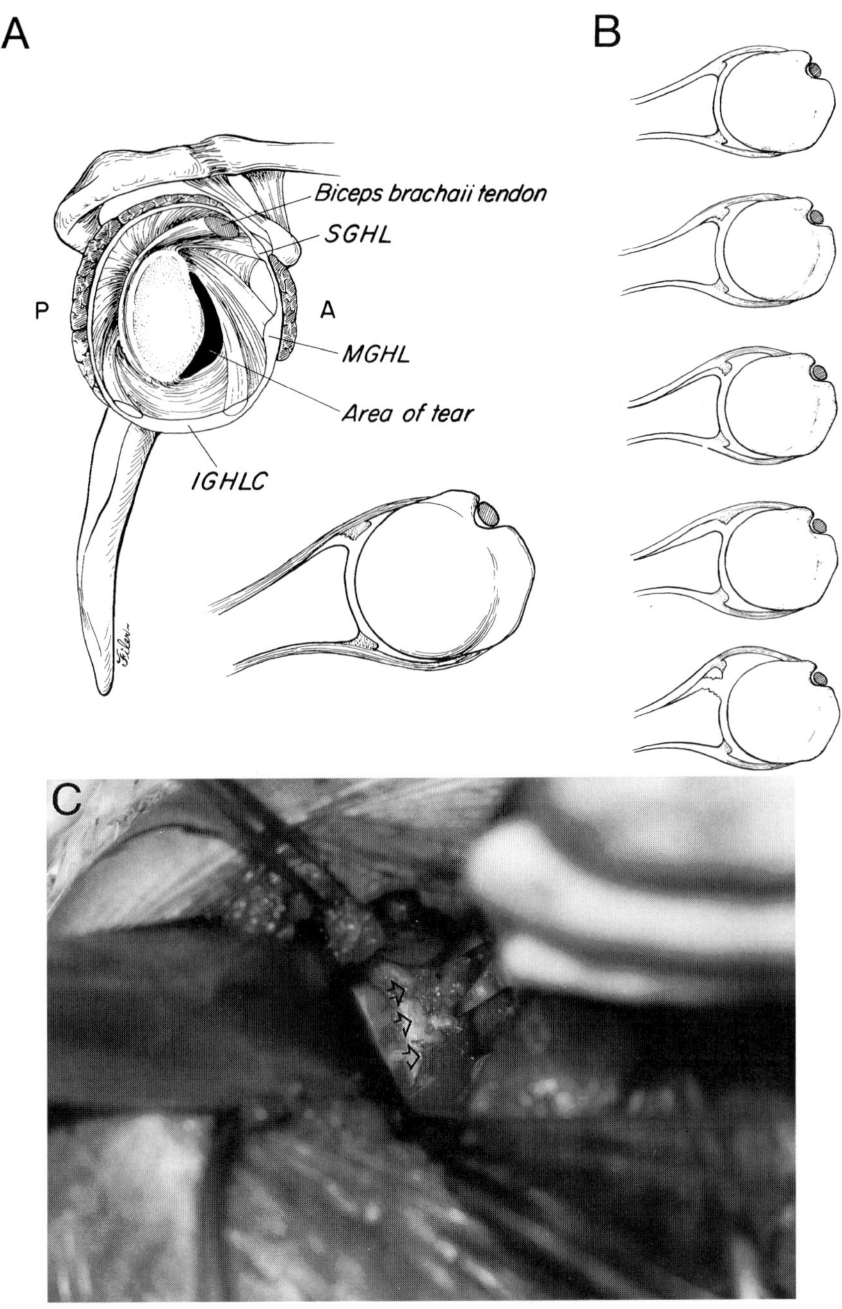

FIGURE 5.

A, a Bankart lesion ("area of tear") is a detachment of the capsuloligamentous structures from the glenoid rim. This usually involves the anterior portion of the inferior glenohumeral ligament complex *(IGHLC)* but may also involve the middle *(MGHL)* and superior *(SGHL)* glenohumeral ligaments. **B,** the Bankart lesion can vary from complete labral detachment with partial periosteal stripping of the anterior scapular neck to extensive periosteal stripping with or without a bony avulsion fracture of the anterior glenoid rim. **C,** anterior exposure demonstrating a Bankart lesion *(arrows)* in a right shoulder. The anterior portion of the glenoid articular surface is visible to the *left*.

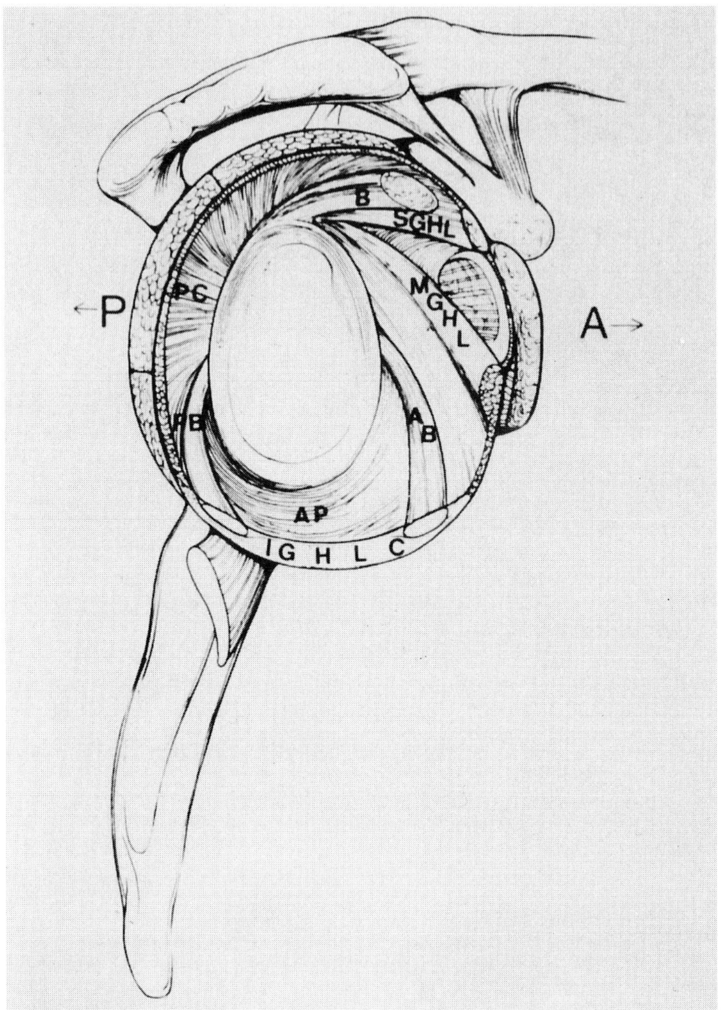

FIGURE 6.

Normal glenohumeral ligament anatomy. This is a right shoulder and the humeral head has been removed to present the glenoid from a lateral view. Anterior *(A)* is to the right and posterior *(P)* to the left. The inferior glenohumeral ligament complex *(IGHLC)* is composed of anterior *(AB)* and posterior *(PB)* bands with an interposed axillary pouch *(AP)*. The middle *(MGHL)* and superior *(SGHL)* glenohumeral ligaments are labeled, as are the biceps *(B)* and posterior capsule *(PC)*. (From O'Brien SJ, Neves MC, Arnoczky SJ, et al: *Am J Sports Med* 18:449–456, 1990. Used by permission.)

Coracohumeral Ligament

The coracohumeral ligament (CHL) originates as a broad band from the base and the lateral border of the coracoid process, and it passes obliquely downward and laterally to the humerus, bridging the rotator interval, between the anterior margin of the supraspinatous tendon and the superior margin of the subscapularis tendon (Fig 7).[33, 44, 45] Laterally, the ligament separates into two major bands that insert into the greater and lesser tuberosities, with a broad insertion over the anatomic neck of the humerus; this creates a tunnel near the bicipital groove through which the biceps

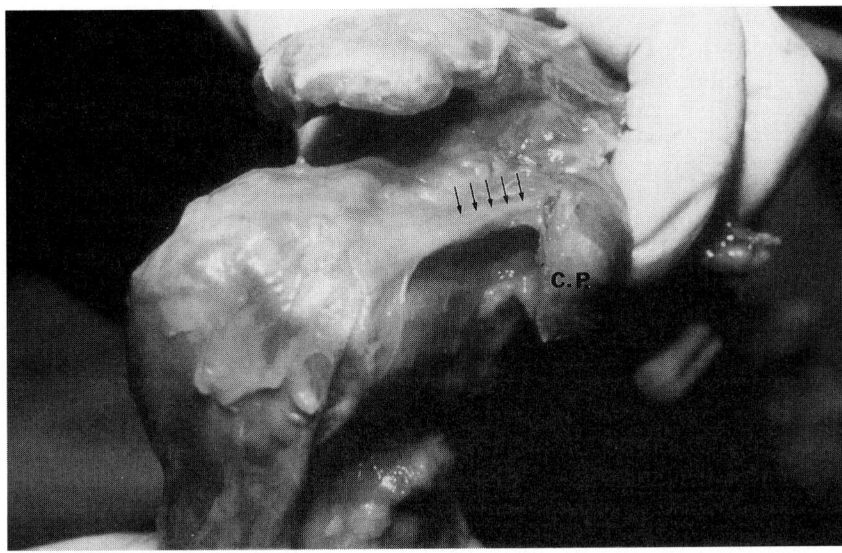

FIGURE 7.
The coracohumeral ligament *(arrows)* in a right shoulder. The coracoid process *(C.P.)* is labeled.

tendon passes. Inferiorly, the CHL blends with the superior glenohumeral ligament (SGHL). Although there is some controversy as to the robustness of this structure, it is generally believed that its major stabilizing role is to passively limit external rotation and inferior translation in the adducted shoulder.[4, 44, 46–51] It has also been shown to be a secondary static stabilizer against posterior translation of the flexed, adducted, and internally rotated shoulder.[52] Lesions of this ligament might be seen in the form of a "rotator interval" defect, and it has been our experience that deficiency of the capsule in this region is often associated with the finding of a large "sulcus sign." Contracture or scarring of this structure has been demonstrated to be one of the principal lesions in adhesive capsulitis.[46, 53]

Superior Glenohumeral Ligament

The SGHL is the most diminutive of the glenohumeral ligaments, although it is present in over 90% of shoulders.[4, 33, 51, 54] The SGHL arises from the labrum along the anterosuperior edge of the glenoid, just inferior to the origin of the tendon of the long head of the biceps, and inserts into the lesser tuberosity of the humerus. Generally it is believed that its function is similar to that of the CHL, although its structural and anatomic characteristics appear to make it less important as a static stabilizer.[4, 47, 51]

Middle Glenohumeral Ligament

The middle glenohumeral ligament (MGHL) has the greatest variation in size of all the ligaments of the shoulder. Furthermore, it is absent or poorly defined in up to 40%. It originates from the supraglenoid tubercle and anterosuperior portion of the labrum, often along with the SGHL, and inserts anteriorly on the base of the lesser tuberosity of the humeral neck, blending with the posterior aspect of the subscapularis muscle. It can be either a discrete band-like structure above the anterior band of the inferior glenohumeral ligament, or it can be sheet-like and confluent with the anterior band of the inferior glenohumeral ligament. It is believed to contribute to stability by acting as a passive restraint to both anterior and inferior translation of the humeral head when the shoulder is in the lower ranges of abduction.[51, 55]

Inferior Glenohumeral Ligament Complex

The inferior glenohumeral ligament complex (IGHLC) is composed of discreet thick anterior and posterior bands with an interposed axillary pouch. O'Brien et al.[1] suggested that this complex functions in a fashion analogous to a hammock: it supports the humeral head in the glenoid during abduction and rotation of the shoulder joint and acts as a barrier against dislocation of the humeral head (Fig 8). This region of the capsule has been shown to have sufficient anatomic, geometric, and structural properties to be a significant static stabilizer.[56, 57] It is generally believed that this ligamentous complex contributes to stability in the abducted shoulder mainly by limiting anterior, posterior, and inferior translation.[8, 51, 52, 55, 58, 59] Its hammock-like arrangement allows for reciprocal movement around the humeral head to act both as a barrier against anterior translation when the shoulder is abducted and externally rotated and as a barrier against posterior translation when the shoulder is abducted and internally rotated.

Posterior Capsule

This is the region of the capsule posterior and superior to the posterior band of the IGHLC.[1] It represents the thinnest region of the joint capsule, and its role is to limit posterior translation when the shoulder is forward-flexed, adducted, and internally rotated.[52]

NEGATIVE INTRA-ARTICULAR PRESSURE

In a normal shoulder joint there is a vacuum effect that is believed to be the result of high osmotic pressure in the interstitial tissues causing water to be drawn out of the glenohumeral joint.[60] This produces an intra-articular pressure within the closed joint compartment that is negative in comparison to atmospheric pressure. This vacuum phenomenon has the effect of resisting displacement of the articular surfaces away from one another.[61] The magnitude of this effect appears to be dependent on arm position and muscle activity. With the arm at the side and the muscles relaxed, this effect is quite important for prevention of inferior stability; however, as the shoulder is abducted and the muscles contract, the magnitude of this negative-pressure effect is minimal.[62–64] Any condition that disrupts the capsule (capsular rupture, "rotator interval" lesion) or increases the volume of the joint compartment (capsular laxity) will reduce the stabilizing vacuum effect of negative intra-articular pressure.

ADHESION-COHESION

Adhesion-cohesion is believed to be a stabilizing mechanism in which the synovial fluid between the opposing articular surfaces allows sliding

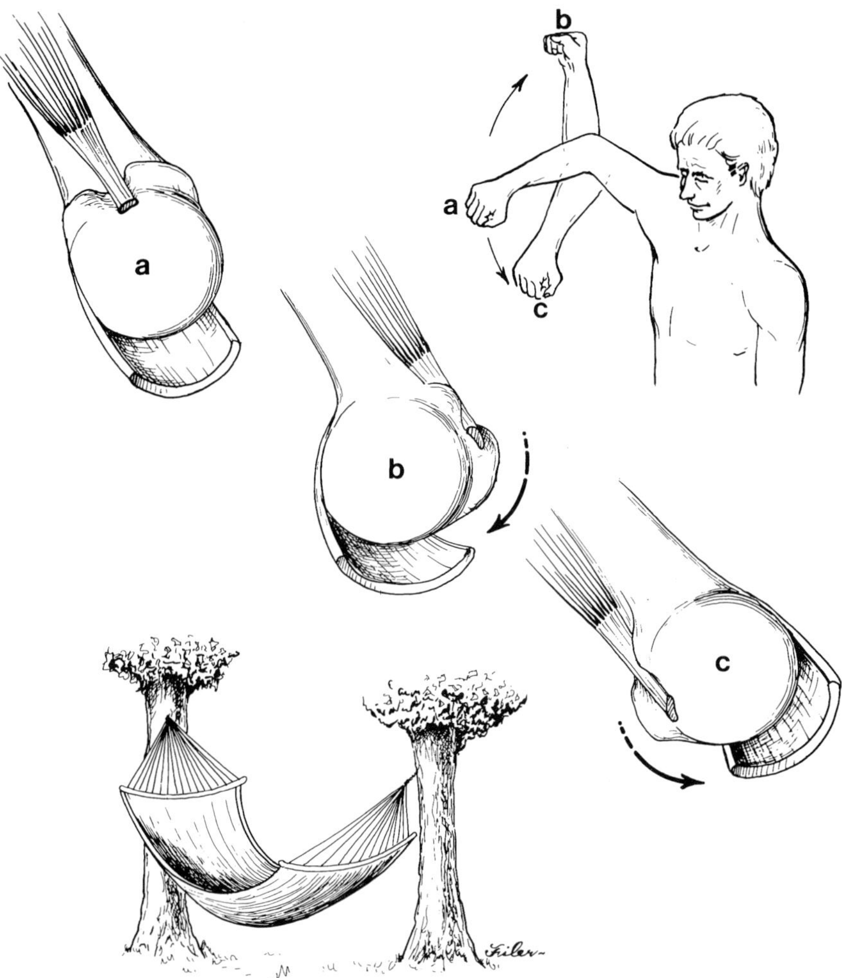

FIGURE 8.

The inferior glenohumeral ligament complex functions in a fashion analogous to a hammock so that in an abducted shoulder it comes underneath the humeral head *(a)*; with external *(b)* and internal *(c)* rotation it moves anteriorly and posteriorly, respectively, thus acting as a barrier to translation of the humeral head in these directions. (Adapted from O'Brien SJ, Neves MC, Arnoczky SJ, et al: *Am J Sports Med* 18:449–456, 1990.)

motion between the two joint surfaces while preventing them from being pulled apart.[60] This is analogous to the situation in which a drinking glass can slide in a film of water on a glass table top but momentarily sticks during attempts to lift the glass off the table top.[60]

DYNAMIC FACTORS

ROTATOR CUFF

The rotator cuff is the musculotendinous complex of four tendons (supraspinatus, infraspinatus, subscapularis, teres minor) that encircle the humeral head and are intricately conjoined with the underlying joint capsule.[65] These structures contribute to stability of the glenohumeral joint dynamically through two mechanisms: (1) the combined action of these muscles results in joint compression creating a concavity-compression fit of the articular surfaces.[38, 39, 66, 67] This joint compression mechanism resists shear and distraction forces tending to displace the humeral head out of the glenoid during forceful shoulder motions (i.e., throwing). (2) Synchronous and coordinated contraction of these muscle units maintains stability by steering the humeral head into the glenoid cavity during shoulder motion.[68–70] The infraspinatus and teres minor have been shown to be especially important in anterior stability when the shoulder is in a position of abduction and external rotation.[71–73]

Injury to the rotator cuff can occur from either a single macrotrauma and cumulative microtrauma, as in overuse injuries. In the former case, a dislocation is not uncommonly associated with a rotator cuff tear in individuals over the age of 40. This is due to the relative age-related attrition of the rotator cuff tendon tissues.[74, 75] In the latter case, repetitive eccentric loading during forceful overhead throwing maneuvers may result in gradual attrition of the supraspinatus insertion. This occurs as the rotator cuff muscles attempt to contain the humeral head in the glenoid.

The importance of normal rotator cuff function to shoulder stability cannot be overemphasized. All therapeutic approaches to shoulder instability emphasize strengthening and conditioning of the rotator cuff as an integral part of the treatment program.[76]

TENDON OF THE LONG HEAD OF THE BICEPS BRACHII

The tendon of the long head of the biceps brachii has been demonstrated to have a major dynamic stabilizing role for the glenohumeral joint. Although electromyography studies have shown that firing of the biceps is most related to elbow function and not to shoulder function,[68] experimental work has also shown that this tendon can significantly increase torsional rigidity of the joint and thus tend to resist external rotation during the late cocking phase of the throwing motion.[77] Furthermore, active contraction of this muscle-tendon unit has been shown to provide significant stability in both the anterior and superior planes.[78–80] This understanding of the normal stabilizing role of the biceps tendon also helps explain the association of SLAP (superior labral detachment anterior and posterior) lesions and anterior shoulder instability.[81, 82]

CLASSIFICATION OF SHOULDER INSTABILITY

We use a classification system for shoulder instability that is based on four factors: the degree of instability, the frequency of occurrence, direction, and etiology of the instability. Categorization of patients according to this format improves our ability to tailor individualized treatment programs for our patients (Table 3).[83–85]

The *degree of instability* is further categorized by the spectrum of injury to the capsulolabral structures. *Dislocation* is defined as complete separation of the glenohumeral articular surfaces, whereas *subluxation* is defined as symptomatic increased humeral head translation on the gle-

TABLE 3.
Shoulder Instability Classification

Frequency
Acute
Recurrent
Fixed (chronic)
Etiology
Traumatic (macrotrauma)
Atraumatic (voluntary, involuntary)
Microtrauma
Congenital
Neuromuscular (Erb's palsy, cerebral palsy, seizures)
Direction
Anterior
Posterior
Inferior
Multidirectional
Degree
Dislocation
Subluxation
Microtrauma (transient)

noid to a degree beyond normal tissue laxity but without complete separation of the glenohumeral articular surfaces. Subluxation of the glenohumeral joint is transient, and the humeral head spontaneously reduces to its normal position in the glenoid fossa.

The *frequency of instability* is described as acute, chronic, or recurrent. An acute episode of glenohumeral instability is one in which the patient is seen within the first 24 hours of the injury. If the glenohumeral joint has been dislocated for a longer period, it is termed a *chronic dislocation. Recurrent instability* describes repeated glenohumeral subluxations, dislocations, or both. A *locked dislocation* describes a chronic glenohumeral dislocation that is irreducible by closed means and is usually seen with an impression defect (Hill-Sachs lesion or reverse Hill-Sachs lesion) of the humeral head.

The *direction of instability* is categorized as anterior, posterior, inferior, or multidirectional instability. Appreciation of the direction of instability is critical to choosing a successful approach to treatment. Although traditionally 95% of all instability has been observed as simple anterior, there has been an increasing recognition of significant posterior instability in athletes. When it occurs, the degree of posterior instability is usually subluxation; however, dislocation occurs with rare, traumatic episodes.

Since Neer and Foster's[86] paper on multidirectional instability, there has been an increasing awareness of both traumatic and atraumatic capsular laxity occurring in more than one direction. The main direction of instability is usually anterior, although inferior instability is the hallmark of this diagnosis. Traditional procedures that treat anterior capsular laxity by Bankart repair or capsular plication may not adequately manage the associated components of inferior and/or posterior instability. In the worst scenario, asymmetrical tightening of the joint capsule may actually lead to fixed subluxation in the opposite direction.[58, 87]

Another dilemma concerning the direction of instability is that some patients may have pain with no knowledge of underlying instability. In fact, many patients with subluxation complain only of pain and have no sense of actual shoulder instability. This can especially be the case in throwing athletes with subtle anterior subluxation and secondary impingement. It also can occur in patients with multidirectional or posterior instability and associated tendonitis.[36, 84, 88]

The *etiology of shoulder* instability may be categorized as traumatic, atraumatic, arising from microtrauma or repetitive overuse, congenital, or neuromuscular. Thomas and Matsen[89] have introduced the acronyms TUBS and AMBRI to aid in classifying the etiology of the majority of patients with instability of the shoulder. The TUBS acronym represents patients who have *t*raumatic instability that is *u*nidirectional in nature, have a *B*ankart lesion, and typically respond well to *s*urgery. The AMBRI acronym represents patients with *a*traumatic instability that is *m*ultidirectional in nature with *b*ilateral shoulder findings; these patients respond best to *r*ehabilitation, but when surgery is necessary in this latter group of patients, it is usually an *i*nferior capsular shift. In our experience, these two acronyms represent each end of a spectrum of pathology. Some patients may have pre-existent constitutional hyperlaxity but experience some type of traumatic event leading to an anterior shoulder dislocation.[90–93] Furthermore, some individuals will have both a Bankart lesion and capsular laxity or rupture following a traumatic dislocation.[94–96]

Clinical instability appears to develop in some patients because of repeated microtrauma or chronic overload, such as in swimmers or throwing athletes.[70] They may have underlying ligamentous laxity, which enables them to excel at their sport, but symptomatic instability may develop from repetitive microtrauma.[90, 97–99a]

A congenital basis for instability may result from developmental anomalies of the proximal portion of the humerus or glenoid. Although these are rare, they can include abnormalities of articular version, dysplasia, and neurologic disorders (i.e., stroke, seizure, Erb's palsy).

It is important to consider whether the dislocation or subluxation is *voluntary* or *involuntary* in nature. With voluntary instability the patient is able to place the shoulder into a position so that with selective muscle contraction and relaxation, he can subluxate or dislocate the shoulder anteriorly, posteriorly, or inferiorly. Voluntary subluxation can be associated with emotional and psychiatric disorders.[100] An important distinction must be made between a patient who is able to dislocate the shoulder on a voluntary basis with muscular contraction and a patient who can dislocate the shoulder by selectively positioning the arm. The first patient may be motivated by secondary gain and should not have surgical treatment. In the second patient, the instability is often disabling to the patient, and although such patients can voluntarily demonstrate instability by positioning their arm, they prefer not to do so. The instability, in fact, impairs their daily activities because they must avoid those positions in which the shoulder dislocates.[84] In our experience, most patients with involuntary posterior instability can demonstrate a voluntary positional type of instability as well. We generally do not exclude these individuals from surgical treatment if conservative measures fail.

NATURAL HISTORY AND NONOPERATIVE TREATMENT

Recurrence is the most common complication of anterior shoulder instability.[42, 94, 101–110] The risk of redislocation is directly proportional to the patient's youth and activity level.[30, 35, 36, 106] Management of a traumatic first-time anterior dislocation remains controversial. Watson-Jones[111] in 1948 advocated immobilization in full internal rotation for at least 4 weeks and stated that he had never seen a recurrence after using this treatment. Subsequent reports have failed to support this claim. McLaughlin and Cavallaro[110] in 1950 reported a 50% recurrence rate but had follow-up on only 18% of 573 patients. Recurrence was 90% in patients less than 20 years old. Rowe and Sakellarides[35] reported an overall recurrence of 58% in a series of 398 patients with follow-up on 53%. Recurrence was strongly related to age, with an incidence of recurrence of 94% in patients under the age of 20, 79% between 20 and 40, and 14% over the age of 40.

The incidence of recurrence after immobilization following the initial dislocation has varied. Rowe and Sakellarides[35] found decreased recurrence after immobilization and recommended 3 weeks in a sling. Henry and Genung,[105] in reviewing 121 high-risk young athletes, found 85% recurrence after no immobilization and 90% recurrence after immobilization for a varied time period.

Hovelius[106,107] reported 2- and 5-year follow-up results of a prospective multicenter study on the effect of immobilization on recurrence, and only those patients who were strictly compliant with the immobilization were included in the comparison. He found that 3 to 4 weeks of immobilization had no effect on the recurrence rate. Again, recurrence correlated highly with the age of the patient. Two or more recurrences had occurred in 55% of the shoulders in patients who were 22 years old or younger, in 37% of the shoulders in patients who were 23 to 29 years old, and in 12% of the shoulders in patients who were 30 to 40 years old. Surgery for the treatment of instability had been performed or was scheduled to be performed in 28%, 18%, and 5%, respectively, of the shoulders in the three age groups. The vast majority of recurrences occur within the first 2 years after the initial dislocation. In the 5-year follow-up study, Hovelius[106, 107] noted that recurrence was only 10% more frequent at the 5-year follow-up as compared with the 2-year follow-up in patients under 30. There was no difference in patients older than 30.

The risk of recurrence following traumatic anterior dislocation in children is especially high. Marans et al.[108] reported a series of 21 patients with open physes and who had radiographic evidence of traumatic anterior dislocation. All 21 patients had one or more recurrent dislocations. Treatment, including immobilization in a sling and swath for as long as 6 weeks, had no effect on the rate of recurrence.

The long-term outcome of voluntary subluxation of the shoulder in children has been reported by Huber and Gerber.[112] Twenty-five patients with 36 affected shoulders were reviewed at skeletal maturity at an average follow-up of 12 years. Nineteen patients (26 shoulders) had no specific treatment. These patients were managed with "skillful neglect." All were employed and had no limitations in their jobs. Two patients required shoulder surgery in adult life but only after trauma. In 18 of the 26 shoulders, voluntary subluxation was still possible, but symptoms were minimal. Seven children (10 shoulders) had undergone stabilizing operations during childhood. Only 3 patients (5 of the 10 shoulders) had good results; 2 shoulders had recurrent instability, 2 were painful and 1 was stiff. In none of the patients in either group did osteoarthritic changes develop.

The effect of a specific rehabilitation program for the shoulder on recurrence of shoulder instability is controversial. Aronen and Regan[101] decreased the prevalence of recurrence of a single anterior traumatic dislocation of the shoulder to 25% with a combination of isometric, isotonic, and isokinetic exercises. However, 4 (20%) of their 20 patients had undergone surgery after 3 years, and this percentage was similar to that in Hovelius' series of patients treated with no formal therapy program.

Burkhead and Rockwood[76] reported the results of a specific shoulder rehabilitation program for 140 shoulders in 115 patients with a diagnosis of traumatic or atraumatic recurrent anterior, posterior, or multidirectional instability. Only 12 (16%) of the 74 shoulders that had traumatic subluxation had a good or excellent result after the exercise program. In the 61 shoulders that had atraumatic subluxation and no psychological illnesses, 53 (87%) had good or excellent results with the rehabilitation program.

Wheeler et al.[113] reported the outcome of acute anterior dislocation of the shoulder in cadets at the U.S. Military Academy. This group of patients, by desire and by necessity, must return to sports and full activity because part of their educational process is a year-round program of physical training, testing, and competitive sports. A nonoperative treatment program was used that consisted of 3 weeks of immobilization, a supervisory rehabilitation program, and restrictions from contact, throwing, and overhead sports for 3 months. The prevalence of recurrent instability was 92% (35 of 38) in cadets treated nonoperatively. Strict adherence to the complete rehabilitation program was inconsistent, but strict adherence to the program was found to have no effect on the recurrence rate.

SURGICAL TREATMENT ALTERNATIVES

ANTERIOR AND MULTIDIRECTIONAL INSTABILITY

All treatment must be formulated on an individualized basis by taking into account the specific need of each patient as well as the pathology encountered during the surgery. This is especially the case in athletes, where the type of sport, age, position, level of ability, laxity, and arm dominance are all factors in decision making. A successful outcome is defined not just as a stable shoulder but also as one that retains a full, pain-free, functional range of motion.

Traditionally, many surgical reports for instability have accepted and even desired some postoperative loss of external rotation. Many of these procedures were "nonanatomic" in the sense that they did not directly restore pathologic anatomy to normal but attempted to substitute changes in surrounding structures to constrain the shoulder joint and prevent instability.[89, 114–125] Currently, most shoulder surgeons perform an anatomic repair that attempts to identify the specific pathology associated with the patient's instability and then correct it. In cases of traumatic anterior instability, the Bankart lesion is the most common finding*; however, intracapsular injury may also be a concomitant finding.[94–96] Moreover, some authors have suggested that inherent or congenital laxity may be a pre-existent risk factor in individuals in whom traumatic anterior instability develops.[90–93] In practice it may be very difficult to distinguish physiologic laxity from pathologic laxity resulting from a capsular injury.[130–133] The senior author (J.P.W.) has had some success in clarifying this issue through the use of examination under anesthesia (EUA) combined with direct arthroscopic inspection.[99, 134, 135] Patients who are found to have a large "sulcus sign" (>2+) in the setting of traumatic dislocation or subluxation are considered to have a significant inferior component to their anterior instability (Fig 9).[86, 97, 136, 137] Some of these individuals have a Bankart lesion in combination with a capsular injury, and some have a capsular injury without a Bankart lesion (Fig 10). In these cases we incorporate a capsular shift into the Bankart repair. These anteroinferior capsular shift techniques have been clearly described in prior publications.[30, 86, 97, 136–140a] The senior author (J.P.W.) has, however, observed that there is a tendency to lose some external rotation with these techniques. Therefore we have attempted to modify our surgical technique in order to preserve as much motion as possible while restoring adequate capsular tension for stability.[141] This is accomplished by selectively shifting the inferior and superior portions of the anterior capsule in a manner that respects their normal anatomic length-tension relationships.[51, 66, 141] Each portion of the capsular shift is performed with the shoulder positioned so that the capsule can be tensioned closed to its maximally lengthened position, thereby avoiding overconstraining the joint. For the inferior capsule this is accomplished by placing the arm in a position of 60 degrees' abduction, 60 degrees' external rotation, and 10 degrees' forward flexion. The superior capsule is then shifted inferiorly and laterally with the shoulder in a position of adduction and 45 degrees' external rotation. The senior author's (J.P.W.) initial experience[141] in the majority of patients has been nearly symmetrical range of motion and a stable shoulder.

In patients with straightforward traumatic anterior instability, a discrete Bankart lesion, no significant inferior laxity on EUA, and a normal-

*References 30, 36, 41, 42, 94, 104, 121, 126–129.

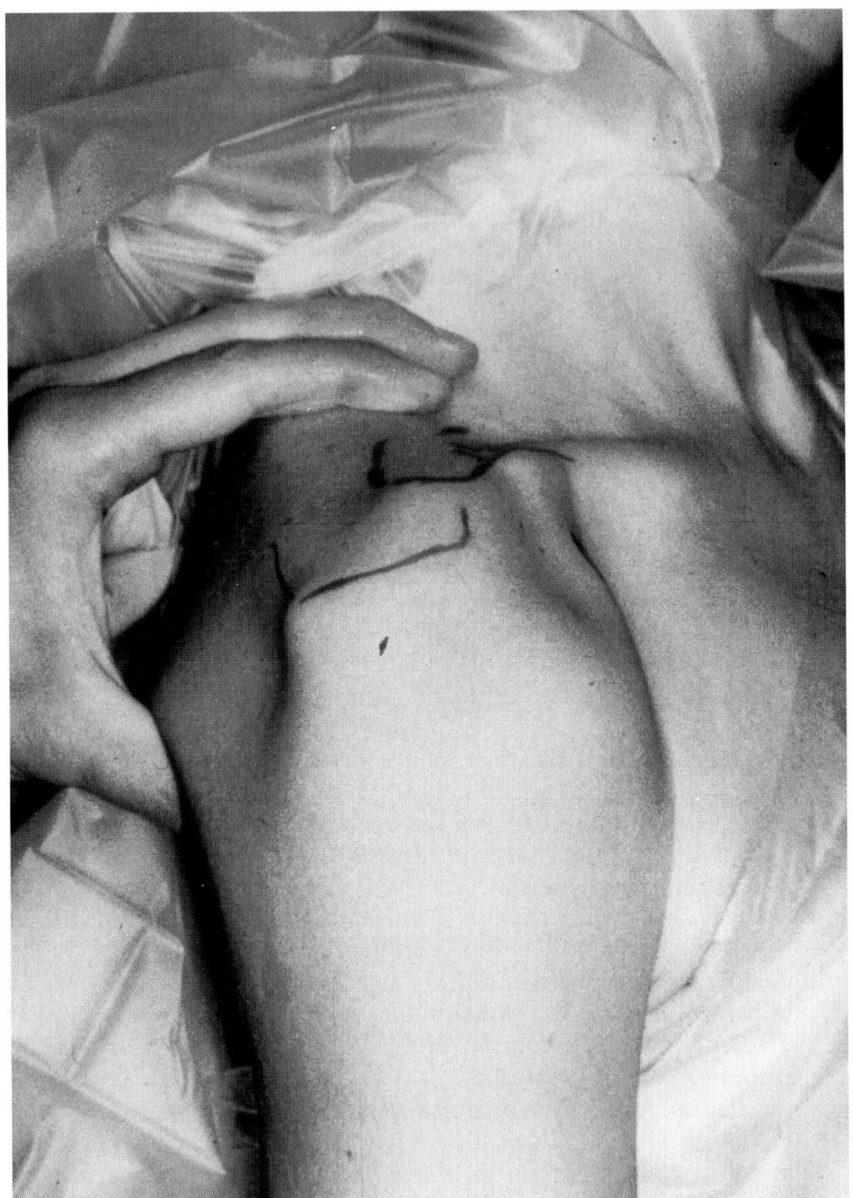

FIGURE 9.
Patient with a large sulcus sign (3+) (see the text for an explanation).

appearing inferior glenohumeral ligament, a classic Bankart repair is very reliable for restoration of stability and preservation of motion. In our hands this is accomplished arthroscopically.[96, 142, 143]

In the case of chronic, atraumatic multidirectional instability with an anteroinferior pattern of laxity that is refractory to conservative treatment, the inferior capsular shift as originally described by Neer and Foster[86] has been a reliable treatment approach. More recent experience by others has supported this approach.[97, 136, 144] However, in the senior author's ex-

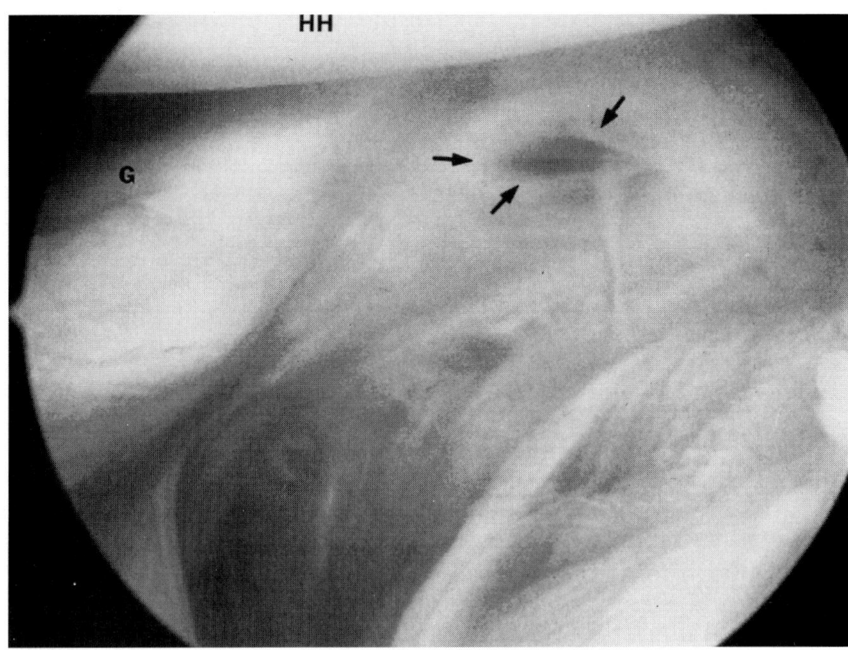

FIGURE 10.
Arthroscopic view through the anterosuperior portal in the left shoulder of a patient with an acute anterior shoulder dislocation. There has been a rupture of the anterior capsule *(arrows)*. The glenoid *(G)* and humeral head *(HH)* are labeled.

perience (J.P.W.) these patients do not usually recover sufficient endurance and tolerance to repetitive overhead motions or heavy lifting.

POSTERIOR INSTABILITY

As stated previously, most posterior dislocations spontaneously reduce, and posterior instability, when it occurs, is more typically recurrent subluxation rather than dislocation.[18, 145–147] Nonoperative or conservative treatment has been the initial approach recommended by most surgeons.[37, 69, 98, 145] Conservative treatment of shoulder instability generally involves strengthening the dynamic muscular stabilizers (rotator cuff and long head of the biceps) of the glenohumeral joint as well as the periscapular muscles (serratus anterior, trapezius, rhomboids). Furthermore, in these patients with posterior shoulder instability, exercises that place the arm in a flexed, relatively adducted position, such as bench press weight lifting, should be avoided.

When nonoperative treatment is unsuccessful and the instability is disabling, most authors recommend operative stabilization. Historically, reconstructions for posterior instability have been reported to be less successful than anterior reconstructions.[144, 147–149] However, because the responsible pathology has been a matter of ongoing debate, there has been no consensus on the optimal method of operative stabilization. Hawkins et al.[144] reported poor results of treatment for posterior instability in 35 patients (50 shoulders); however, this series was suboptimal since 41 of these patients had voluntary instability and only 11 were attributed to trauma. Furthermore, in 26 shoulders, a variety of procedures were performed by many different surgeons. These included 17 glenoid osteotomies, 6 reverse Putti-Platt procedures, and 3 biceps transfers, with an associated recurrence rate of 41%, 83%, and 33%, respectively. Overall, there was a 50% recurrent rate with operative treatment. Similarly, Norwood and Terry[149] reported that only 10 of 19 patients (53%) were stable at follow-up after glenoid osteotomy. Tibone and Ting[147] reported a 30% recurrence rate after posterior staple capsulorraphy with a 40% complication rate and only 1 of 20 patients returning to throwing.

Several other surgeons have reported a much more favorable outcome of surgery for posterior instability.[145, 150, 151] The consistent factor in these studies is the recognition of posteroinferior capsular laxity or excessive redundancy and its treatment by a posteroinferior capsular shift. Fronek et al.[145] reported the results of 27 patients with posterior subluxation. Sixteen of the 27 patients had not had a major single causative traumatic event and were successfully treated with rehabilitation alone. Eleven patients with a traumatic episode or major disability caused by instability were treated surgically with a 91% successful outcome. Bone block procedures were rarely necessary, and the ability to voluntarily sublux the shoulder by positioning it did not affect the result. Surgery was successful in returning several professional football players to their previous level of play.

Bigliani et al.[150] reported similar results when a posteroinferior capsular shift was used to address the posterior and inferior capsular redundancy. Their preliminary results with this procedure were a good to excellent outcome in 22 of the 25 shoulders. All but 2 patients returned to work, and most could resume their sporting activities. At long-term follow-up evaluation[133] (average, 5 years) of 38 shoulders treated with the posterior capsular shift procedure, the results were satisfactory in 80%. When only primary cases were included, the success rate increased to 96% (24 of 25 shoulders).

A posteroinferior capsular shift can be combined with a labral repair when there is a concomitant reverse Bankart lesion. Augmentation with a bone graft harvested from the scapular spine is used only in rare cases, such as when significant glenoid hypoplasia is present or in certain revision situations in which there is frank loss of the posterior glenoid surface.

Tibone and Ting[147] reported the results of posterior capsulorraphy in athletes with posterior subluxation. Seventy percent of the patients improved enough with a conservative program to the point that they were able to participate in their sport without problems. In patients treated operatively with posterior capsulorraphy, the rate of recurrence of instability after surgery was high (27.5%). However, in the patients in this series, posterior instability most commonly developed after overuse of the shoulder or a minor traumatic injury followed by insidious symptoms, so-called microtrauma rather than macrotrauma. Gross trauma was an uncommon cause of posterior instability in this athletic population. Success as measured by return to throwing was poor in that only 28% (4 of

14) of elite throwers returned to throwing whereas 50% of the competitive and 60% of the recreational athletes returned to their sports.

Our approach to patients with refractory chronic posterior instability is a posteroinferior capsular shift similar to the method described by Fronek,[145] Bigliani,[150] and their coworkers. The procedure is performed through a 5- to 6-cm skin incision centered over the posterior aspect of the glenohumeral joint and in Langher's lines. The deltoid muscle is split in line with its fibers, beginning at the scapular spine and extending distally 5 to 6 cm. Care is taken to not split the deltoid muscle distally beyond the teres minor muscle because this might injure the axillary nerve. The interval between the infraspinatus and the teres minor is identified. This interval is developed by blunt dissection, and the capsule is freed from the overlying muscles. We try to detach only several centimeters of the rotator cuff tendons from their insertions. Careful sharp and blunt dissection allows mobilization of the interval between the rotator cuff tendons and the capsule so that a T-plasty type of shift can be performed at the glenoid rim. When the inferior and superior capsular flaps are closed, the shoulder is positioned in slight abduction and neutral rotation. We have actually seen several cases in which there was loss of internal rotation after this procedure, so we try to avoid shifting the posterior capsule with the arm in external rotation. The senior author (J.P.W.) has not used a posterior bone block in a 5-year experience of 36 cases, and posterior glenoid osteotomy is reserved only for those rare cases with documented excessive retroversion.

Postoperatively, the patient is placed in a prefabricated "gunslinger" brace with the shoulder positioned in neutral rotation and 10 degrees' abduction and extension. The brace is worn full-time for 6 weeks.

The senior author's (J.P.W.) 5-year experience with 36 cases has been good to excellent results in 33 cases. One patient had recurrent instability and 2 patients experienced symptomatic loss of internal rotation and forward flexion that required a second procedure to restore motion. Five patients have been able to continue playing competitive football at the high school or collegiate level.

THE ROLE OF ARTHROSCOPIC SHOULDER STABILIZATION

Over the past decade there has been growing enthusiasm for arthroscopic approaches in the treatment of shoulder instability. This has developed as a result of advancements in instrumentation and techniques, as well as a more sound appreciation of the spectrum of pathology that accompanies shoulder instability. Furthermore, it has been recognized that some open approaches have the drawbacks of requiring inpatient stay, causing surgical morbidity by dissection through otherwise normal tissue planes, having the potential for limitation external rotation, and resulting in a less than satisfactory cosmetic scar.[87] The potential advantages of an arthroscopic repair of shoulder instability are the ability to identify concomitant intra-articular pathology (i.e., SLAP lesions, Hill-Sachs lesions, rotator cuff tears), selectively repair the Bankart lesion in an outpatient setting, create less postoperative pain for the patient, achieve better cosmesis, and permit more full return of motion.* Furthermore, direct arthroscopic inspection has been very helpful in the identification of concomitant capsular injuries. In addition, depending on the experience of the surgeon, an arthroscopic approach may be easier and faster than an open repair technique.[143, 157]

Despite these theoretical advantages, the recurrence rate after most arthroscopic stabilization procedures remain over twice that of a standard open capsulolabral repair technique.[152–157] In addition, staple repair techniques have had the major drawbacks of loosening and breakage of implants with articular injury.[159] The transosseous suture techniques have their own disadvantages of risk to neurovascular structures from pin placement and the necessity of an accessory posterior incision through which the sutures must be tied.

Despite all these drawbacks, enthusiasm continues for these approaches. Recent developments in bioabsorbable fixation techniques and refined patient selection and surgical technique offer the promise of improving the reliability of this type of surgical approach.

The senior author (J.P.W.) reserves an arthroscopic approach for individuals with recurrent, post-traumatic anterior instability who are found on examination to have anterior instability without significant inferior laxity and on arthroscopic inspection to have a discrete Bankart lesion with no evidence of capsular injury. In our hands this technique has been applied to 104 patients over the past 4 years with a recurrence rate of 7%.[96]

SUMMARY

Advances in our understanding of the factors that maintain stability and the spectrum of pathology associated with instability have led to a more organized and quantitative approach to the treatment of these clinical conditions. Open surgical techniques for the treatment of anterior instability are very reliable for achieving stability; however, return to forceful overhead athletics is less ensured. In general, the success rate for surgical treatment of atraumatic and multidirectional instability as well as posterior instability is less than that for approaches to anterior instability. However, these surgical procedures are also relatively reliable. Arthroscopic techniques continue to develop but the long-term efficacy of these techniques has not yet been established.

REFERENCES

1. O'Brien SJ, Neves MC, Arnoczky SJ, et al: The anatomy and histology of the inferior glenohumeral ligament complex of the shoulder. *Am J Sports Med* 18:449–456, 1990.
2. Soslowsky LJ, Flatow EL, Bigliani LU, et al: Articular geometry of the glenohumeral joint. *Clin Orthop* 285:181–190, 1992.
3. Doos SP, Ray GS, Saha AK: Observation of the tilt of the glenoid cavity of the scapula. *J Anat Soc India* 15:114, 1966.

*References 82, 96, 102, 113, 134, 142, 143, 152–158.

4. Ovesen J, Nielsen S: Stability of the shoulder joint: Cadaver study of stabilizing structures. *Acta Orthop Scand* 56:149–151, 1985.
5. Saha AK: *Theory of Shoulder Mechanism: Descriptive and Applied.* Springfield, Ill, Charles C Thomas, 1961.
6. Saha AK: Dynamic stability of the glenohumeral joint. *Acta Orthop Scand* 42:491–505, 1971.
7. Sarrafian SK: Gross and functional anatomy of the shoulder. *Clin Orthop* 173:11–19, 1983.
8. Schwartz R, O'Brien SJ, Warren RF, et al: Capsular restraints to anterior-posterior motion of the abducted shoulder. *Orthop Trans* 12:727, 1988.
9. Basmajian JV, Bazant FJ: Factors preventing downward dislocation of the adducted shoulder joint. *J Bone Joint Surg Am* 41:1182–1186, 1959.
10. Bestard EA, Schuene HR, Bestard EH: Glenoplasty in the management of recurrent shoulder dislocation. *Contemp Orthop* 12:47, 1986.
11. Galinat BJ, Howell SM, Kraft TA: The glenoid-posterior acromion angle: An accurate method of evaluating glenoid version. *Orthop Trans* 12:727, 1988.
12. Hill HA, Tkach L: The study of glenohumeral orientation in patients with anterior recurrent shoulder dislocations. *Orthop Trans* 9:47–48, 1986.
13. Hurley JA, Anderson TE, Dear W, et al: Posterior shoulder instability. Surgical versus conservative results with evaluation of glenoid version. *Am J Sports Med* 20:346–400, 1992.
14. Itoi E, Motzkin NE, Morrey BF, et al: Scapular inclination and inferior stability of the shoulder. *J Shoulder Elbow Surg* 1:131–139, 1992.
15. Mallon WJ, Brown HR, Vogler JB, et al: Radiographic and geometric anatomy of the scapula. *Clin Orthop* 277:142–154, 1992.
16. Randelli M, Gambrioli PL: Glenohumeral osteometry by computed tomography in normal and unstable shoulders. *Clin Orthop* 208:151–156, 1986.
17. Scott DJ Jr: Treatment of recurrent posterior dislocations of the shoulder by glenoplasty. Report of three cases. *J Bone Joint Surg Am* 49:471–476, 1967.
18. Brewer BJ, Wubber RC, Carrera GF: Excessive retroversion of the glenoid cavity. A cause of non-traumatic posterior instability of the shoulder. *J Bone Joint Surg* 68:724, 1986.
19. Chaudhuri GK, Sengupta A, Saha AK: Rotational osteotomy of the shaft of the humerus for recurrent dislocation of the shoulder: Anterior and posterior. *Acta Orthop Scand* 45:193, 1974.
20. Cyprien JM, Vasey HM, Burdet A, et al: Humeral retrotorsion and glenohumeral relationship in the normal shoulder and in recurrent anterior dislocation. *Clin Orthop* 175:8–17, 1983.
21. Inman VT, Saunders JR, Abbott LC: Observations on the function of the shoulder joint. *J Bone Joint Surg* 26:1–30, 1944.
22. Kronberg M, Brostrom L-A, Soderlund V: Retroversion of the humeral head in the normal shoulders and its relationship to normal range of motion. *Clin Orthop* 253:113–117, 1990.
23. Kronberg M, Brostrom L-A: Humeral head retroversion in patients with unstable humeroscapular joints. *Clin Orthop* 260:207–211, 1990.
24. Surin V, Blader S, Boras GM, et al: Rotational osteotomy of the humerus for posterior instability of the shoulder. *J Bone Joint Surg Am* 72:182–186, 1990.
25. Weber BG, Simpson LA, Hardegger F: Rotational osteotomy for recurrent anterior dislocation of the shoulder associated with a large Hill-Sachs lesion. *J Bone Joint Surg Am* 66:1443–1450, 1984.
26. Weber BG: Recurrent dislocation of the shoulder. Treatment with subcapital rotational osteotomy. *Acta Orthop Scand* 45:986–988, 1974.

27. Calandra JJ, Baker CL, Uribe JW: The incidence of Hill-Sachs lesions in initial anterior shoulder dislocations. *Arthroscopy* 5:254–257, 1989.
28. Eve FS: A case of subcoracoid dislocation of the humerus with the formation of an indentation on the posterior surface of the humeral head. *Medicochir Trans Soc London* 63:317–321, 1880.
29. Pavlov H, Warren RF, Weiss C, et al: The roentgenographic evaluation of certain surgical conditions. *Clin Orthop* 184:153–158, 1985.
30. Rowe CR, Patel D, Southmayd WW: The Bankart procedure: A long-term end-result study. *J Bone Joint Surg Am* 60:1–16, 1978.
31. Rowe CR, Zarins B, Ciullo JV: Recurrent anterior dislocation of the shoulder after surgical repair. *J Bone Joint Surg Am* 66:159–168, 1984.
32. Conolly JF: Humeral head defects associated with shoulder dislocation. The diagnostic and surgical significance. *Instr Course Lect* 21:42–52, 1972.
33. DePalma AF, Callery G, Bennett GA: Variational anatomy and degenerative lesions of the shoulder joint, in Blount WP (ed): *American Academy of Orthopaedic Surgeons Instructional Course Lectures.* Ann Arbor, Mich, JW Edwards, 1949, pp 225–281.
34. Hermodsson I: Rontgenologische Studern uber due Traumatischen und Habituellen Schultergelenk-Verrenhungen. Nach vorn un Nach Unten. *Acta Radiol Suppl* 20:1–173, 1934.
35. Rowe CR, Sakellarides HT: Factors related to recurrences of anterior dislocation of the shoulder. *Clin Orthop* 20:40–47, 1961.
36. Rowe CR, Zarins B: Recurrent transient subluxation of the shoulder. *J Bone Joint Surg Am* 63:863–872, 1981.
37. Neer CS II: *Shoulder Reconstruction.* Philadelphia, WB Saunders, 1990.
38. Howell SM, Galinat BJ: The glenoid-labral socket. A constrained articular surface. *Clin Orthop* 243:122–125, 1989.
39. Lippitt SB, Vanderhooft JE, Harris SL, et al: Glenohumeral stability from concavity-compression: A quantitative analysis. *J Shoulder Elbow Surg* 2:27–35, 1993.
40. Cooper DE, Arnoczky SP, O'Brien SJ, et al: Anatomy, histology and vascularity of the glenoid labrum. *J Bone Joint Surg Am* 74:46–52, 1992.
41. Bankart ASB: The pathology and treatment of rcurrent dislocation of the shoulder joint. *Br J Surg* 26:23–29, 1938.
42. Bankart ASB: Recurrent or habitual dislocation of the shoulder joint. *BMJ* 2:1132–1133, 1923.
43. Moseley HF, Overgaard B: The anterior capsular mechanism in recurrent anterior dislocation of the shoulder: Morphological and clinical studies with special reference to the glenoid labrum and glenohumeral ligaments. *J Bone Joint Surg Br* 44:913–927, 1962.
44. Cooper DE, O'Brien SJ, Arnoczky SP, et al: The structure and function of the coracohumeral ligament: An anatomic and microscopic study. *J Shoulder Elbow Surg* 2:70–77, 1993.
45. Soslowsky LJ, An CH, Johnston SP, et al: Geometric and mechanical properties of the coracoacromial ligament and their relationship to rotator cuff disease. *Trans Orthop Res Soc* 18:139, 1993.
46. Harryman DT, Sidles JA, Harris SL, et al: The role of the rotator interval capsule in passive motion and stability of the shoulder. *J Bone Joint Surg Am* 74:53–66, 1992.
47. Helmig P, Sojbjerg JO, Sneppen O, et al: Glenohumeral movement patterns after puncture of the joint capsule: An experimental study. *J Shoulder Elbow Surg* 2:209–215, 1993.
48. O'Connell PW, Nuber GW, Mileski RA, et al: The contribution of the glenohumeral ligaments to anterior stability of the shoulder joint. *Am J Sports Med* 18:579–589, 1990.

49. Terry GC, Hammon D, France P, et al: The stabilizing function of passive shoulder restraints. *Am J Sports Med* 19:26–34, 1991.
50. Warner JJP, Caborn DNM, Bergen R, et al: Dynamic capsuloligamentous anatomy of the glenohumeral joint. *J Shoulder Elbow Surg* 2:115–133, 1993.
51. Warner JJP, Deng X, Warren RF, et al: Static capsuloligamentous restraints to superior-inferior translation of the glenohumeral joint. *Am J Sports Med* 20:675–685, 1992.
52. Warren RF, Kornblatt IB, Marchand R: Static factors affeting posterior shoulder stability. *Orthop Trans* 8:89, 1984.
53. Neer CS II, Satterlee CC, Dalsey RM, et al: The anatomy and potential effects of contracture of the coracohumeral ligament. *Clin Orthop* 280:182–185, 1992.
54. Ferrari DA: Capsular ligaments of the shoulder: Anatomical and functional study of the anterior superior capsule. *Am J Sports Med* 18:20–24, 1990.
55. Turkel SJ, Panio MW, Marshall JL, et al: Stabilizing mechanisms preventing anterior dislocation of the glenohumeral joint. *J Bone Joint Surg Am* 63:1208–1217, 1981.
56. Bigliani LU, Pollock RG, Soslowski LJ, et al: Tensile properties of the inferior glenohumeral ligament. *J Orthop Res* 10:187–197, 1992.
57. Ticker JB, Flatow EL, Pawluk RJ, et al: The inferior glenohumeral ligament: A correlative biomechanical, biochemical and histological investigation. *Trans Orthop Res Soc* 39:313, 1993.
58. Bigliani LU, Flatow EL, Kelkar R, et al: Effect of anterior tightening on shoulder kinematics and contact. Presented at the Second World Congress of Biomechanics, Amsterdam, July 10–15, 1994, p 304.
59. Bowen MK, Deng X, Warren RF, et al: Role of the inferior glenohumeral ligament complex in limiting inferior translation of the glenohumeral joint. *Trans Orthop Res Soc* 38:497, 1992.
60. Matsen FA, Thomas SC, Rockwood CA: Anterior glenohumeral instability, in Rockwood CA, Matsen FA (eds): *The Shoulder*. Philadelphia, WB Saunders, 1990.
61. Gibb TD, Sidles JA, Harryman DT, et al: The effect of capsular venting on glenohumeral laxity. *Clin Orthop* 268:120–127, 1991.
62. Browne AO, Hoffmeyer P, An KN, et al: The influence of atmospheric pressure on shoulder stability. *Orthop Trans* 14:259, 1990.
63. Kumar VP, Balasubramaniam P: The role of atmospheric pressure in stabilising the shoulder. An experimental study. *J Bone Joint Surg Br* 67:719–721, 1985.
64. Warner JJP, Deng X, Warren RF, et al: Superior-inferior translation in the intact and vented glenohumeral joint. *J Shoulder Elbow Surg* 2:99–125, 1993.
65. Clark J, Sidles JA, Matsen FA: The relationship of the glenohumeral joint capsule to the rotator cuff. *Clin Orthop* 254:29–34, 1990.
66. Bowen MK, Deng XH, Warner JP, et al: The effect of joint compression on stability of the glenohumeral joint. *Trans Orthop Res Soc* 17:289, 1992.
67. Vanderhooft E, Lippitt S II, Matsen FA III: Glenohumeral stability from concavity compression: A quantitative analysis. Presented at the annual meeting of the American Shoulder and Elbow Surgeons, Washington, DC, Feb 23, 1992, p 14.
68. Bradley JP, Tibone JE: Electromyographic analysis of muscle action about the shoulder. *Clin Sports Med* 10:789–805, 1991.
69. Jobe FW: The shoulder in sports, in Rockwood CA, Matsen FA (eds): *The Shoulder*. Philadelphia, WB Saunders, 1990.
70. Richardson AB, Jobe FW, Collins HR: The shoulder in competitive swimming. *Am J Sports Med* 8:159–163, 1980.

71. Cain PR, Mutschler TA, Fu FH: Anterior stability of the glenohumeral joint. A dynamic model. *Am J Sports Med.* 15:144–148, 1987.
72. Itoi E, Newman SR, Kuechle DK, et al: Dynamic stabilizers of the shoulder with the arm in abduction. *J Bone Joint Surg Br* 76:834–836, 1994.
73. Blasier RB, Goldberg RE, Tothman ED: Anterior shoulder stability: Contributions of rotator cuff forces and the capsular ligaments in a cadaveric model. *J Shoulder Elbow Surg* 1:140–150, 1992.
74. Kaltsas DS: Comparative study of the properties of the shoulder joint capsule with those of other joint capsules. *Clin Orthop* 164:20–25, 1982.
75. Reeves B: Experiments on the tensile strength of the anterior capsular structures of the shoulder in man. *J Bone Joint Surg Br* 50:858–865, 1968.
76. Burkhead WZ, Rockwood CA: Treatment of instability of the shoulder with an exercise program. *J Bone Joint Surg Am* 74:890–896, 1992.
77. Rodosky MW, Harner CD, Fu FH: The role of the long head of the biceps muscle and superior glenoid labrum in anterior stability of the shoulder. *Am J Sports Med* 22:121–130, 1994.
78. Itoi E, Motzkin NE, Morrey BF, et al: The stabilizing function of the long head of the biceps with the arm in a hanging position. *J Shoulder Elbow Surg* 3(suppl):32, 1994.
79. Itoi E, Kuechle DK, Newman SR, et al: Stabilizing function of the biceps in stable and unstable shoulders. *J Bone Joint Surg Br* 75:546–551, 1993.
80. Warner JJP, McMahon PJ: The role of the long head of biceps brachii in superior stability of the glenohumeral joint. *J Bone Joint Surg Am* 77:366–372, 1995.
81. Snyder SJ, Karzel RP, DelPizzo W, et al: SLAP lesions of the shoulder. *Arthroscopy* 6:274–279, 1990.
82. Warner JJP, Kann S, Maddox L: Arthroscopic repair of combined Bankart and superior labral detachment anterior and posterior lesions: Technique and preliminary results. *Arthroscopy* 10:383–391, 1994.
83. Cooper DE, Warren JP, Warren RF: Complications of shoulder instability in the competitive athlete, in Bigliani LU (ed): *Complications of Shoulder Surgery*. Baltimore, Williams & Wilkens, 1993.
84. Silliman JF, Hawkins RJ: Classification and physical diagnosis of instability of the shoulder. *Clin Orthop* 291:7–19, 1993.
85. Zarins B, McMahon MS, Rowe CR: Diagnosis and treatment of traumatic anterior instability of the shoulder. *Clin Orthop* 291:75–84, 1993.
86. Neer CS II, Foster CR: Inferior capsular shift for involuntary inferior and multidirectional instability of the shoulder. *J Bone Joint Surg Am* 62:897–907, 1980.
87. Lusardi DA, Wirth MA, Wurtz D, et al: Loss of external rotation following anterior capsulorrhaphy of the shoulder. *J Bone Joint Surg Am* 75:1185–1192, 1993.
88. Garth WP, Allman FL, Armstrong WS: Occult anterior subluxations of the shoulder in noncontact sports. *Am J Sports Med* 15:579–585, 1987.
89. Thomas SC, Matsen FA III: An approach to the repair of the glenohumeral ligaments in the management of traumatic anterior glenohumeral instability. *J Bone Joint Surg Am* 71:506–513, 1989.
90. Dowdy PA, O'Driscoll SW: Shoulder instability. An analysis of family history. *J Bone Joint Surg Br* 75:782–784, 1993.
91. Emery RJH, Mullaji MB: Glenohumeral joint instability in normal adolescents. Incidence and significance. *J Bone Joint Surg Br* 73:406–408, 1991.
92. O'Driscoll SW, Evans DC: Contralateral shoulder instability following anterior repair. *J Bone Joint Surg Br* 73:941–946, 1991.
93. Uthoff HK, Piscopo M: Anterior capsular redundancy of the shoulder: Congenital or traumatic? *J Bone Joint Surg Br* 67:363–366, 1985.

94. Bost FC, Inman VT: The pathological changes in recurrent dislocation of the shoulder: A report of Bankart's operative procedure. *J Bone Joint Surg* 24:595–613, 1942.
95. Speer KP, Derg X, Torzilli PA, et al: A biomechanical evaluation of the Bankart lesion. *Trans Orthop Res Soc* 39:315, 1988.
96. Warner JJP, Miller MD, Marks PH, et al: Arthroscopic Bankart repair with the Suretac device. Part I: Clinical observations. *Arthroscopy* 11:2–13, 1995.
97. Altchek DW, Warren RF, Skyhar MJ, et al: T-Plasty modification of the Bankart procedure for multidirectional instability of the anterior and inferior types. *J Bone Joint Surg Am* 73:102–112, 1991.
98. Fu FH, Burkhead WZ, Flatow EL, et al: Symposium: Controversies in reconstruction of the unstable shoulder: Mobility versus instability. *Contemp Orthop* 26:407–427, 1993.
99. Warner JJP, Micheli LJ, Arslanian LE, et al: Patterns of flexibility, laxity, and strength in normal shoulders, and shoulders with instability and impingement. *Am J Sports Med* 18:366–375, 1990.
99a. Dubs L, Gschwend N: General joint laxity, quantification and clinical relevance. *Arch Orthop Trauma Surg* 107:65–72, 1988.
100. Rowe CR, Pierce DS, Clarke JG: Voluntary dislocation of the shoulder. *J Bone Joint Surg Am* 55:445–460, 1973.
101. Aronen JG, Regan K: Decreasing the incidence of recurrence of first time anterior shoulder dislocations with rehabilitation. *Am J Sports Med* 12:283–291, 1984.
102. Baker CL, Uribe JW, Whitman C: Arthroscopic evaluation of acute initial anterior shoulder dislocations. *Am J Sports Med* 18:25–28, 1990.
103. Codman EA: *The Shoulder: Rupture of the Supraspinatus Tendon and Other Lesions in or About the Subacromial Bursa.* Boston, Thomas Todd, 1934.
104. Dickenson JW, Devas MB: Bankart's operation for recurrent dislocation of the shoulder. *J Bone Joint Surg Br* 39:114–119, 1957.
105. Henry JH, Genung JA: Natural history of glenohumeral dislocation—revisited. *Am J Sports Med* 10:135–137, 1982.
106. Hovelius L: Anterior dislocation of the shoulder in teenagers and young adults. Five-year prognosis. *J Bone Joint Surg Am* 69:393–399, 1987.
107. Hovelius L, Eriksson K, Fredin H, et al: Recurrences after initial dislocation of the shoulder. Results of a prospective study of treatment. *J Bone Joint Surg Am* 65:343–349, 1983.
108. Marans HJ, Angel KR, Schemitsch EH, et al: The fate of traumatic anterior dislocation of the shoulder in children. *J Bone Joint Surg Am* 74:1242–1244, 1992.
109. McLaughlin HL: Recurrent anterior dislocation of the shoulder. I: Morbid anatomy. *Am J Surg* 99:628–632, 1960.
110. McLaughlin HL, Cavallaro WU: Primary anterior dislocation of the shoulder. *Am J Surg* 80:615, 1950.
111. Watson-Jones R: Recurrent dislocation of the shoulder. *J Bone Joint Surg Br* 30:6, 1948.
112. Huber H, Gerber C: Voluntary subluxation of the shoulder in children. A long-term follow-up study of 36 shoulders. *J Bone Joint Surg Br* 76:118–122, 1994.
113. Wheeler JH, Ryan JB, Arciero RA, et al: Arthroscopic versus nonoperative treatment of acute shoulder dislocations in young athletes. *Arthroscopy* 5:213–217, 1989.
114. Ahmadain AM: The Magnuson-Stack operation for recurrent anterior dislocation of the shoulder. *J Bone Joint Surg Br* 69:111–114, 1987.
115. Barry TP, Lombardo SJ, Kerlan RK: The coracoid transfer for recurrent an-

terior instability of the shoulder in adolescence. *J Bone Joint Surg Am* 67:383–387, 1985.
116. Ferlic DC, DiGiovine NM: A long-term follow-up retrospective study of the modified Bristow operation. *Am J Sports Med* 16:469–474, 1988.
117. Gerber C, Terrier F, Ganz R: The Trillat procedure for recurrent anterior instability of the shoulder. *J Bone Joint Surg Br* 70:130–134, 1988.
118. Hill JA, Lombardo SJ, Kerlan RK: Modified Bristow-Helfet procedure for recurrent anterior shoulder subluxations and dislocations. *Am J Sports Med* 9:283–287, 1981.
119. Leach RE, Corbett M, Schepsis A, et al: Results of a modified Putti-Platt operation for recurrent shoulder dislocations and subluxations. *Clin Orthop* 164:20–25, 1982.
120. Lombardo SJ, Kerlan RK, Jobe FW, et al: The modified Bristow procedure for recurrent dislocations of the shoulder. *J Bone Joint Surg Am* 58:256–261, 1976.
121. Morrey BF, Janes JM: Recurrent anterior dislocation of the shoulder. Long-term follow-up of the Putti-Platt and Bankart procedures. *J Bone Joint Surg Am* 58:252–256, 1976.
122. Rao JP, Francis AM, Daczkewyez HH: Treatment of recurrent anterior dislocation of the shoulder by duToit staple capsulorraphy. *Clin Orthop* 204:169–176, 1986.
123. Torg JS, Balduini FC, Ronci C: A modified Bristow-Helfet procedure for recurrent dislocation and subluxation of the shoulder. *J Bone Joint Surg Am* 69:904–913, 1987.
124. Truchly G, Thompson WAL: Simplified Putti-Platt procedure. *JAMA* 179:859–862, 1962.
125. Varmakarken JE, Jensen CH: Recurrent dislocation of the shoulder: A comparison of the results after the Bankart and Putti-Platt procedures. *Orthopedics* 12:453–455, 1989.
126. Berg EE, Ellison AE: The inside-out Bankart procedure. *Am J Sports Med* 18:129–133, 1990.
127. Cave EF, Rowe CR: Capsular repair for recurrent dislocation of the shoulder: Pathologic findings and operative technique. *Surg Clin North Am* 27:1289–1294, 1947.
128. duToit GT, Roux D: Recurrent dislocation of the shoulder. Twenty-four year study of the Johannesburg staple operation. *J Bone Joint Surg Am* 37:633, 1955.
129. Loomer R, Fraser J: A modified Bankart procedure for recurrent anterior/inferior shoulder instability. A preliminary report. *Am J Sports Med* 17:374–379, 1989.
130. Harryman DT, Sidles JA, Clark JM, et al: Translation of the humeral head on the glenoid with passive glenohumeral motion. *J Bone Joint Surg Am* 72:1288–1298, 1990.
131. Harryman DT, Sidles JA, Clark JM, et al: Laxity of the normal glenohumeral joint: A quantitative in vivo assessment. *J Shoulder Elbow Surg* 1:66–76, 1992.
132. Hawkins RJ: The assessment of glenohumeral translation using manual and fluoroscopic techniques. *Orthop Trans* 12:728–729, 1988.
133. Maki NJ: Cineradiographic studies with shoulder instability. *Am J Sports Med* 16:362–364, 1988.
134. Adolfsson L, Lysholm J: Arthroscopy and stability testing for anterior shoulder instability. *Arthroscopy* 5:315–320, 1989.
135. Gerber C, Ganz R: Clinical assessment of instability of the shoulder (with special reference to anterior and posterior drawer tests). *J Bone Joint Surg Br* 66:551–556, 1984.

136. Bigliani LU, Kurzweil PR, Schwartzbach CC, et al: Inferior capsular shift procedure for anterior-inferior shoulder instability in athletes. *Orthop Trans* 13:560, 1989.
137. Neer CS II, Fithian TE, Hansen PE, et al: Reinforced cruciate repair for anterior dislocation of the shoulder. *Orthop Trans* 9:44–45, 1985.
138. Bigliani LU, Kurzweil PR, Schwartzbach CC, et al: Inferior capsular shift procedure for anterior-inferior shoulder instability in athletes. *Orthop Trans* 13:560, 1989.
139. Jobe FW, Giangarra CE, Kuitne RS, et al: Anterior capsulolabral reconstruction of the shoulder in athletes in overhead sports. *Am J Sports Med* 19:428–434, 1991.
140. Protzman RR: Anterior instability of the shoulder. *J Bone Joint Surg Am* 62:909–918, 1980.
140a. Rubenstein DL, Jobe FW, Glousman RE, et al: Anterior capsulolabral reconstruction of the shoulder in athletes. *J Shoulder Elbow Surg* 1:229–237, 1992.
141. Warner JJP, Johnson D, Miller M, et al: The concept of a "selective capsular shift" for anterior-inferior instability of the shoulder. *J Shoulder Elbow Surg*, 1995, in press.
142. Warner JJP, Miller MD, Marks P: Arthroscopic Bankart repair with the Suretac device. Part II: Experimental observations. *Arthroscopy* 11:14–20, 1995.
143. Warner JJP, Warren RF: Arthroscopic Bankart repair using a cannulated absorbable fixation device. *Operative Techniques Orthop* 1:192–197, 1991.
144. Hawkins RJ, Koppert G, Johnson G: Recurrent posterior instability (subluxation) of the shoulder. *J Bone Joint Surg Am* 66:169, 1984.
145. Fronek J, Warren RF, Bowen M: Posterior subluxation of the glenohumeral joint. *J Bone Joint Surg Am* 71:205, 1989.
146. Mowery CA, Garfin SR, Booth RE, et al: Recurrent posterior dislocation of the shoulder: Treatment using a bone block. *J Bone Joint Surg Am* 67:777, 1985.
147. Tibone J, Ting A: Capsulorrhaphy with a staple for recurrent posterior subluxation of the shoulder. *J Bone Joint Surg Am* 72:999, 1990.
148. Boyd HB, Sisk TD: Recurrent posterior dislocation of the shoulder. *J Bone Joint Surg Am* 54:779–786, 1972.
149. Norwood AL, Terry GC: Shoulder posterior subluxation. *Am J Sports Med* 12:25–30, 1984.
150. Bigliani LU, Endrizzi DP, McIlveen SJ, et al: Operative management of posterior shoulder instability. *Orthop Trans* 13:232, 1989.
151. Pollock RG, Bigliani LU: Recurrent posterior shoulder instability. Diagnosis and treatment. *Clin Orthop* 291:85–96, 1993.
152. Hawkins RJ: Arthroscopic stapling repair for shoulder instability: A retrospective study of 50 cases. *Arthroscopy* 5:122–128, 1989.
153. Johnson LL: Arthroscopic management for shoulder instability: Stapling. Presented at the American Association of Nurse Anesthetists Specialty Day Meeting, Atlanta, February 1988.
154. Maki NJ: Arthroscopic stabilization: Suture technique. *Operative Techniques Orthop* 1:180–183, 1991.
155. Matthews LS, Vetter WL, Oweida SJ, et al: Arthroscopic staple capsulorraphy for recurrent anterior shoulder instability arthroscopy. *Arthroscopy* 4:106–111, 1988.
156. Morgan CD, Bodenstub AB: Arthroscopic Bankart suture repair: Technique and early results. *Arthroscopy* 3:111–122, 1987.
157. Snyder SJ, Strafford BB: Arthroscopic management of instability of the shoulder. *Orthopedics* 16:993–1002, 1993.

158. Wolf EM, Wilk RM, Richmond JC: Arthroscopic Bankart repair using suture anchors. *Operative Techniques Orthop* 1:184–191, 1991.
159. Zuckerman JD, Matsen FA: Complications about the glenohumeral joint related to the use of screws and staples. *J Bone Joint Surg Am* 66:175–180, 1984.

Current Concepts in Shoulder Rehabilitation

W. Ben Kibler, M.D.
Medical Director, Lexington Clinic Sports Medicine Center, Lexington, Kentucky

Beven Livingston, P.T., A.T.C.
Clinical Specialist, Lexington Clinic Sports Medicine Center, Lexington, Kentucky

Robin Bruce, P.T.
Physical Therapist, Lexington Clinic Sports Medicine Center, Lexington, Kentucky

Proper rehabilitation of the shoulder requires a comprehensive program that includes understanding the demands placed on the shoulder by athletic activity, functions of the shoulder in athletic activity, pathophysiology of shoulder pathology and its evaluation, goals and methods of rehabilitation, timing and usage of rehabilitation modalities, and criteria for assessment of outcomes. This current-concepts chapter will review present knowledge in these areas and will provide a framework of principles that will allow the construction of rehabilitation protocols to allow efficient restoration of shoulder function after injury. Specific protocols that are used in our clinic will be presented in Appendix A, but most emphasis will be placed on understanding the framework for evaluation of dysfunction and restoration of function.

Restoration of shoulder function is important because of the shoulder's importance in athletic activities and its relatively high rate of injury. The shoulder is the third most frequently injured joint in college athletes,[1] the most commonly injured area in baseball players,[2] and the first or second most commonly injured area in tennis players.[3] Failure to properly restore functional ability at the shoulder will result in subpar performance, repeat injury in the shoulder, or overload and possible injury at other anatomic points in the athlete.[4]

In summary, shoulder rehabilitation involves more than *how* modalities or methods should be used. It also involves knowledge of *why* there is an injury, *what* is injured or altered, and when the athlete may return to play. Effective rehabilitation must address all of these questions.

DEMANDS ON THE SHOULDER

Descriptive biomechanical analysis of the shoulder reveals large motions, forces, and loads during an overhead motion, either in tennis or baseball.

Advances in Operative Orthopaedics, vol. 3

Rotational velocities have been recorded as high as 7,000 degrees/sec in baseball[5, 6] and 1,500 degrees/sec in tennis.[7] An angular velocity of 1,150 degrees/sec was recorded as the shoulder adducts.[8] Total rotation of 165 degrees is seen in tennis[7] and 185 degrees in baseball.[6] Anterior translatory forces at the glenohumeral joint in acceleration may be as high as 40% of body weight in baseball,[8] whereas distraction forces at the glenohumeral joint in deceleration approximate 90% of body weight.[6] At the moment of ball impact in tennis, shoulder internal rotation contributes 30% of the total racquet momentum, whereas horizontal adduction contributes 13%.[9] The scapula rotates through an arc of 65 degrees and translates up to 15 cm on the thorax.[3]

These motions are developed rapidly and peak quickly, ranging from 0.11 to 0.29 seconds, depending on the direction, the skill level, and the sport.[3] Similarly, they must be decelerated and regulated over a short period of time to minimize injury.[8]

In summary, analysis shows that the shoulder is exposed to large motions, high forces, and large loads in the course of normal overhead throwing activity. These forces and loads are of short duration and high intensity and must be repeated many times in a match, game, or practice. The data that have been collected and reported are mainly from professional athletes and therefore represent the high end of the spectrum, but forces in recreational athletes are probably not extremely far below these values. Rehabilitation of the shoulder should focus on returning shoulder function to its maximum ability to withstand these inherent demands for all levels of play.

FUNCTIONS OF THE SHOULDER

The shoulder functions most effectively in a relatively limited set of anatomic conditions that create a balance between the *mobility* to achieve the wide ranges of motion and disparate positions necessary in throwing and the *stability* necessary to allow a normal path of the instant center of rotation in the face of the need to generate large forces and the presence of the translatory and distraction loads that occur in throwing.[10]

The glenohumeral joint is highly mobile and can achieve over 16,000 positions for the arm.[11] This mobility is allowed by the "large-ball/small-socket" bony anatomy and the rather voluminous capsule of the glenohumeral joint that does not restrain rotation in the mid ranges[12] and the minimally constrained but well-guided scapula.[13] The scapula must retract and protract on the thorax to follow the humerus and must elevate to avoid glenohumeral impingement with abduction and rotation.

Local stability to offset the translatory and distraction loads is conferred by interaction of the bony, ligamentous, and muscular constraint systems that control the path of the instant center of motion of the glenohumeral joint.[14–16] Most of the alterations in athletic performance and the signs and symptoms of clinical pathology can be related to changes in this normal path. This normal path has been demonstrated in several studies.[12, 17, 18] They show that glenohumeral translation is only 1 to 2 mm in the midranges of motion but may be as much as 5 to 10 mm in an anterior/posterior direction or 4 to 5 mm in an inferior/superior direction.

These data indicate that the glenohumeral joint, despite its outward anatomic appearance, really does function as a ball-and-socket joint in the large majority of positions the shoulder assumes in throwing. This means that the constraint systems work through a "circle of stability"[14, 19, 20] by which opposing structures on each side of the joint are active to control motion.

This circle of stability is necessary because the bony constraint system alone is inadequate to allow inherent stability.[127] However, the geometry of the surfaces, aided by the glenoid labrum, allows a "concavity-compression" or suction-like effect that increases bony stability.[21, 22] This effect is maximized by proper positioning of the scapula and its glenoid in relation to the moving humerus.[12, 23] Since this relationship is constantly changing as the arm moves, the scapular muscles must be balanced and strong.[24]

The capsuloligamentous constraint system contributes to the circle of stability by stabilizing glenohumeral motion at the extremes of motion and by controlling abnormal translations, either in anterior/posterior or superior/inferior directions.[14, 19, 20, 25–27] Different components of the capsuloligamentous system are the main restraints in different positions, but they work in concert so that no component is the sole restraint.[25, 26] These structures work both by themselves in a static fashion and as part of a dynamic system in association with active muscular contraction.[22, 28] Both rotator cuff firing[29] and biceps activity[30] have been shown to stiffen the capsule and decrease glenohumeral translation.

The muscular constraint system contributes to the circle of stability by several mechanisms. The first is the previously mentioned contribution to dynamic capsuloligamentous stability. The second is by the muscles acting as dynamic ligaments in which their passive elements are used to limit joint excursion.[31] The third and most important is coordinated contraction of muscles as force couples to position the bones or control a motion.[32] Coactivation, or simultaneous contraction of agonist and antagonist muscles, will create low net torque around the joint but will create increased control of the joint. Reciprocal activation of the agonist with inhibition of the antagonist muscles will increase torque and motion. In either situation, muscle activity compresses the glenohumeral joint and allows smooth motion.[33, 34]

There are many examples of force couples around the shoulder joint. Scapular rotation is controlled by an upper component consisting of the upper trapezius and levator scapulae and a lower component consisting of the lower trapezius and serratus anterior.[35] Scapular retraction/protraction is controlled by the trapezius and rhomboids paired with the serratus.[3, 36] This muscular activity allows the scapula to perform its four roles. They are acromial elevation, a socket for the moving humerus, providing a stable muscular anchor, and allowing motion from full retraction in cocking to full protraction in follow-through.[13] Glenohumeral rotation within the normal range of motion is controlled by the deltoid, an extrinsic humeral head elevator, paired with the supraspinatus and infraspinatus of the rotator cuff, which are intrinsic humeral head depressors.[35, 36] Glenohumeral motion in the transverse plane is stabilized by the subscapularis paired with the infraspinatus/teres minor.[35]

This rather complex mechanism of muscular activity for joint control is dependent on afferent and efferent neurologic input for maximal efficiency. Afferent sensory input is mainly from proprioceptive fibers in muscle and capsule[37, 38] and improves the fine-tuning regulation of coactivation.[14] Efferent motor input is by both cortical pathways and the development of learned motor programs of specific muscle activation patterns to allow a more rapid response at the spinal cord level.[32, 39, 40]

In addition to joint control for stability, muscle activity is necessary to generate the torques that are required for athletic activity. This is traditionally thought to be the most important role of shoulder muscular activity. However, studies have shown that the cross-sectional area of the shoulder muscles is not sufficient to generate the observed torques,[41, 42] optimum velocity is not related to shoulder muscle strength,[43] and peak torques and maximal velocities of the shoulder or of thrown objects decrease to about 50% of maximum as other body parts are restricted.[42, 44, 45] Preliminary quantitative analysis demonstrates that the shoulder contributes only 13% of the total kinetic energy of the tennis serve.[46] The largest part of the velocity—and therefore the kinetic energy, torque, and acceleration that is seen at the shoulder—is developed through a sequential activation of links in a kinetic chain.[15, 47–49] This chain allows the generation, summation, and transfer of forces from the proximal segments of the legs and back through the shoulder to the hand. These segments are efficient in this process, as indicated by the large velocities and rotations. The shoulder functions as a funnel in the kinetic chain by transferring and concentrating the velocity and energy, thereby adding force by the concentration. Preliminary quantitative analysis shows that the shoulder link contributes 21% of the total force in the tennis serve as compared with only 13% of the total kinetic energy.[46] Shoulder muscle activity in the kinetic chain, is therefore primarily concerned with joint stability to regulate the forces and minimize turbulence (abnormal translation) through the funnel and secondarily with torque and velocity generation.[15, 36] This mode of operation implies coordinated muscle coactivation by force couples.

In summary, the shoulder functions locally as a ball-and-socket joint with a predictable, but small path of the instant center of motion, even in the face of large velocities, large forces, and large displacement vectors. It also functions as a link in the kinetic chain by acting as a stable base for the arm to move and funneling velocities and accelerations from the legs to the hand. All three constraint systems are integrated to allow these functions. Although the bony and ligamentous constraint systems are important in these functions, the muscular constraint system has the largest role. It maximizes the role that the bony constraints can play, and it improves and extends the effectiveness of the ligamentous system. It works as an agonist/antagonist force couple to generate forces and motion, but it primarily works as a coactivation force couple to provide glenohumeral joint compression, guide the instant center of rotation, stabilize the position of the scapula, and regulate the translatory and distractive forces and motions developed through the shoulder joint complex. This is the reason that muscle activity is large and complex in overhead activity, whether it be in baseball,[50, 51] swimming,[52, 53] tennis,[3, 54] or javelin throwing.[55] It is doubtful that cortical or reflex mechanisms are quick or responsive enough or are so finely tuned to allow the high degree of precision necessary for optimum shoulder function. Learned motor programs, with or without sensory input, that position the body links in certain predetermined ways and activate muscles in agonist/antagonist or coactivation patterns may be the most important avenue for fine control of these rapid movements.[32, 51, 56] It appears that these motor patterns may be improved with training and skill acquisition because firing patterns are more coordinated, shorter in duration, and higher in amplitude in skilled athletes.[57]

Rehabilitative efforts around the shoulder must take into account how these functions have been altered by sporting activity, injury, and surgery or other treatment. Specific rehabilitation programs can be tailored to restore the physiologic or biomechanical functions that are not allowing normal shoulder function.

PATHOPHYSIOLOGY OF SHOULDER INJURY

Concepts about shoulder pathology are evolving as more knowledge accumulates about shoulder physiology and biomechanics. The traditional method of anatomically based, discrete diagnosis (rotator cuff tendinitis, anterior glenohumeral dislocation) is not as helpful or precise in light of more recent knowledge. Just as normal shoulder function has been shown to be largely the result of an integration of several different constraint systems, pathology is more likely to involve a failure of more than one of the systems. There will probably be one that is more involved or prominent clinically, but others may be contributing factors in shoulder dysfunction or symptoms.

Shoulder pathology results from acute macrotrauma or chronic repetitive microtrauma. Acute macrotrauma implies an *event*—a one-time incident that instantly converts an anatomically normal structure into an abnormal structure. Examples of this mechanism would be a fracture or an acute traumatic dislocation. This mechanism is relatively infrequent in sports and causes less than 20% of the shoulder pathology. Repetitive microtrauma represents a *process*—a chronic series of events that produce cellular degeneration and subsequent tissue alterations.[58–60] These alterations may result in clinical symptoms, tissue damage, or alterations in flexibility or strength and may cause biomechanical alterations as athletes continue to compete in the face of tissue abnormalities.[4, 8, 14, 61] The onset of symptoms may be distant in time from the initiation of the pathologic process, and the clinical symptoms may be the "tip of the iceberg" of the entire pathologic process.[62, 63] Examples of this pathologic mechanism would be chronic rotator cuff tendinitis, attritional labral tears, and nontraumatic capsuloligamentous instability.

In either situation, the pathologic process alters the constraint systems so that the circle of stability is lost and the instant center of rotation is not contained.

Bony constraint failure is usually due to acute macrotrauma. This would include glenoid fractures causing loss of concavity-compression or bony Bankhart lesions causing loss of capsuloligamentous attachment.

However, other systems could be involved as well. Examples would include inferior glenohumeral ligament strain with bony Bankhart lesions, inhibition of the serratus anterior or supraspinatus associated with pain from a fracture, or capsular stiffness caused by immobilization following a dislocation.

Capsuloligamentous failure can occur through macrotrauma or microtrauma. Macrotrauma injuries include acute superior labral (SLAP) injuries caused by falls on outstretched arms[64] or acute capsular strains or ligamentous Bankhart lesions in acute dislocations. Microtrauma-induced capsuloligamentous failure is a common cause of pathology in athletes performing high-demand overhead activities.[65, 66] This may be a primary ligamentous failure, or it may be secondary to failure or imbalance in the muscular constraints, either the supraspinatus, biceps, or subscapularis/infraspinatus.[28, 30, 65, 67] Another capsuloligamentous deficiency is glenohumeral internal rotation deficit.[3, 14, 68, 69] This tightness has been documented after injury[68] and has been demonstrated in relation to the opposite shoulder,[69] published norms,[70] or other types of athletes.[70, 71] It is seen in both males and females to a similar degree[70] and appears to be present at an early age as a result of intense athletic participation.[71] This is often associated with excessive amounts of glenohumeral external rotation in baseball pitchers[14] and less commonly in tennis players.[7] This internal rotation deficit has been shown to cause increased anterior and anterior-superior translation of the instant center of rotation in the midranges of motion, thereby increasing anterior shear forces.[12] In addition, this lack of internal rotation alters the normal internal rotation necessary for maximum performance[9] and shifts this function to other links in the kinetic chain. Internal rotation deficits or external rotation deficits secondary to overtightening at surgery or prolonged immobilization may also be associated with bony deficits as a result of excessive shear.[72, 73]

Muscular constraint failure is common in shoulder pathology. Weakness can be due to direct or indirect trauma, fatigue, or pain-induced inhibition or can be seen with ligamentous failure or tightness. This weakness will adversely affect the generation of velocity, kinetic energy, and force in the shoulder link, but it is more important as a cause of force couple imbalance, thereby affecting the circle of stability.

Scapular muscle failure is a frequent finding in shoulder pathology.[13, 14, 74, 75] This appears to be a nonspecific response to glenohumeral pain, injury, or pathology and appears in 68% to 100% of cases. This is not associated with long thoracic nerve paralysis. Disruption of the force couples causes abnormalities of scapular position and motion that have been termed lateral scapular slide[13] or scapulothoracic dyskinesis.[75] These abnormalities have deleterious effects on shoulder function by affecting the four purposes of the scapula in overhead activities. Lack of acromial elevation caused by upper trapezius weakness increases impingement. Trapezius, rhomboid, and serratus anterior weakness impairs the scapula's ability to position itself as a congruent socket for the moving humerus; stabilize itself as an anchor for insertions of the rotator cuff, deltoid, biceps and triceps; and move smoothly and fully into retraction and protraction during the throwing motion.[13] This dyskinesis will also serve as a break in the kinetic chain that disrupts funneling of velocity and force and does not allow a stable base for the arm to work.

Rotator cuff tears, either partial or full thickness, are also examples of muscular constraint failure. Rotator cuff injury results in failure of energy and force production, but its most deleterious effects are on the position and stabilization of the glenohumeral joint. Supraspinatus weakness decreases capsular stiffness[30] and decreases concavity/compression.[22] Infraspinatus weakness alters the deltoid force couple and leads to excessive superior translation.[35] Subscapularis weakness can lead to overstretching of the anterior capsular structures and cause anterior translation.[76]

Strength imbalances may also play a role in altering muscular constraints by creating force couple alterations. Several studies have shown that absolute peak torque values and peak torque ratios are altered in both baseball players[77, 78] and tennis players.[79, 80] These studies document increased internal rotation torque as compared with external rotation torque at several speeds. The etiology of this acquired imbalance is not known. It may be an advantageous training effect, it may be the result of "plyometric-like" activity of cocking and acceleration, or it may be selective inhibition of the posterior muscles. The major problem with this force couple imbalance is that it decreases concavity/compression and accentuates anterior translation because of the internal rotation deficit.

Proprioceptive deficits are also seen in shoulder pathology. Abnormalities in shoulder joint kinesthesia have been demonstrated after shoulder joint dislocation.[81, 82] These types of deficits have been demonstrated to be deleterious to the function of other joints by altering muscle firing patterns,[83, 84] and these deficits would be expected to play an even larger role in a muscle-dependent joint like the shoulder.

Pathology in other areas of the body can also cause or contribute to shoulder pathology. Since the shoulder is dependent on proximal muscle activity and movement to produce most of the velocity, energy, and force that go to the hand, biomechanical flaws or anatomic injuries in these segments may impose larger demands on the shoulder for force and velocity generation. Examples would be ankle sprains, knee pathology, and back pain, inflexibility, or weakness.[41] This kinetic chain failure creates a "catch-up" situation if the distal links are called upon to increase their energy or force production to maintain normal force production. The arm muscles, with their smaller cross-sectional area, cannot initiate or sustain this activity well, thereby putting them more at risk of fatigue or injury. Our studies have shown that in the professional tennis player model, a decrease of 10% in trunk/leg kinetic energy requires an 18.5% increase in shoulder velocity, or 40% increase in shoulder mass, to achieve the same resultant energy at the hand.[15] Since the shoulder link is already operating at extremely high velocities, increases of this magnitude can be expected to cause further shearing or translatory forces in addition to fatiguing the muscles and placing the joint at higher risk of injury.

In summary, pathology at the shoulder can be described as a failure of the circle of stability caused by failure of the constraint mechanisms. The types of failure are many and varied but are basically caused by macrotrauma or more commonly microtrauma. Since the constraint systems work together, failure of one system may lead to failure or compromise of the others. The constraint mechanisms may fail individually, concurrently, or consecutively. Whether shoulder pathology is due to macrotrauma or microtrauma, associated alterations in flexibility, strength, strength balance, or proprioception can be expected either because of direct injury, treatment, or the process of injury. Also, since the shoulder is a key link in the kinetic chain of throwing activities, biomechanical flaws or injuries in other links can have major or minor effects on shoulder function and pathology. Therefore, diagnostic or evaluation systems for shoulder pathology cannot focus solely on one site of pathology or one specific clinical finding but must evaluate the shoulder in the context of its total function.

EVALUATION OF SHOULDER PATHOLOGY

Several examination frameworks for shoulder pathology are available in the literature.[85–87] The goal of any comprehensive framework is to make a complete and accurate diagnosis of the shoulder pathology. This includes not only the clinical symptoms and signs but also the anatomic, biomechanical, and physiologic alterations that may accompany the clinical symptoms. These alterations affect and magnify the symptoms, alter athletic performance, and affect the completeness and efficiency of rehabilitation. They may be local, or they may be distant in the kinetic chain.

In developing the evaluation framework we use in our clinic[85] we have categorized these alterations into four broad groups.[88] The first group (tissue injury complex) is those tissues that are directly injured with overt or clinically apparent pathologic changes. Examples would be labral tears, rotator cuff pathology, or fractures. The second group (tissue overload complex) consists of those tissues that are altered because of repetitive microtrauma overload, with nonovert or subclinical pathologic change but measurable change in tissue characteristics. Examples would be glenohumeral internal rotation deficit, scapular stabilizer muscle weakness, or contralateral hip rotational deficit. The third group (functional biomechanical deficit complex) consists of biomechanical inefficiencies caused by tissue alterations or treatment that create increased demand on the shoulder structures. Examples would be force couple imbalance around the shoulder, scapular dyskinesis, shoulder stiffness from immobilization, or kinetic chain breakage caused by back rotational inflexibility. The fourth group (subclinical adaptations) includes the changes in mechanics or physiology that the athlete adopts in the face of tissue alterations in trying to maintain peak performance. Examples would be dropping the shoulder from the overhead position in throwing to avoid impingement, "short arming" in the face of instability, "opening up" or leading with the body when the leg or back muscles are weak, or excessive wrist snap when the kinetic chain is broken at the shoulder.

For macrotrauma situations, the evaluation may be relatively simple because there may be few associated alterations. However, for repetitive microtrauma situations, which account for most pathologic problems around the shoulder, these alterations are common and may be quite widespread.

As can be seen, the complete evaluation process may need to be quite lengthy and involved. The depth of the evaluation will depend on the athlete's skill level, level of participation, and desire to return to maximal competition. For elite-level or intensely competitive athletes, it will involve a comprehensive history of symptoms and athletic dysfunction or any "transition elements"[62] that may have imposed extra sports demands, a physical examination including the shoulder and the entire kinetic chain, and possible demonstration of throwing, hitting, or running mechanics.[85] Facilities and equipment should be available for this type of examination. For less competitive athletes, a less inclusive examination may be possible. The goals of the evaluation, however, remain the same. Enough information should be gathered to assess all of the anatomic and functional alterations that are contributing to shoulder pathology.

The examination findings should be recorded on forms so that an accurate baseline record is established. This will allow comparisons to be made as treatment and rehabilitation progress and can serve as a large database for research or for outcomes analysis.

In summary, a complete and accurate diagnosis can give a comprehensive view of the whole spectrum of anatomic and biomechanical abnormalities the athlete has that must be corrected in treatment. This diagnosis is then used as the basis for the exercise prescription for functional treatment and rehabilitation. Examples of the use of this framework for evaluation of an elite tennis player and a college basketball player will illustrate these principles.[15]

CASE EXAMPLES

CASE 1

History.—A 24-year-old right-handed professional tennis player was evaluated for a 4-month history of pain in the dominant shoulder. The pain was first noted while athlete was trying to develop a new, harder service motion. Pain occurred at the top of the serve motion around ball impact, hurt on follow-through, and increased as the match progressed. Physical therapy modalities and nonsteroidal anti-inflammatory drugs (NSAIDs) afforded only temporary relief. Rotator cuff impingement was diagnosed. Subacromial injection provided no relief, and rotator cuff exercises increased the symptoms. Two months ago the athlete felt a pop on service motion with increased symptoms. Pain started in the first game, he could not hit high groundstrokes, and he changed his serve to a three-quarters serve with more sidespin. His performance was rated 50% at best.

Physical Examination.—Physical examination revealed the following: (1) normal posture of the back and shoulders except for a prominence of the right scapula; (2) normal quadriceps and hamstring strength bilaterally; (3) bilateral hamstring tightness—hip flexion of 55 degrees with the knees extended; (4) Left hip range of motion, 25 degrees' internal/55 degrees' external rotation; right hip range of motion, 45 degrees' internal/50 degrees' external rotation; (5) back sit and reach, (−) 3 cm; (6) scapular slide asymmetry,[13] 2.6 cm lateral slide on the right; (7) right glenohumeral rotation, 15 degrees' internal/95 degrees' external rotation; left glenohumeral rotation, 50 degrees' internal/95 degrees' external rotation; (8) muscle strength, 4/5 serratus anterior, 4/5 upper trapezius, 4−/5 infraspinatus, 4/5 supraspinatus, 5/5 deltoid, 5/5 biceps and triceps, and 5/5 subscapularis; (9) positive impingement sign; (10) positive anterior slide[13] and "clunk"[86] tests; and (11) no apprehension sign, a negative sulcus sign, and no anterior-inferior instability.

Imaging.—Plain radiographs were negative, but a computed tomographic (CT) arthrogram detected a defect in the anterior-superior glenoid labrum and dye extravasation into the rotator cuff tendon.

Complete and Accurate Diagnosis.—The method of injury involved chronic repetitive microtrauma. The clinical symptom complex included rotator cuff impingement, pain in service motion, and decreased performance; the tissue injury complex consisted of an articular side, partial rotator cuff tear, and an anterior-superior glenoid labral tear; and the tissue overload complex consisted of hamstrings (inflexibility), contralateral hip external rotators (inflexibility), lumbar paraspinals (inflexibility), scapular stabilizers (weakness), the posterior rotator cuff (weakness, inflexibility), and the posterior capsule (inflexibility). Functional biomechanical deficits included kinetic chain breakage at the hip and trunk, scapular dyskinesis, and loss of internal/external rotation and humeral head depression force couples. Among the subclinical adaptations were opening up on the serve at the three-quarters arm position and excessive wrist snap. The constraint systems involved were the capsuloligamentous (anterior-superior glenoid labrum and posterior capsule) and muscular systems (posterior cuff [local], scapular [regional], and hip and trunk [distant]). The instant center of rotation abnormality consisted of excessive anterior/superior and superior translation. The transition element[62] involved a new service motion superimposed on an inflexible and weak musculoskeletal base.

CASE 2

History.—A 20-year-old college basketball player fell on his dominant arm during a game and sustained an abduction external rotation injury with acute anterior glenohumeral dislocation. He had no prior history of shoulder problems. The dislocation was reduced in the locker room, and radiographs showed no fracture or other pathology. After the treatment options were outlined, the patient opted for surgical stabilization. Open surgery consisted of repair of a large Bankhart lesion with anchor fixation. Sling and swathe postoperative immobilization was employed for 2 weeks, with Codman exercises for 2 weeks. One month postoperatively the patient was cleared for formal rehabilitation.

Physical Examination.—The following findings were noted: (1) normal posture; (2) no pain to palpation; (3) range of motion: active, 25 degrees' internal/30 degrees' external rotation; passive, 45 degrees' internal/40 degrees' external rotation; abduction, 60 degrees with a scapular tilt; glenohumeral abduction, 40 degrees; and flexion, 80 degrees; (4) strength: deltoid, 4+/5; supraspinatus, 4+/5; infraspinatus, 4−/5; and subscapularis, 4−/5; and, (5) no back, trunk, or hip inflexibility.

Complete and Accurate Diagnosis.—The method of injury involved acute macrotrauma with repair. The clinical symptom complex consisted of stiffness and decreased strength; the tissue injury complex involved the anterior capsulolabral complex, which was repaired, and the subscapularis muscle, also repaired; and there was no tissue overload complex. The functional biomechanical deficit complex consisted of global shoulder muscle weakness and stiffness as a result of injury, surgery, and immobilization. The subclinical adaptation complex consisted of trapezius substitution in abduction. Among the constraint systems involved were the capsuloligamentous (tear with repair) and muscular (weakness) systems. The instant center of rotation abnormality was decreased rotation, but there was no problem with translation.

This evaluation framework is helpful in identifying how different pathologic processes affect the anatomy, physiology, and biomechanics of the athlete and allow the clinician to set up an exercise prescription to resolve the injuries and symptoms and restore function as completely as possible.

GOALS OF REHABILITATION

The ultimate goal of rehabilitation is maximal restoration of function for an anatomic area or a specific athletic activity. For the shoulder in overhead athletic activity, locally this means restoration of the constraints that comprise the circle of stability and, distantly, restoration of the links of the kinetic chain. There are many methods that can be used to accomplish these goals, including modalities, rest, medication, surgery, flexibility exercises, and strength exercises. To be most efficacious, they must be used in a logical and scientifically based sequence in line with their benefit to tissue healing and function.

METHODS OF REHABILITATION

Rest should be used to relieve soreness and pain, prevent further injury, prevent the development of subclinical adaptations, and allow the body to start the healing process. This is actually relative rest. The kinetic chain can still be exercised, aerobic endurance is maintained, and some limited motion may be allowed. Strict immobilization is kept to a minimum because of deleterious neurologic and tissue effects.[89] Periods of rest may also be necessary during the later stages of rehabilitation to allow recovery from exercise.

Medication should be used for specific purposes, mainly pain relief. Pain, which is a potent inhibitor of muscle activation and coactivation, is especially deleterious around a muscle-dependent joint like the shoulder. There is very little evidence for inflammation as a major source of pain in chronic athletic shoulder conditions, but in acute overload situations such as tendinitis caused by excessive throwing, inflammation may contribute substantially.[90] A stronger case can be made for anti-inflammatory medication, either oral NSAIDS or oral or injectable corticosteroids, in the acute phase of shoulder pathology. Nonsteroidal anti-inflammatory agents should be used for their analgesic rather than their anti-inflammatory properties in the more common chronic microtrauma situations. Medications should be viewed as adjunctive rather than curative and should be prescribed with all of the known dangers to the tendons, stomach, and kidneys in mind. None of the NSAIDS appear to have any special benefit or better benefit-risk ratio.[91] Long-acting crystalline corticosteroid suspensions provide the fastest relief and are preferred over aqueous preparations.[90] After injection, exercises should be avoided for 2 to 3 days.

Surgery may be required to relieve clinical symptoms and heal the tissue injury complex. This may range from arthroscopic decompression to repair of torn labra or internal fixation of fractures. The surgical procedure should create conditions for optimal rehabilitation. Fixation should be secure enough to start early protected motion, and the soft tissues should be tensioned to allow mobility with stability. Overtightening or overimmobilization should be avoided because this creates undesirable biomechanics.

Ultrasound, high-frequency mechanical vibrations, produces thermal and nonthermal physiologic effects for therapeutic purposes.[92] Mechanical energy is transmitted to organic molecules in longitudinal waves. Tissues with high protein content such as muscle and nerve absorb ultrasound more readily. An increased thermal response and possible tissue damage can occur at heterogeneous tissue interfaces such as bone-muscle. Ultrasound is the most effective deep-heating modality; it reaches muscles and deep-seated joints such as the hip and shoulder.[93, 94] Thermal effects result in increased peripheral blood flow, increased tissue metabolism, and greater tissue extensibility.[95, 96] Nonthermal effects of ultrasound on membrane stability have been advocated to treat pain and inflammation.[97] However, experimental studies have been contradictory. Some showed no benefit when compared with controls,[98] whereas others demonstrated an incompletely understood effect to reduce inflammation.[99–101] Ultrasound does have analgesic effects because of its action on membrane stability, presynaptic inhibition, and increased cortisol levels.[102] Phonophoresis is a technique that uses mechanical energy to drive whole molecules of medication, usually corticosteroids, into tissue. Although some symptomatic relief is reported with phonophoresis as compared with placebo,[103] there is incomplete evidence that the corticosteroid molecules can be driven into deep symptomatic areas such as the rotator cuff.[104]

Electrical stimulation has been used in the treatment of both acute and chronic shoulder injuries. There is considerable anecdotal and empirical support for its use in modifying pain and inflammation, but no scientific studies of its efficacy have been performed.[105] High-voltage galvanic stimulation has been used for relaxing muscle spasm, reducing edema, increasing local blood flow, and maintaining range of motion.[106, 107] Iontophoresis, which uses differences in electrical potential to deliver medication to deep tissues, allows medications to penetrate to tissues with reduced vascularity such as bursae and tendon.[108]

Cryotherapy, the therapeutic use of cold, is used to decrease tissue temperature, inflammation, the metabolic rate, circulation, and muscle spasm. These all combine in an acute injury to reduce secondary hypoxic injury around the primary injury, decrease pain, and decrease swelling in chronic injuries. The main effects are reduction in postinjury, postoperative, or postexercise pain or swelling. Cellular effects to reduce swelling and hypoxia are due to decreased prostaglandin-mediated inflammation[109] and decreased histamine-mediated membrane permeability.[110] Effects on pain and spasm are due to decreased nerve conduction and decreased spindle activity.[108] Methods of delivery vary from ice bags to cold compression devices. The depth of penetration also varies. Cold must be used carefully to avoid skin problems caused by overexposure.

The methods of rehabilitation described thus far have all been advocated to help treat shoulder problems. Scientific studies showing their efficacy are lacking.[105] Most appear to have a role early in the pathologic process in decreasing some of the symptoms of pain, spasm, and inflammation. They appear to have less of a role in chronic problems that are not particularly painful or inflamed but are mainly dysfunctional. Rehabilitation beyond the resolution of symptoms requires the achievement of proper flexibility and dynamic muscle stability, both locally and in the kinetic chain.

Flexibility exercises can be used to restore the mobility of the glenohumeral joints. They may be tight as a result of repetitive microtrauma overload, disuse due to pain, or immobilization. The exercises can also help improve flexibility to a certain extent in postoperative shoulders that are too tight. They work by reducing connective tissue adhesions,[105] reducing collagen cross-links,[89] and reducing tissue stiffness. Stretching also improves the viscoelastic properties of muscle.[111] The net result is tissues that are pliable, pain free as a result of a lack of excessive tension, balanced inflexibility, and not prone to abnormal translations.

Flexibility exercises may be passive, in which gravity or a therapist facilitates the stretching, assistive, in which the other arm or a wand is used to move the injured arm, or active, in which the involved arm is self-powered.[105] They are usually started in short arcs of motion in positions that are not harmful or painful and are then progressed by stages to full ranges. The motions are controlled in regard to position, time, and speed. Moderate tension should be developed so that the viscoelastic properties of tension relaxation and creep are used to maximize tissue pliability.[111, 112]

Flexibility exercises are usually started early in the rehabilitation program and should be continued throughout the phases of rehabilitation. Flexibility is traditionally very slow to return to normal, especially if it is due to repetitive microtrauma. The key point in stretching is that the muscle or joint area that is tight must be isolated with the particular exercise so that it is selectively stressed. Body mechanics can adapt to produce an integrated movement that masks a tight joint or muscle. A cross-body stretch for a tight posterior shoulder capsule can be achieved by excessive scapular mobility and never putting tensile stress on the posterior aspect of the shoulder. Stabilizing the scapula on a table or against a wall will allow stress across the shoulder. Also, touching the toes may be accomplished by trunk flexion, with no stress on the tight hamstrings or hip extensors. Keeping the back straight eliminates this adaptation.

Manual mobilization and manual capsular stretching, as well as cross-friction massage, can also be used to restore flexibility.[113] They must obviously be done carefully in order to not disrupt internal repairs, create new damage, or reinjure the damaged tissue.

Muscle strengthening exercises are the key to complete functional rehabilitation of the shoulder. Generation and summation of forces through the kinetic chain, position and motion of the scapula and glenoid, proper stiffness of the capsule, and torque production at the shoulder are possible only by restoration of the mechanical and neurologic properties of the muscle.

The mechanical properties of muscle may be improved by loading a muscle so that it hypertrophies. This is usually done by isolating it and then progressively loading it isometrically, concentrically, and eccentrically as the muscle's ability to contract increases. The best ways to work isolated muscles are with rubber tubing or free weights. As the muscles get stronger, machines, which are less specific for individual muscles, may be added. However, the targeted muscles must have some strength to benefit from the machines. With the combined movement patterns that are created by the machines, strong muscles may compensate for weak ones and may retard development of the weaker muscles.[14] These methods may selectively strengthen certain muscles that can be identified on examination, thereby creating the possibility of normal force generation and force couple balance. They have disadvantages in that muscle hypertrophy is often a slow process, especially in chronic injuries, and isolated muscle activities are not functional around the shoulder. This type of training becomes a prelude to normal shoulder muscle activity.

Neurologic control of muscle activity is the final method of muscle function. Alterations in muscle firing patterns[67] and "neural drive"[89] as a result of fatigue, pain, altered proprioception, or disuse are commonly seen in shoulder problems. Most of the early strength gains seen in rehabilitating muscle are due to improvement in firing patterns, motor unit recruitment, and a decreased threshold for firing.[114] Therefore, early emphasis should be placed on making muscles safely and painlessly contract. This may be done through isometrics, very short arc isotonics, or mild cocontraction activities with the joint in a safe position. As more joint flexibility is achieved, more positions for muscle cocontraction in single planes of movement can be gained. More resistance can be added through the tubing, weights, or machines to allow for optimal strength gains. Emphasis does not have to be on maximal strength gains, but balance of agonist and antagonists.

Neurologic training can then progress to re-establishment of the motor patterns that are necessary for the fine control of shoulder movement in multiple planes. The major programs to facilitate this process are proprioceptive neuromuscular facilitation (PNF) and other proprioceptive drills, closed-chain exercises, and open-chain exercises.

Proprioceptive neuromuscular facilitation exercises are combined movement patterns that use specific sensory input from a therapist to the patient to bring about a specific activity or movement.[115] Rhythmic stabilization techniques may be applied at various positions of flexion and abduction. The alternating stimulus requires neurologic activation of stretch receptors and enhances the motor patterns that provide the dynamic stabilizing activity of the shoulder muscles. Proprioceptive neuromuscular facilitation patterns may be used for the trunk and scapula as well as the shoulder. Other kinesthetic exercises include the use of unstable boards[116] or active and passive shoulder repositioning.[117]

CLOSED KINETIC CHAIN EXERCISES FOR THE SHOULDER

Steindler first noted that there are differences in muscle recruitment and joint motion when the distal end of the arm or leg meets considerable resistance as with when it is free to move.[118] These differences are summarized in Table 1.[119] He coined the term *closed kinetic chain* to describe situations in which the distal end meets considerable resistance. The operational definition we use states that a closed kinetic chain is a sequential combination of joints in which the distal segment meets considerable resistance and translation of the instant centers of motion of the joints occurs in a predictable manner that is secondary to the distribution of forces through a base of support.

Closed kinetic chain exercise has been used in lower extremity reha-

TABLE 1.
Characteristics of Open- vs. Closed-Chain Muscle Patterns*

Characteristic	Open	Closed
End segment	Free	Not free
Axis of motion	Motion distal to the axis of the joint	Motion both distal and proximal to the joint
Muscle contraction	Primarily concentric	All types
Movement	Usually isolated	Predomination of certain muscle groups
Loads	Artificial and abnormal	Normal
Velocity	Predetermined	Variable
Stress/strain	Inconsistent	Consistent
Stabilization	Artificial	Postural
Planes	Occurs in 1 of the cardinal planes	Combination of motion in all 3
Proprioception	Foreign, erroneous	Normal
Techniques	Limited to equipment, done to failure	Unlimited, done to substitution
Reaction	More of an action, isolated	Both reaction and action, integrated
Muscle-firing patterns	Agonist/antagonist	Coactivation

*Adapted from Gray G: Rehabilitation of running injuries—biomechanical and proprioceptive considerations, in *Topics in Acute Care and Trauma Rehabilitation*. Rockville, Md, Aspen, 1986.

bilitation with good results.[120–122] These exercises are beneficial in rehabilitation because they decrease strain and shear on the anterior cruciate ligament (ACL) by coactivation of the quadriceps and hamstrings; allow specificity of training in that most athletic activities are done with the foot on the ground; allow concurrent shift, the pattern of agonist/antagonist muscle activity that occurs in locomotion; and stimulate proprioception.

Although most overhead throwing functions seem to involve mainly open-chain activities, there are several reasons to use closed-chain exercises in shoulder rehabilitation. First, the shoulder's function as a funnel transferring forces from the stable base of the trunk in a predictable manner satisfies the definition of a closed kinetic chain activity. Second, these exercises, by promoting coactivation force couples, enhance dynamic joint stability, which appears to be the primary role of the shoulder muscles. Third, by fixing the hand, these exercises promote scapular stability, the base from which the shoulder and arm can function. Fourth, strengthening of the shoulder in a closed-chain function will decrease tensile stress on the capsular ligaments, decrease tensile stress on the supraspinatus tendon, and decrease the effect of the deltoid component of the abduction force couple.[123] Fifth, because the exercises emphasize stability, muscle coactivation, and scapulohumeral rhythm, proprioceptive activity is enhanced. Finally, closed-chain exercises may be done at loads that are safe enough to use early in rehabilitation. Preliminary work with normal volunteers in our laboratory has demonstrated that these exercises can be done with muscle responses of 10% to 40% of maximal firing capacity, well within safety limits (see Table 4).

In summary, closed-chain exercises should be employed in shoulder rehabilitation because they simulate and enhance most of the important functions of the shoulder joint, recreate the motor patterns for joint stability, and are safe to use. They should be used throughout the rehabilitation process but are particularly suited for the earlier stages, when neurologic retraining is stressed, when a stable scapular base is important, and when minimal tension and shear are applied across injured or healing tissues. By using these exercises in this fashion, we have been able to move most shoulder-injured athletes more rapidly through the early stages of rehabilitation and with earlier return of scapuloglenohumeral rhythm and force couple strength.

The five types of progression in closed-chain exercise include (1) weight or load distribution, minimal to maximal; (2) stable to unstable surface; (3) intensity, i.e., resistance, work/rest ratio, and contact area; (4) eyes open vs. eyes closed; and (5) static dynamic loading-movement patterns. Each will be described in the stages of rehabilitation.

OPEN KINETIC CHAIN EXERCISES FOR THE SHOULDER

Although the shoulder does act as a stable base for the transfer of forces and for movement of the hand and wrist, it also has large amounts of rotational movement and does supply kinetic energy and force to the moving hand, which in most sports has little resistance to movement. Thus there is a role for open-chain exercises to restore this aspect of shoulder function. All of these open-chain activities require a preparation (cocking) phase, an acceleration (ball release, racket impact) phase, and a deceleration (follow-through) phase. Muscles are working as agonist/antagonist force couples, but they also need to reverse roles between the acceleration and deceleration phases. Because of the very short time between each of these phases, these patterns must be preprogrammed. Also, the function of the shoulder in throwing places one component of the force couple in a prestretch, or tensilely loaded, position in the cocking phase. This position facilitates the rapid concentric contraction needed to power the joint forward in the acceleration phase. This is seen not only at the shoulder but throughout the kinetic chain as well, from knee flexion/extension through hip-lumbopelvic rotation to scapular retraction/protraction. Therefore, open-chain exercises should emphasize large ranges of motion, rapid joint activity, and prestretching followed by forceful agonist/antagonist force couple firing. These activities can only be conducted by tissues that are anatomically sound and neurologically activated and have a good base of closed-chain function. They are to be used in the preparation-to-play phase.

Plyometric exercises are the best type of exercises to achieve these functional goals. They all involve a prestretch, which tensions the muscles and stores elastic energy, and then a rapid explosive contraction. They should be employed throughout the kinetic chain to replicate the activities and generate the force needed to move the hand.

TIMING AND USAGE OF REHABILITATION MODALITIES

The tools of rehabilitation must be used in a logical, diagnosis-specific way to achieve maximum efficacy. The goals of rehabilitation of every shoulder pathologic problem may be the same, but the starting point for rehabilitation varies widely, depending on the pathologic process, type of treatment, and complicating alterations. This point reinforces the need for a complete and accurate diagnosis as a starting place for rehabilitation.

The functional shoulder program that we use is based on the basic science that has been presented. It is divided into three phases, each based on the resolution of certain aspects of the tissue injuries or alterations noted and using the basic tools outlined (Table 2). There are specific goals, activity progressions, and criteria for movement to the next phase. Within each phase, the specific activities will be classified by type, duration, frequency, intensity, and duration. Since this is a function-based program, all of the protocols tend to progress to some common end points in the later phases, regardless of the starting point. Most of the variability in the protocols is in the acute phase.

ACUTE PHASE

The acute phase begins with the onset of clinical symptoms of injury or when the patient is seen for rehabilitation. Patient injuries will vary widely, from acute fracture or dislocation, to a postoperative rotator cuff repair, to an overload tendinitis. However, in each instance attention will focus on resolving the clinical symptom complex and the tissue injury complex that have been identified in the evaluation.

The goals of the acute phase are listed in Table 3.

TABLE 2.
Phases of Rehabilitation and Complexes Addressed in Each Phase

Acute phase
Clinical symptom complex
Tissue injury complex
Recovery phase
Tissue injury complex
Tissue overload complex
Functional biomechanical deficit complex
Functional phase
Functional biomechanical deficit complex
Subclinical adaptation complex

Tissue healing will be promoted by a combination of rest, short-term immobilization, medication, injections, or surgery, based on the clinical findings. Pain symptoms should be aggressively addressed by the proper use of medications, modalities, and rest because pain is a potent inhibitor of normal shoulder function. Early control of pain will decrease inhibition-based muscle atrophy and allow better scapular control by counteracting serratus inhibition. Range-of-motion exercises should be started in pain-free arcs and may be passive or active-assisted. They may be progressed to larger arcs as healing progresses. Muscle strengthening may be started with isometric activity, which allows some strength gains without much joint motion. Scapular PNF patterns may be started early to restore stability to the base of arm activity.

Closed kinetic chain exercises begin with weight shifts from one arm to the other while standing with arms on a table (Fig 1) and progress by increasing the amount of weight distributed through the hands to the shoulders by leaning more forward. Further progressions in the standing position use unstable objects such as balls, tilt boards, or BAPS boards (Fig 2). Finally, the patient can be loaded dynamically by pushing from several different directions (Fig 3). These exercises are usually done in glenohumeral positions with less than 60 degrees of flexion and less than 45 degrees of abduction. This allows minimal shear and evokes low-level (10% to 30%) muscle activity in the deltoid and rotator cuff (Table 4).

Exercise for the rest of the kinetic chain should be emphasized in this

TABLE 3.
Goals of the Acute Phase of Rehabilitation

Create conditions for tissue healing
Reduce pain and inflammation
Re-establish nonpainful range of motion
Retard muscle atrophy of the entire upper extremity complex
Neuromuscular control of the scapula in neutral glenohumeral positions
Maintain fitness of the rest of the kinetic chain

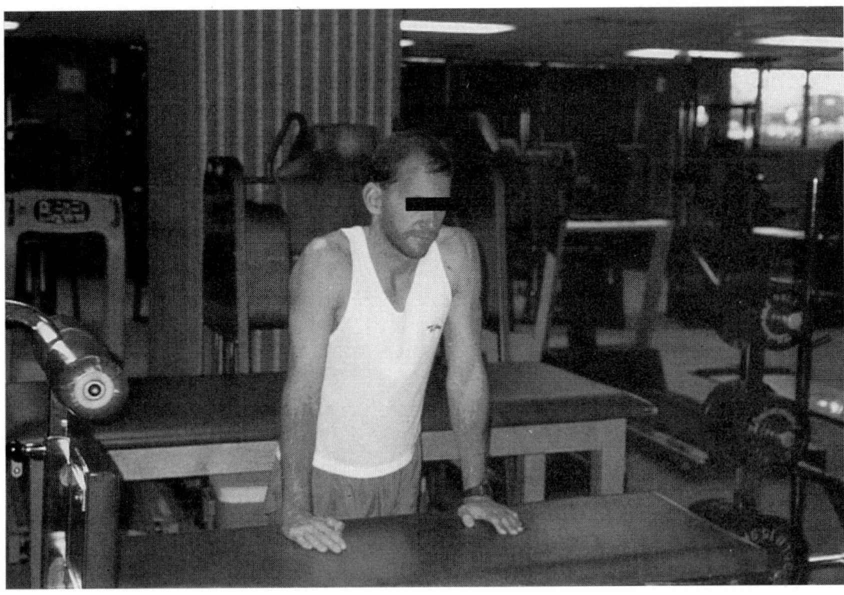

FIGURE 1.
Acute phase—position for initiation of standing stationary closed-chain activities.

phase. Aerobic exercises such as running, bicycling, or stepping can be done with minimal adaptation. Lower extremity strengthening, by either open- or closed-chain methods, can be done. Elbow, wrist, and hand exercises may be done within safe limits. Flexibility exercises for all parts of the kinetic chain, especially those found to be tight, should be performed.

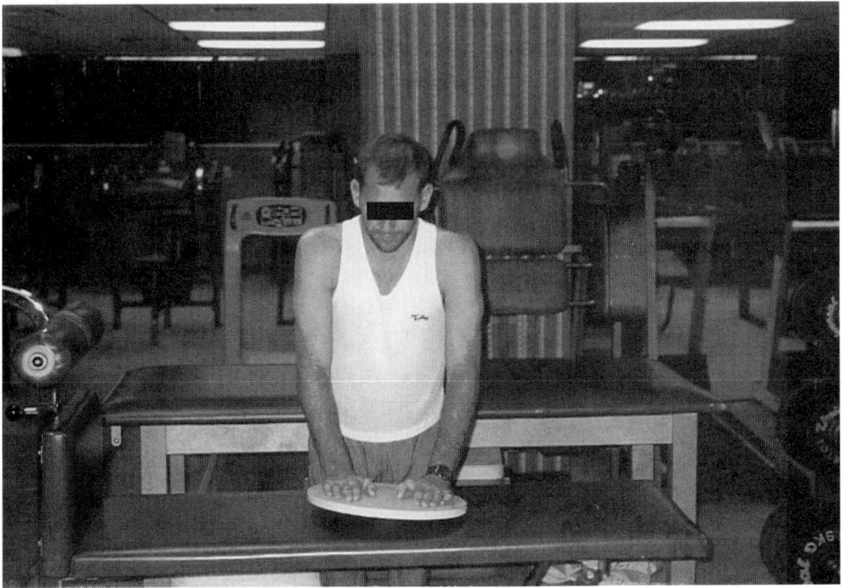

FIGURE 2.
Acute phase—progression to unstable surfaces.

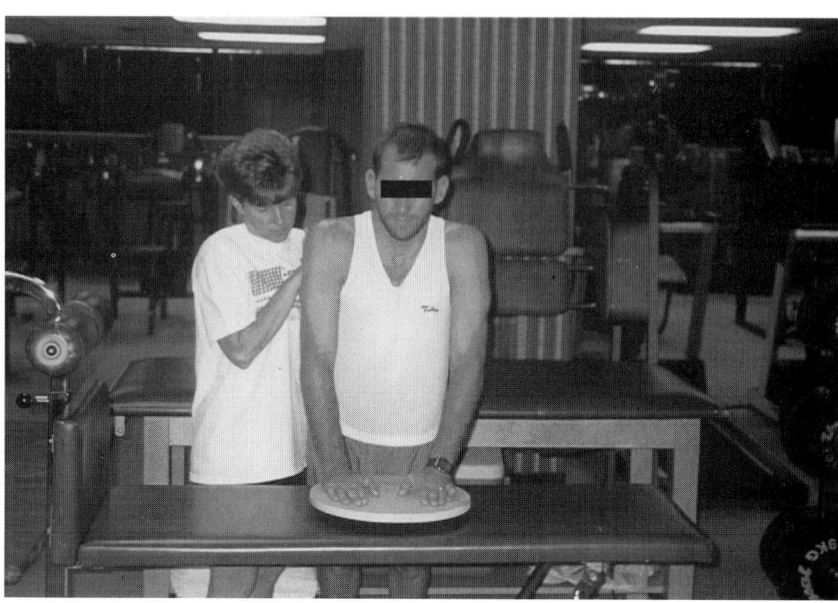

FIGURE 3.
Acute phase—dynamic stabilization responding to external pressures in several directions.

This phase of rehabilitation will be the most diverse because of the wide spectrum of clinical symptoms and tissue injuries and the variety of early treatments. The basic objective is the same: create stable, healing tissues and improve joint health to allow more advanced rehabilitation. By establishing specific goals rather than time tables, these criteria allow safe and predictable progression to the next phase.

Criteria for progression out of the acute phase include the following:

1. Progression of tissue healing (healed or sufficiently stabilized for active motion)
2. Passive range of motion 75% of the opposite side
3. Minimal pain or tenderness
4. Manual muscle test strength in nonpathologic areas 4+/5
5. Scapular control (scapular slide less than 1.5 cm)
6. Continued kinetic chain function

RECOVERY PHASE

The recovery phase will continue rehabilitation of the tissue injury complex but will also address the tissue overload and functional biomechanical deficit complexes. The goals are listed in Table 5. Entry into this phase assumes that the injured tissues may be loaded in tension and compression so that normal strength and flexibility may be reached. Exercises should be first done in safe arcs and single planes of motion (flexion/extension at 45 degrees' abduction and abduction/adduction at 0 to 60 degrees) and then proceed to larger arcs (0 to 90 degrees, 90 degrees' abduction) as tissue tolerance allows.

TABLE 4.
Muscle Firing as a Percentage of the Maximal Muscle Activity for Different Closed-Chain Patterns

Activity	Serratus Anterior	Supra-spinatus	Infra-spinatus	Rhomboid	Upper Trapezius	Lower Trapezius	Anterior Deltoid	Posterior Deltoid
Standing weight shift	<10	<10	<10	<10	<10	<10	<10	<10
Standing rocking board	<10	<10	<10	<10	<10	<10	<10	<10
Four-point weight shift	30	<10	<10	<10	<10	<10	30	<10
Four-point rocking board	30	<10	<10	<10	<10	<10	30	<10
Clock flexion	20	20	20	20	20	<10	20	<10
Clock abduction	20	20	20	40	20	<10	20	<10
Standard push-up	25	20	20	35	35	10	70	30
Angled push-up	25	20	20	35	35	10	45	30

TABLE 5.
Goals of the Recovery Phase of Rehabilitation

Regain and improve upper extremity muscle flexibility, strength, balance, and endurance
Improve neuromuscular control of scapuloglenohumeral movement
Normalize arthrokinematics of the shoulder in single planes of motion
Establish normal kinetic chain velocity and force generation patterns

Adequate joint range of motion is very important. Active assisted exercises with wands should be pushed toward normal motions (Fig 4). Scapular mobilization should be continued if there is still any dyskinetic or restricted movement of the scapula. Glenohumeral internal rotation is usually the most resistant motion to normalize. Some of the most common techniques for shoulder stretching such as the cross-body stretch are not successful in stretching the posterior capsule and muscles because of excessive scapular displacement. The scapula must be stabilized on a table, floor, or wall before rotational movements at the glenohumeral joint are done (Figs 5 to 7).

Strength, strength balance, and endurance gains in this phase are due to both muscle hypertrophy and improved neurologic firing patterns. Isotonic and isometic exercises can be used to facilitate these gains. Progression can be achieved by the following:

1. Increasing the speed of movement
2. Changing the resistance
3. Altering the number of repetitions
4. Increasing the frequency and duration of exercise sessions

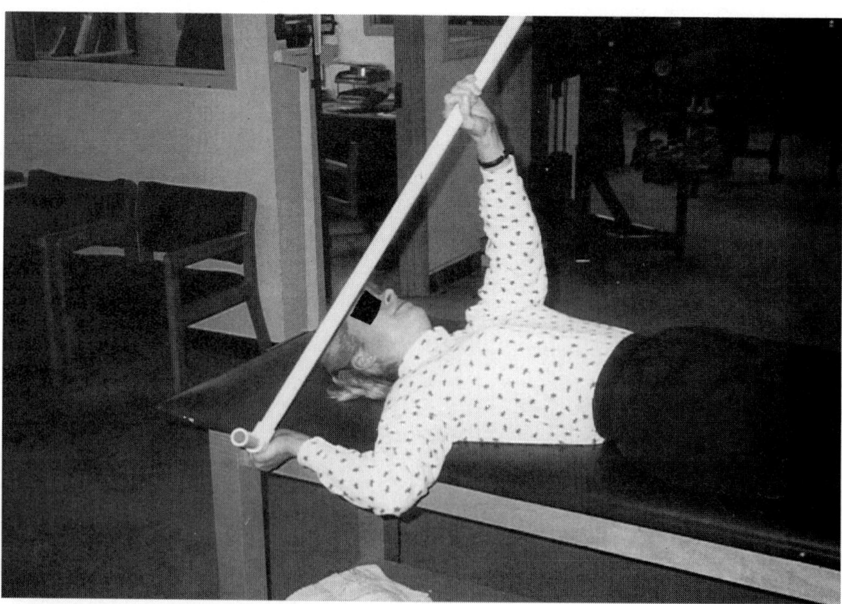

FIGURE 4.
Active assisted wand exercises for shoulder rotation.

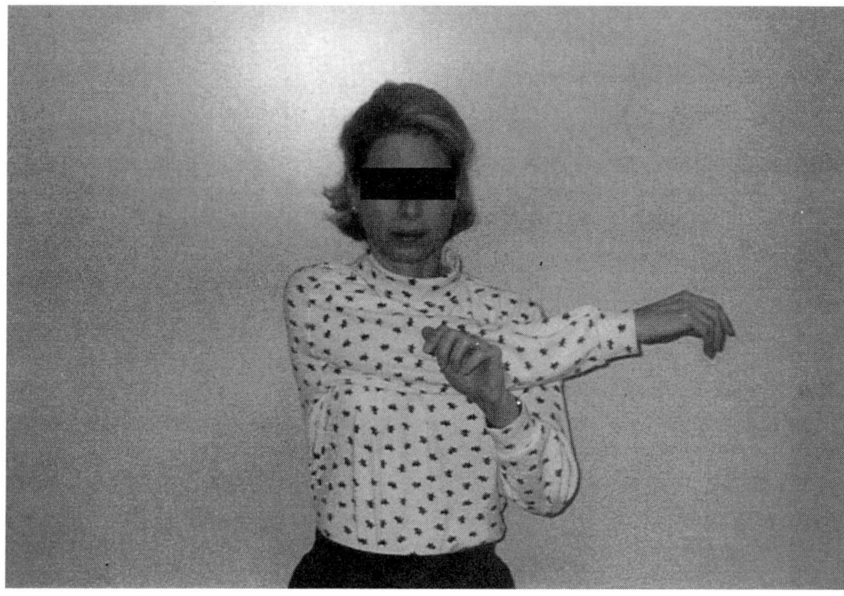

FIGURE 5.
Improper shoulder rotation. Cross-body stretch affects the scapulothoracic joint rather than the posterior glenohumeral joint.

5. Altering the pattern of exercise as to open or closed chain
6. Altering the range of motion through which the muscle works

Strength activities usually start with relatively light resistance moved slowly through relatively small arcs. As the muscles adapt, more resistance, more speed, and larger arcs are possible. Eventually, however,

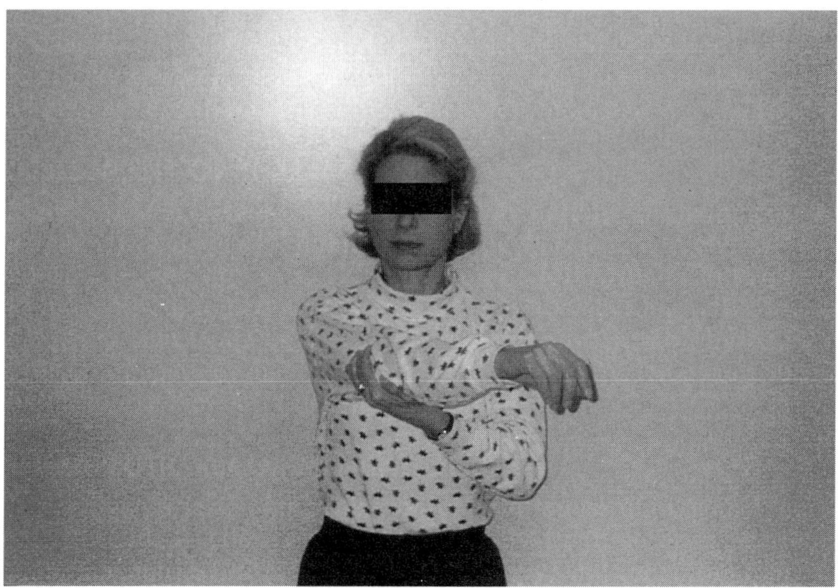

FIGURE 6.
Scapula stabilized against a wall. Stretch now affects the posterior glenohumeral joint.

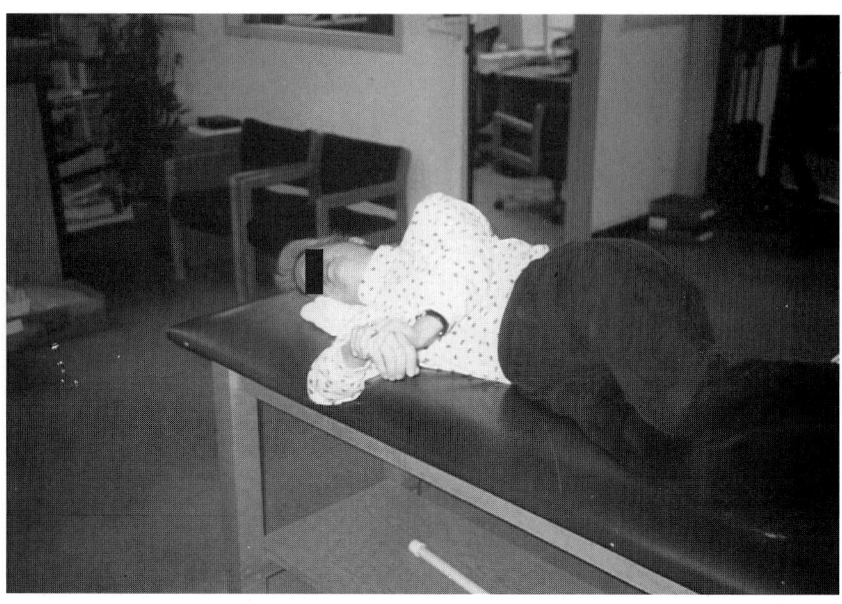

FIGURE 7.
Scapula stabilized on a table. Rotation affects the glenohumeral joint.

muscles need to be trained for sport- or activity-specific resistance, speeds, and motions. Shoulder muscle function for a football lineman will be rehabilitated differently from that of a baseball pitcher.

Many types of resistance are possible for shoulder rehabilitation, among them body resistance (push-ups, pull-ups), manual PNF, free weights, surgical tubing or Theraband, and many types of isotonic or isokinetic machines. All of these may be used in the program. Machines are helpful to isolate and improve specific uniplanar motions, but they are also limited because shoulder function is multiplanar. Tubing, PNF, and free weights involve multiple muscles and several directions of motion.

The strengthening program should move from proximal to distal and from large force-generating muscles to smaller regulating muscles. We start at the spine and scapular muscles, work to the extrinsic shoulder muscles, and then focus on the intrinsic muscles of the rotator cuff. Proprioceptive neuromuscular facilitation patterns, scapular pinches, shoulder shrugs, back extensions, and seated long rows allow posterior stability.

Closed-chain exercises are a safe way to work on the deltoids, biceps, and triceps without putting shear or tensile stresses on the joint structures. They also work very well to load the rotator cuff muscles at low levels of activity (see Table 4). Progression in this phase will include putting more weight on the shoulder by doing modified push-ups (Fig 8) or moving from quadriped to triped to biped stances (Fig 9). As soon as flexibility to 90 degrees can be achieved, the arm can be placed at 90 degrees' abduction either against the wall or a movable object, and scapular movement, humeral rotation, and humeral depression activities may be started. These have the advantage of working the muscles at low levels of activity, eliminating deltoid activity and rotator cuff inhibition, work-

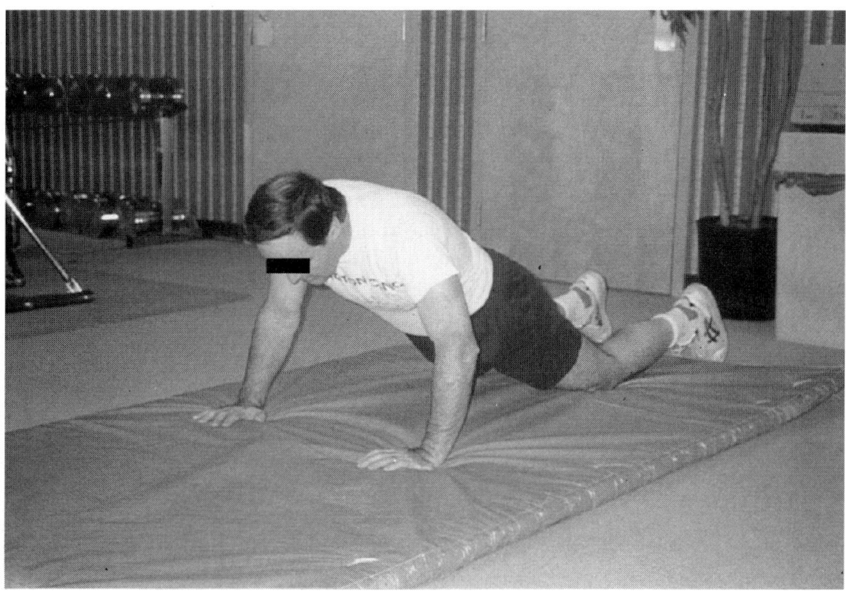

FIGURE 8.
Recovery phase—modified push-up position to increase the load in closed-chain activities.

ing the muscles in a cocontraction force couple, and working them in positions more closely approximating functional positions (Figs 10 to 12). Scaption exercises have been demonstrated to be effective at this stage.[50] Finally, dynamic movement patterns may be started (Fig 13).

Open-chain strengthening can build upon this base of strength and

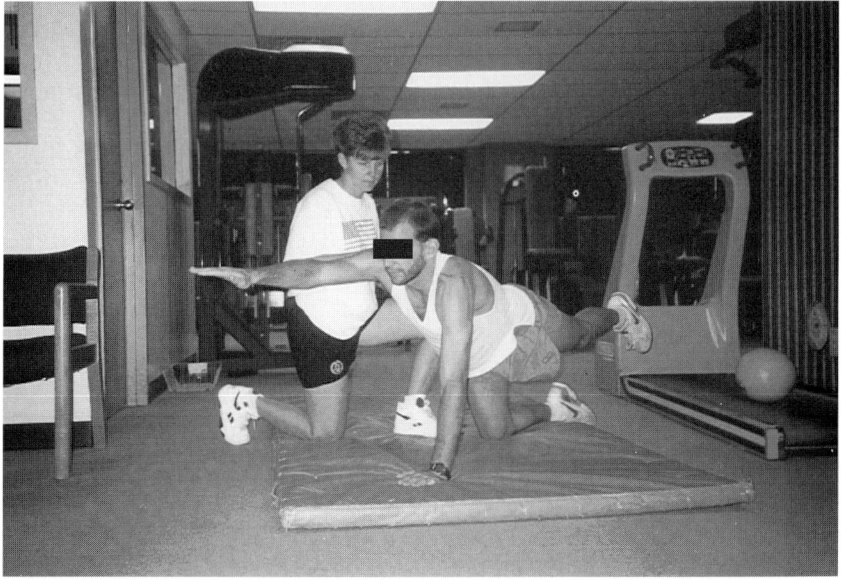

FIGURE 9.
Recovery phase—progression to a biped stance.

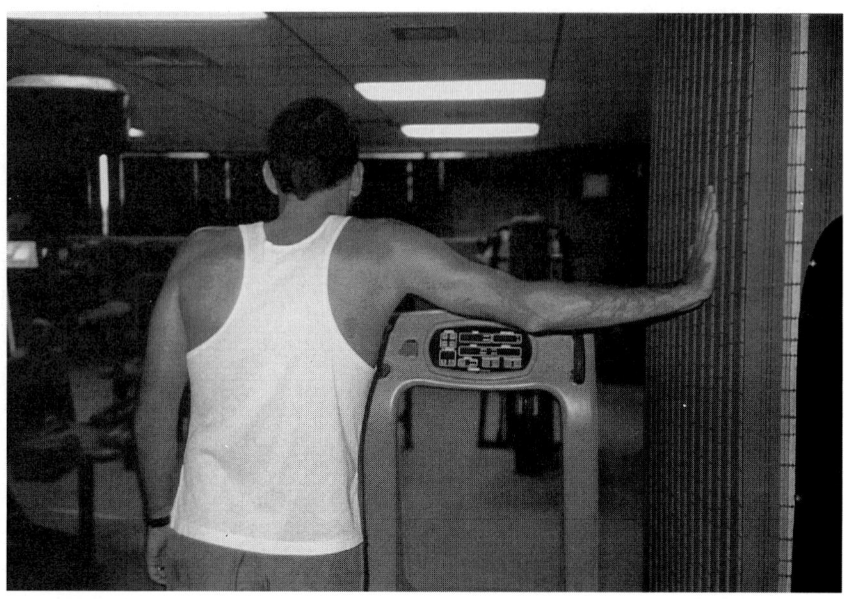

FIGURE 10.
Recovery phase—hand stabilized on a wall with deltoid firing decreased. Scapular movement and humeral head depression are started from this position.

balance. Increased resistance, more repetitions, and work-rest ratios of 1:1 will increase muscle function. Generally, maximum strength can be achieved by lifting a maximum amount of resistance relatively slowly for 4 to 6 repetitions per set, power is achieved by lifting about 75% of the maximum quickly for 5 repetitions per set, and endurance is achieved by

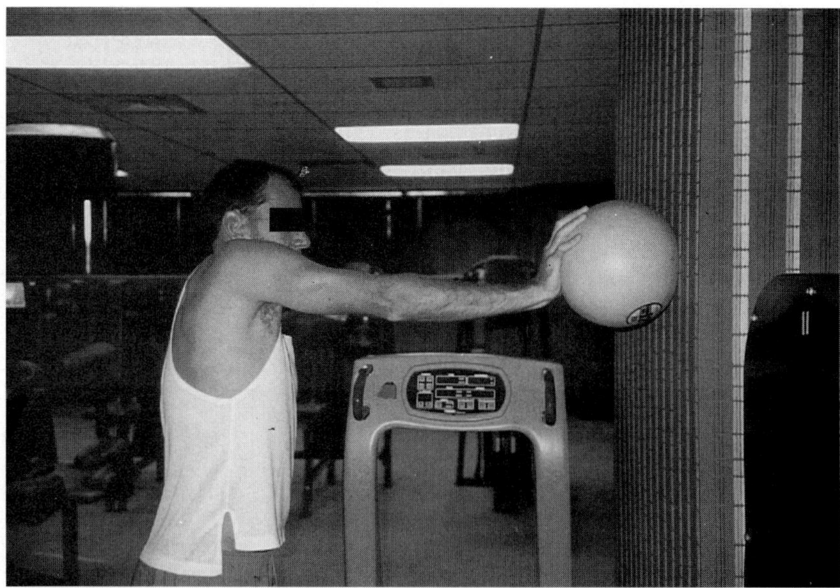

FIGURE 11.
Recovery phase—progression to an unstable surface. Arm rotations can be added.

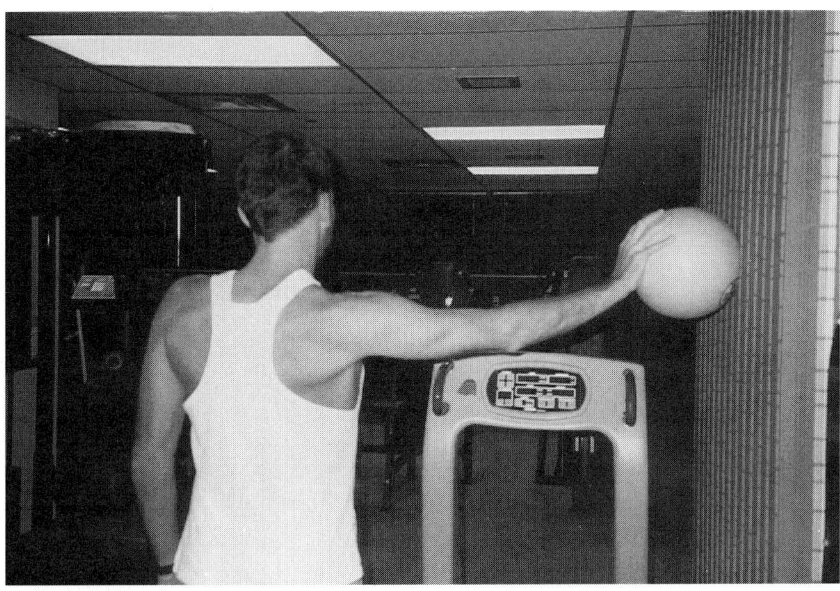

FIGURE 12.
Recovery phase—humeral head depression.

lifting 50% to 60% of the maximum rapidly for 8 to 15 repetitions per set.[124] Many different exercises can be used, but it does not appear that one specific set or type of exercises is most beneficial. Several strengthening protocols have been published and can be used.*

Strengthening will help re-establish neuromuscular control by stimulating neurologic firing patterns, but specific proprioceptive activity also

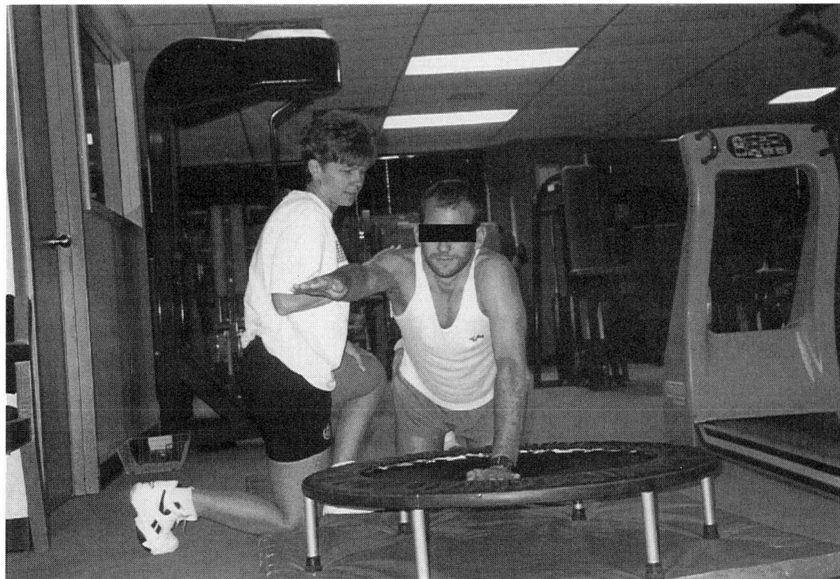

FIGURE 13.
Recovery phase—progression to dynamic stabilization.

*References 8, 14, 15, 51, 68, 74, 79, 117.

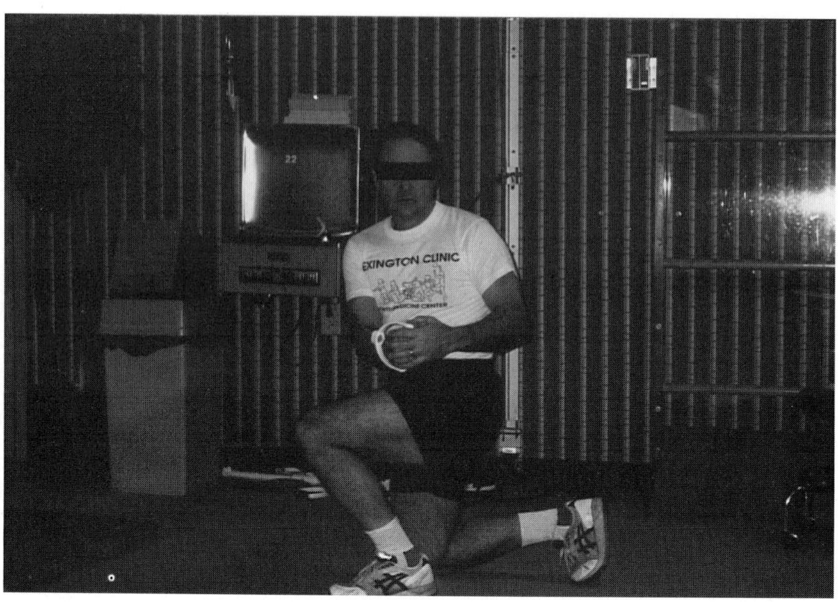

FIGURE 14.
Trunk rotation exercises for strength.

needs to be done.[117] Proprioceptive neuromuscular facilitation patterns, by stimulating the sensory receptors for stretch and enhancing coordinated firing patterns, are the major influences in establishing efficient motor control. Closed-chain activities, by causing axial loading and joint compression, also simulate and facilitate the return of normal motor firing patterns.

The kinetic chain should be totally rehabilitated in the recovery phase. All of the areas of decreased flexibility should be normalized, and sport- or activity-specific strength and endurance in the legs and trunk should be obtained.[2] Agonist/antagonist force couples for velocity generation may be developed in the legs by squats, plyometric depth jumps, or alternation of leg extension and leg curls. Hip extensions and abductions, or one-legged squats, will improve gluteal function. Trunk rotation exercises (Fig 14) are integral to rehabilitation for tennis or baseball. Trunk strengthening and balance are facilitated by "Swiss ball" exercises, which employ resisted movements over a large ball. These provide proprioceptive and movement challenges in addition to resistance (Fig 15).

The recovery phase of rehabilitation is the longest and most complex because of the large amount of work required to restore all of the disordered components, both locally and distantly. As has been mentioned, many protocols have been recommended for this type of rehabilitation. This probably reflects the lack of precise knowledge as to the best progression in this phase. However, the general principles outlined for this phase do serve as reasonable guidelines for choosing exercises and progressions to efficiently move through this phase. We have found that the

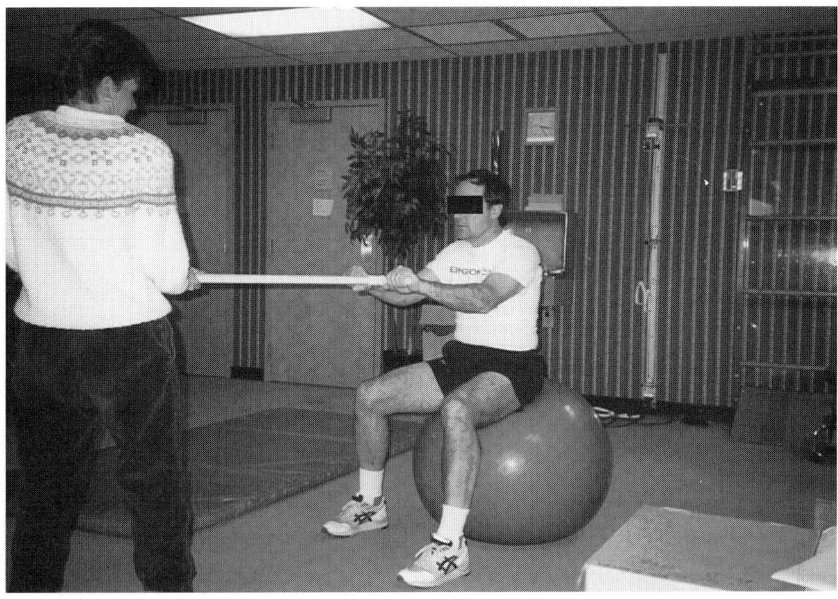

FIGURE 15.
"Swiss ball"—dynamic stabilization and proprioception exercises.

addition of closed-chain activities, especially the ones that allow rotator cuff and scapular activity at 90 degrees' abduction without activating the deltoid, has allowed much more rapid progression through the sometimes difficult stage of initiating muscle strength and balance production.

By the end of the recovery phase, most of the protocols will be merging toward the common goals of gaining full motion and muscular balance. The major differences will be in the sport-specific activities.

Criteria for progression out of the recovery phase include (1) full nonpainful active and passive range of motion of the scapula and glenohumeral joint, (2) no pain or tenderness, (3) strength at 80% of the opposite side with good force couples, (4) scapular asymmetry less than 0.5 cm, and (5) a normal kinetic chain.

FUNCTIONAL PHASE

The functional phase will address any of the remaining functional biomechanical deficits, correct any subclinical adaptations that may have developed, and use functional progressions to return to play. This is the final common pathway of all of the protocols. The goals are to do the following:

1. Increase the power of the scapular and shoulder muscles
2. Increase neuromuscular control in multiple planes of motion
3. Return to sport- and activity-specific functions.

Power is the rate of doing work. Work may be done to move the joint and the extremity, or it may be done to absorb a load and stabilize the joint or extremity. Power has a time component, and for shoulder function, quick movements and quick reactions are the dominant ways of doing work. Methods to improve sport-specific shoulder power should include fast-speed (300 degrees/sec) isokinetics; fast-speed isotonics using light weights or tubing in multiple planes such as diagonals, crosses, or circles (Fig 16); plyometrics; using tubing or medicine balls; and advanced closed-chain activities.

Plyometric exercises are especially important in this phase of rehabilitation because they activate the stretch-shortening cycles of muscle activity that are common in all shoulder activities.[14] This is best seen in the baseball pitch or tennis serve, in which the preparation or cocking

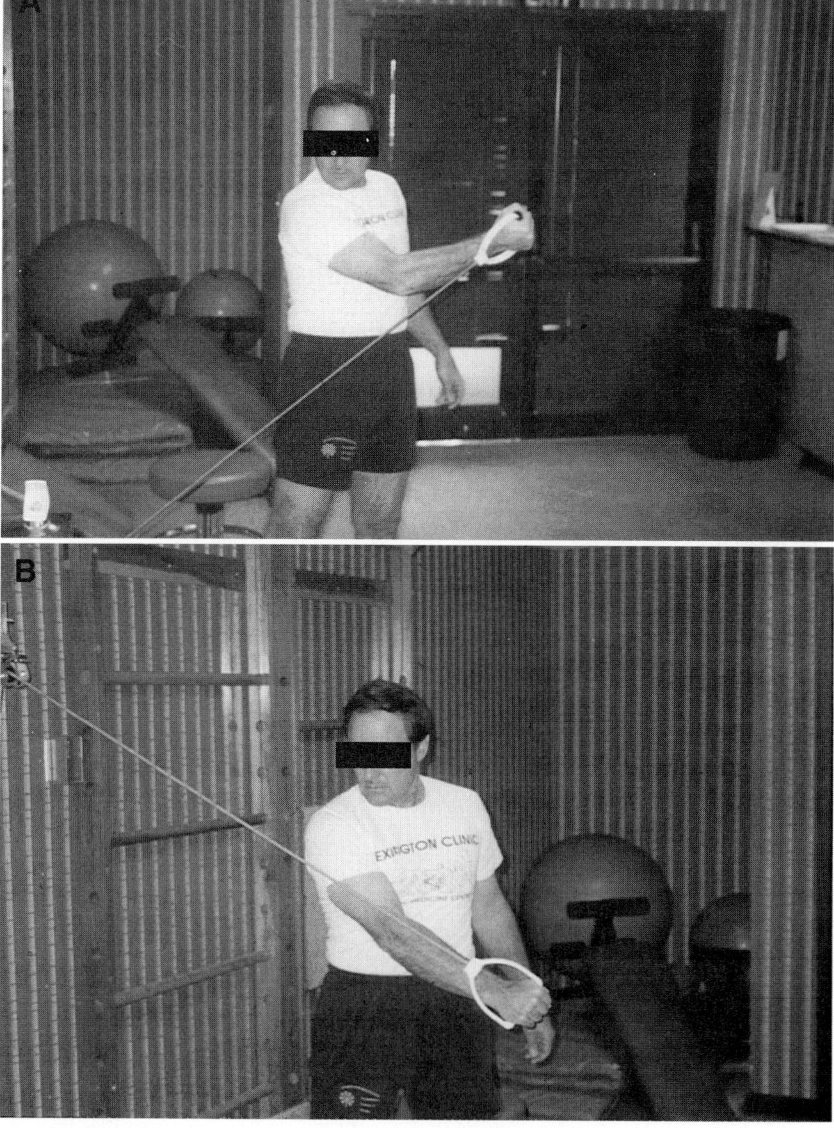

FIGURE 16.
A and **B**, diagonal, multiplanar exercises with rubber tubing. Concentric and eccentric patterns should be used.

phase prestresses and stretches the anterior musculature of the shoulder. This phase is immediately followed by a forceful concentric contraction when the arm is brought forward. It appears that this stretch, in addition to placing the actin-myosin cross-links at an advantageous position, also stimulates muscle spindle activity and improves the amount and efficiency of the muscle contraction.[14, 125]

Plyometric-based rubber tubing exercises may be used to mimic any of the motions in tennis, baseball, or other throwing sports. Different levels of resistance can be applied as the exercises progress.

Medicine balls are particularly effective plyometric tools. The weight of the ball creates a prestretch, creates a resistance, and demands a powerful contraction to be propelled forward. Progression can go from two-handed chest passes, to overhead throws, to rotational passes (Figs 17 and 18), and to one-handed throws (Fig 19).[126, 127] The ball may be initially held in the hands, with progression to catching and returning the throw. Rotational movements at the hips and trunk are very important for sports-specific activities and should be included in the medicine ball drills. Advanced closed-chain activities play a role in the functional phase but are probably less important in preparing the athlete for throwing since throwing has such a large open-chain component. However, these exercises, which can include push-ups, uneven-surface push-ups (Fig 20), and dynamic resistance activities (Fig 21), require shoulder muscle firing activity at 30% to 70% of maximum, which is very similar to their activity observed during throwing. Therefore we include these types of activities for competitive athletes who will place maximum demands on their shoulders.

The patient is usually playing with some modifications, such as the number of pitches or matches, or is ready to play sometime during the

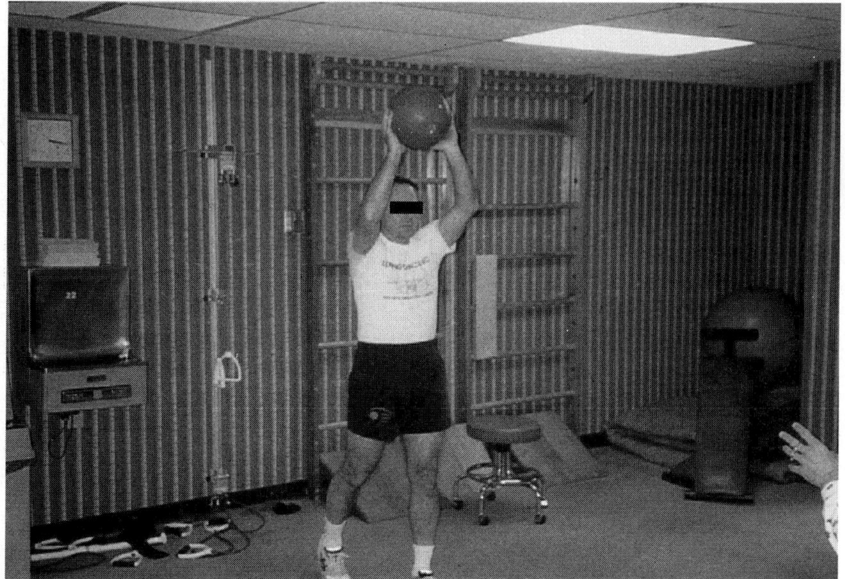

FIGURE 17.
Two-handed overhead medicine ball toss.

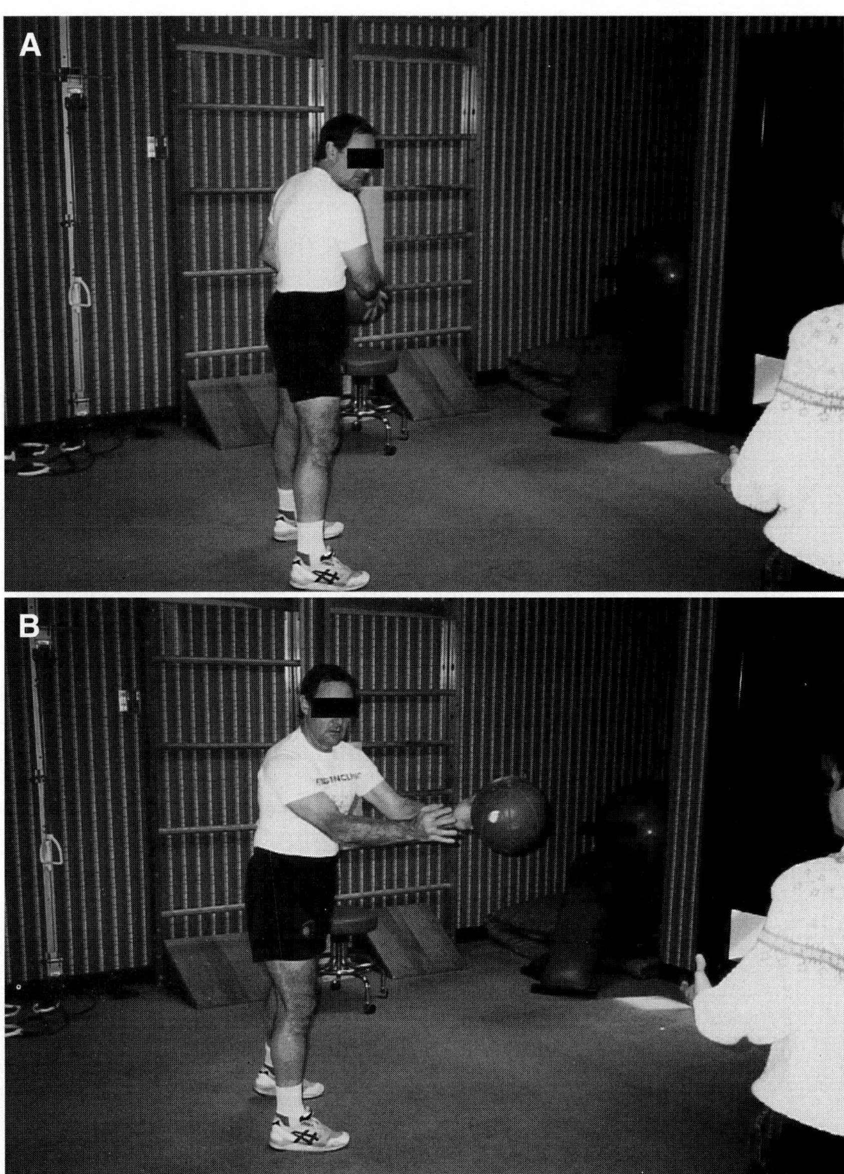

FIGURE 18.
A and **B,** Two-handed rotational medicine ball toss. This should be done in both directions of rotation.

functional phase. Functional progressions of throwing, hitting, or serving need to be completed before full competition is allowed. These progressions test all of the mechanical parts of the normal overhead motion. Very few deviations from the normal parameters should be allowed since these will work against the athlete's ability to respond to the normal demands inherent in the sport. The most common of these is the "long-toss–short-toss" program for baseball throwers (Table 6).[127] Others would include progressions of serving (Table 7). The athlete may progress through the progressions as rapidly as possible.

The functional phase is also the perfect time to instruct the athlete in

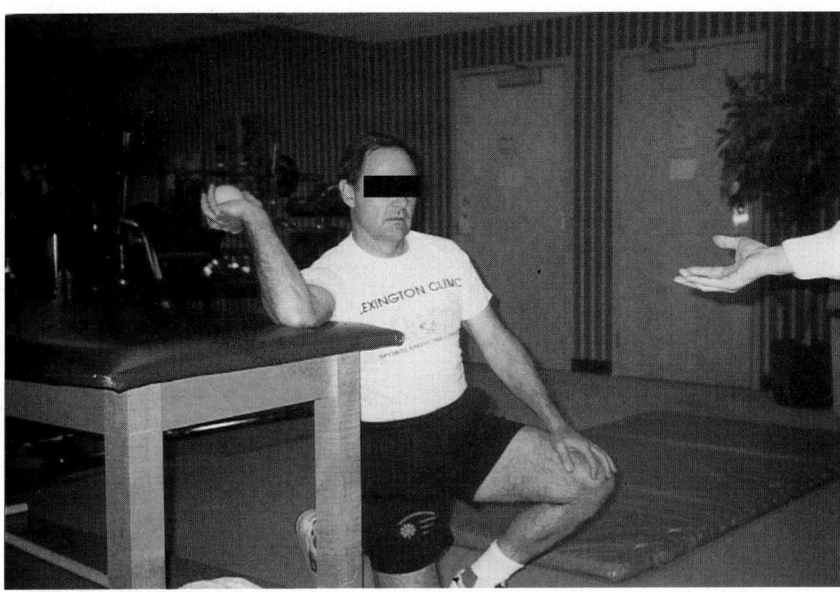

FIGURE 19.
One-handed medicine ball toss. The arm should rotate externally and then forcefully rotate internally.

preventive activities or "prehabilitation." A maintenance program of stretching, muscle balance exercises, power exercises, and kinetic chain exercises is the best way to condition to prevent the overload injuries that are common around the shoulder.[128] These should be sport specific and based on the periodization principle of conditioning.[129]

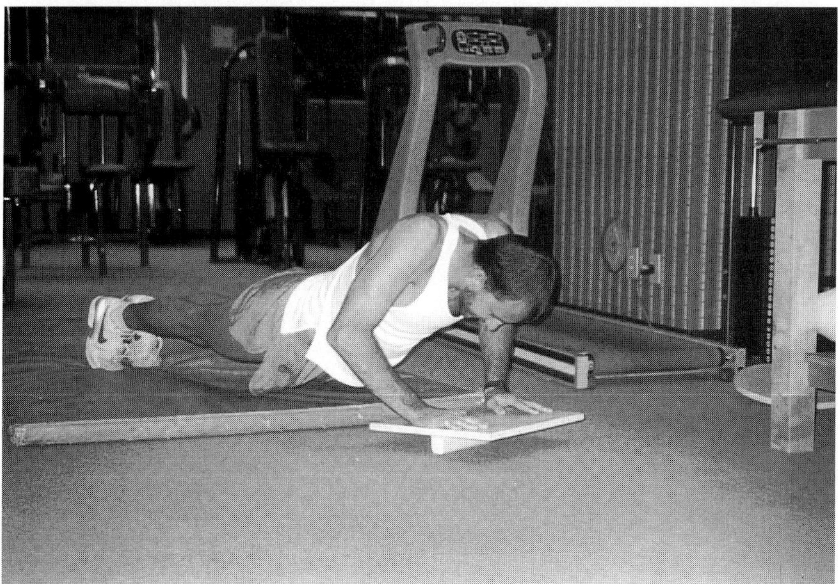

FIGURE 20.
Functional phase—push-ups on an unstable surface. One hand may also be placed on a stable surface.

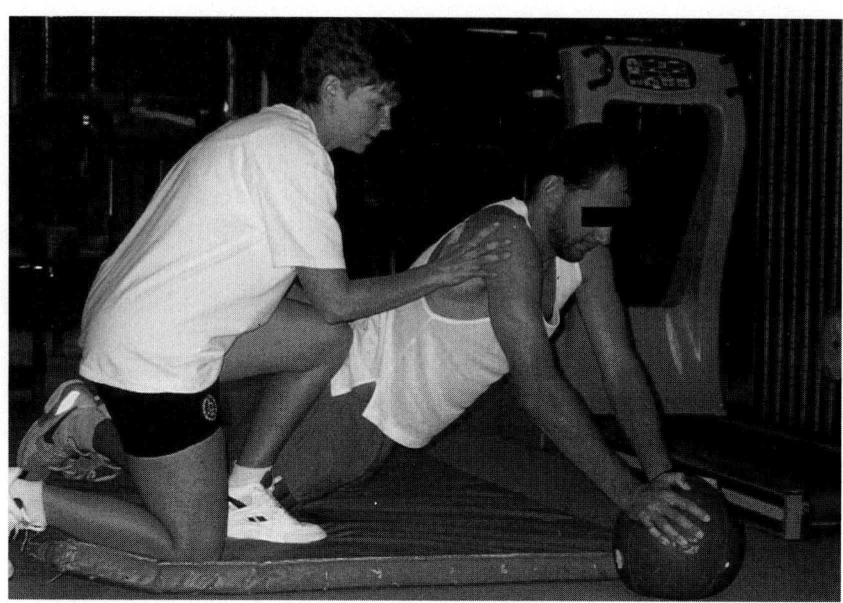

FIGURE 21.
Functional phase—progression to dynamic resistance.

There is a tendency, after the hard work and effort involved in the recovery phase, to skip over the functional phase. However, any deficits not cleared in this phase will continue to create biomechanical inefficiencies. Force couple deficits will put extra stress on the rest of the kinetic chain. Subclinical adaptations such as throwing with an extra wrist snap, opening the hip up too soon, or hitting the serve with three-quarters motion all impose extra inherent demands on structures that are barely tolerating the "normal" demands. In addition, the extra power and smooth mechanics developed in this phase allow better performance.

TABLE 6.
Long-Toss–Short-Toss Program for Return to Pitching*

45 ft: Warm-up; throws, normal motion (25 × 2) (25 × 3)
60 ft: Warm-up; throws, normal motion (25 × 2) (25 × 3)
90 ft: Warm-up; throws, normal motion (25 × 2) (25 × 3)
120 ft: Warm-up; throws, normal motion (25 × 2) (25 × 3)
60 ft off the mound: Throws at 50% (15–30–45) fastball
60 ft off the mound: Batting practice at 50% (30–45–60) fastball
60 ft off the mound: Batting practice at 75% (15–30–45) fastball
60 ft off the mound: Batting practice at 75% (45–60–75) fastball, 50% breaking ball
60 ft off the mound: Batting practice (60–90) at 75% both
Simulated game (75–90–105)

*Adapted from Wilk KE: Internal throwing program for baseball players, in Wilk KE (ed): *Preventative and Rehabilitative Exercises for the Shoulder and Elbow*. Birmingham, Ala, ASMI, 1991.

TABLE 7.
Functional Progression for Serving

Arm movement in a serve motion—no racquet
Upward ball toss, arm movement in a serve motion—no racquet, then with racquet
Hitting a ball with a racquet, standing at the net
Hitting a ball with a racquet, standing at the service line
Hitting a ball with a "second-serve" motion, standing at the base line
Hitting a ball with a flat serve motion, standing at the baseline
Aiming a serve into the proper court
Full activity

The criteria for movement out of this phase into full competition are (1) normal arthrokinematics in multiple-plane activities; (2) isokinetic strength, balance, and work at 90% of normal; (3) completion of functional progressions, and (4) satisfactory clinical examination.

SUMMARY

The timing and usage of the tools and methods of rehabilitation of the shoulder are evolving. There is no "best way" at this time, and many programs appear to achieve good results. Adherence to basic principles appears to be the best framework for constructing a good program. The specific rehabilitation programs that were used for the 2 case examples are presented in Appendices A and B, and a specific program for scapular control is presented in Appendix C. In the future, outcomes analysis will determine the most efficacious programs.

OUTCOMES ASSESSMENT

Evaluation tools for the assessment of outcomes of clinical problems allow an evaluation of the quality and appropriateness of the care rendered for the problem.[130] Without some valid evaluation there is little way to decide (1) whether rehabilitation affects the clinical course of the problem, (2) which rehabilitation tools and methods are best for a given problem, and (3) which protocol is most efficacious (quality/cost) for a problem. These large evaluation tools need to be very detailed to give the comprehensive focus that will supply larger answers to these problems.[130] However, for smaller clinical situations, a more compact, narrow-focus review can serve as an evaluation instrument for the appropriateness of the treatment. We are currently using a narrow-focus evaluation instrument to do in-house reviews of certain pathologic problems or treatment protocols.

Outcomes analysis is really a form of refined clinical analysis.[130] The general outline of the evaluation is shown in Table 8. A specific, well-definable aspect of care is first identified (superior labral tears, rotator cuff tears less than 2 cm, or traumatic anterior instability with a Bankhart lesion). Then objective indicators (range of motion, pain rating scales, normal scapulohumeral rhythm) are established as guidepoints. The vicious-

TABLE 8.
General Guide for Narrow-Focus Outcomes Analysis Tool

- Identify aspect of care to be addressed
- Indicators
  - Make indicators objective and measurable
  - Set a specific time frame for each indicator
  - Indicators can be broken down into different phases of rehabilitation for more specificity (i.e., the different phases for rehabilitation postoperatively, different phases for ankle sprain rehabilitation, general diagnosis)
- Choose a specific data source
  - This can be patient charts, rehabilitation notes, flow sheets, etc.
- Choose a specific sampling for the indicators
  - Athletes
  - Nonathletes
  - Age specific
  - All patients in the specific aspect of care being studied seen in a 1- or 2-month period
- Choose a method
  - Chart review
  - Cybex test results

cycle complexes and the rehabilitation phases are useful reference points as well. General times for achievement of the guidepoints should be used. Prospective data keeping on standardized forms allows a reproducible data source. The method of review, in terms of sample, personnel, and technique should be established prospectively. An example of a clinical outcome analysis of a rehabilitation protocol for operatively stabilized superior glenoid labral tears is presented in Table 9. Through these methods we are trying to design a rehabilitation protocol that will achieve the desired goals with the most efficient use of time and resources.

CONCLUSIONS

Rehabilitation of the shoulder is a subcategory of general sports rehabilitation. It shares the same needs for complete and accurate diagnosis, knowledge of the athletic context in which the rehabilitation is given, knowledge of the proper usage of rehabilitation tools, and outcomes analysis. It also shares the same goals of functional restoration. However, several unique characteristics of the shoulder demand special techniques and knowledge for appropriate rehabilitation. These include the large variety of pathologic problems, the mobility/stability equilibrium, the shoulder's position in the kinetic chain, and the presence of both open- and closed-chain functional patterns.

This chapter has attempted to summarize current knowledge of these areas and suggest general principles that are founded on this scientific base. Specific programs have been suggested in certain areas, but because there is little outcomes analysis to suggest the efficacy of one protocol

TABLE 9.
Sample Outcome Analysis Monitor

Aspect of care
- Rehabilitation of the shoulder for 1 month after glenoid labral repair

Indicators
- Phase I (within 2–3 wk postoperatively)
  - Active range of motion of the shoulder at 75% of the uninvolved side
  - Initiation of concentric strengthening exercises at home
  - Ability to actively depress the involved scapula and humeral head
  - Alleviation of all edema at the involved shoulder
- Phase II (3–6 wk postoperatively)
  - Active range of motion pain free and 100% vs. the uninvolved side
  - Subjective complaint of pain with movement of the involved shoulder decreased by 75%
  - No lateral displacement of the scapula with the shoulder in a neutral glenohumeral posture
  - 3+/5 to 4−/5 grade strength of the scapular stabilizer and rotator cuff muscles
- Phase III (6–10 wk postoperatively)
  - Performing a periodization/training program
  - Pain-free sport-specific activities
  - 4/5 to 4+/5 grade strength of the glenohumeral and scapular stabilizer muscles
  - Normal scapulohumeral rhythm
  - Negative lateral scapular slide with movement of the involved arm as compared with the uninvolved arm

Data source
- Rehabilitative services patient charts for labral repairs done during the month of August 1994.

Sample
- Twenty-five computerized randomly selected charts to be reviewed

Method
- Patient chart reviewed by specified personnel with mathematic computation done to indicate the percentage of patients who met the goals of the above indicators

Reason for monitoring
- To assess the quality of treatment and care rendered to patients after glenoid labral repair by the physical therapists in the sports medicine department
- To identify areas of improvement and update care for this diagnosis
- To review the appropriateness of the documentation
- To help stimulate new ideas to make rehabilitation of this diagnosis more efficient and effective

over another, they are only suggestions about what works for us in a large clinical practice with a shoulder emphasis. The expectation that more advances will certainly be made in the understanding and implementation of rehabilitation for the shoulder will make this area one of the most exciting in sports medicine in the years to come.

REFERENCES

1. Jackson DS, Furman WK, Benson BL: Patterns of injuries in college athletes. *Mt Sinai J Med* 47:423–430, 1980.
2. Kibler WB, Chandler TJ: Rehabilitation for tennis and baseball, in Griffin L (ed): *Rehabilitation of the Injured Knee*. St Louis, Mosby, 1994, pp 219–227.
3. Kibler WB: Evaluation of sports demands as a diagnostic tool in shoulder disorders, in Matsen FA, Fu FH, Hawkins RJ (eds): *The Shoulder: A Balance of Mobility and Stability*. Rosemeont, Ill, American Academy of Orthopedic Surgeons, 1994, pp 379–399.
4. Herring SA: Rehabilitation from muscle injury. *Med Sci Sports Exerc* 22:453–456, 1990.
5. Pappas AM, Zawacki RM, Sullivan TJ: Biomechanics of baseball pitching. A preliminary report. *Am J Sports Med* 13:216–222, 1985.
6. Fleisig GS, Dillman CJ, Andrews JR: The biomechanics of proper throwing, in Andrews JR, Wilk KE (eds): *The Athlete's Shoulder*. New York, Churchill-Livingstone, 1994, pp 335–354.
7. Kibler WB: Racquet sports, in Fu F, Stone D (eds): *Sports Injuries—Mechanisms, Prevention and Treatment*. Baltimore, Williams & Wilkins, 1994, pp 531–551.
8. Andrews JR: Biomechanics of throwing. AAOS/AOSSM Shoulder Course Syllabus, Orlando, Fla, December 1994.
9. Spriginis E, Marshall R, Elliott B: A three dimensional kinematic method for determining the effectiveness of arm segment rotations in producing racquet head speed. *J Biomech* 27:245–254, 1994.
10. Woo SLY, McMahon PJ, Debski RE: Factors limiting and defining shoulder motion: What keeps it from going farther? in Matsen FA, Fu FH, Hawkins RJ (eds): *The Shoulder: A Balance of Mobility and Stability*. Rosemont, Ill, American Academy of Orthopedic Surgeons, 1994, pp 141–159.
11. Perry J: Normal upper extremity kinesiology. *Phys Ther* 58:265–278, 1978.
12. Harryman DT, Sidles JA, Clark JM: Translation of the humeral head on the glenoid with passive glenohumeral motions. *J Bone Joint Surg Am* 72:1334–1343, 1990.
13. Kibler WB: Role of the scapula in the overhead throwing motion. *Contemp Orthop* 22:525–532, 1991.
14. Wilk KE, Arrigo C, Andrews JR: Current concepts in the rehabilitation of the athlete's shoulder. *J South Orthop Assoc* 3:216–231, 1994.
15. Kibler WB: Current concepts of shoulder biomechanics—pathology and treatment. *J South Orthop Assoc* 3:254–271, 1994.
16. Dempster WT: Mechanism of shoulder movement. *Arch Phys Med Rehabil* 46:49–70, 1965.
17. Howell SM, Galinat BJ, Renzi AJ: Normal and abnormal mechanics of the glenohumeral joint in the horizontal motion plane. *J Bone Joint Surg Am* 70:227–232, 1988.
18. Hawkins RJ, Schutte JP, Huckell GJ: The assessment of glenohumeral translation using manual and fluoroscopic techniques. *Orthop Trans* 12:727–728, 1988.
19. Bowen MK, Warren RF: Ligamentous control of shoulder stability based on selective cutting and static translation experiments. *Clin Sports Med* 10:757–782, 1991.
20. Schwartz RE, O'Brien SJ, Warren RF: Capsular restraints to anterior-posterior motion of the abducted shoulder; a biomechanical study. *Orthop Trans* 12:727, 1988.
21. Howell SA, Galinat BJ: The glenoid labral socket. A constrained articular surface. *Clin Orthop* 243:122–135, 1986.

22. Matsen FA, Harryman DT, Sidles JA: Mechanics of glenohumeral instability. *Clin Sports Med* 10:783–788, 1991.
23. Moseley JB, Jobe FW, Pink M: EMG analysis of the scapular muscles during a shoulder rehabilitation program. *Am J Sports Med* 20:128–134, 1992.
24. Rowe CR, Zarins B: Recurrent transient subluxation of the shoulder. *J Bone Joint Surg Am* 63:863–872, 1981.
25. Warren RF, Kornblatt IB, Marchano R: Static factors affecting posterior shoulder stability. *Orthop Trans* 8:89–93, 1984.
26. Warner JJP, Deng XH, Warren RF: Static capsuloligamentous restraints to superior inferior translation of the glenohumeral joint. *Am J Sports Med* 20:675–685, 1992.
27. O'Brien SJ, Neues MC, Arnoczky SJ: The anatomy and histology of the inferior glenohumeral ligament complex of the shoulder. *Am J Sports Med* 18:449–456, 1990.
28. Cain PR, Mutschler TA, Fu FH: Anterior stability of the glenohumeral joint, a dynamic model. *Am J Sports Med* 15:144–148, 1987.
29. Warner JJP, Caborn DNM, Berger R: Dynamic capsulo-ligamentous anatomy of the glenohumeral joint. *J Shoulder Elbow Surg* 2:115–133, 1993.
30. Rodosky MN, Harner CD, Fu FH: The role of the long head of the biceps muscle and superior glenoid labrum in anterior stability of the shoulder. *Am J Sports Med* 22:121–130, 1994.
31. Hill AV: The mechanics of voluntary muscle. *Lancet* 261:947–951, 1951.
32. Speer KP, Garrett WE: Muscular control of motion and stability about the pectoral girdle, in Matsen FA, Fu FH, Hawkins RJ (eds): *The Shoulder: A Balance of Mobility and Stability*. Rosemont, Ill, American Academy of Orthopedic Surgeons, 1994, pp 159–173.
33. Poppen NK, Walker PS: Normal and abnormal motion of the shoulder. *J Bone Joint Surg Am* 58:195–201, 1976.
34. Vanderhooft E, Lippit S, Harris S: Glenohumeral stability from concavity-compression: A quantitative analysis. *Orthop Trans* 16:774, 1992.
35. Inman VT, Saunders CM, Abbott LC: Observations on the function of the shoulder joint. *J Bone Joint Surg Am* 26:1–30, 1944.
36. Perry J, Glousman R: Biomechanics of throwing, in Nicholas JA, Hershman EB (eds): *The Upper Extremity in Sports Medicine*. St Louis, Mosby, 1990, pp 725–748.
37. Lephart SM, Fu FH, Warner JJP: Normal shoulder proprioception measurements in college age individuals. Presented at the American Orthopedic Society for Sports Medicine annual meeting, Sun Valley, Idaho, 1992.
38. Lephart SM: Proprioceptive findings in athletes with shoulder instability. Presented at the American College of Sports Medicine annual meeting, Indianapolis, 1994.
39. Basmajian JV, Deluca CJ: *Muscles Alive: Their Functions Revealed by Electromyography*. Baltimore, Williams & Wilkins, 1985, pp 223–289.
40. Fuchs AF, Anderson ME, Binder MD: The neural control of movement, in Patton HD, Fuchs AF, Hille B (eds): *The Textbook of Physiology*. Philadelphia, WB Saunders, 1989, pp 503–509.
41. Young JL, Herring SA, Press JM: The Influence of the spine on the shoulder in the throwing athlete. *Med Sci Sports Exerc*, in press.
42. Alexander RM: Optimum timing of muscle activation for simple models of throwing. *J Theor Biol* 150:349–372, 1991.
43. Bartlet LR, Storey MD, Simons BD: Measurements of upper extremity torque production and its relationship to throwing speed in the competitive athlete. *Am J Sports Med* 17:89–91, 1989.
44. Toyoshima S, Hoshikawa T, Miyashita M: Contribution of body parts to throwing performance, in *Biomechanics IV*. Baltimore, University Park Press, 1974, pp 169–174.

45. Whiting WC, Puffer JC, Finerman G: Three dimensional cinematographic analysis of water polo throwing in elite performers. *Am J Sports Med* 13:95–98, 1985.
46. Kibler WB: Biomechanical analysis of the shoulder during tennis activities. *Clin Sports Med* 14:79–85, 1995.
47. Elliott BC: Tennis strokes and equipment, in Vaughn CL (ed): *Biomechanics of Sport*. Boca Raton, Fla, CRC Press, 1989, pp 263–288.
48. Groppel JL: Biomechanics of the kinetic chain in throwing. *Med Sci Sport Exerc*, in press.
49. Hong O, Roberts EM: A three dimensional six segment chain analysis of forceful overarm throwing. *Proceedings of Nacob IL, The Second North American Congress on Biomechanics*, Chicago, 1992, pp 55–56.
50. Jobe FW, Tibone JE, Jobe CM: The shoulder in sports, in Rockwood CA, Matsen FA (eds): *The Shoulder*. Philadelphia, WB Saunders 1990, pp 961–990.
51. Bradley JP, Tibone GE: Electromyographic analysis of muscle action about the shoulder. *Clin Sports Med* 10:789–805, 1991.
52. Perry J: Anatomy and biomechanics of the shoulder in throwing, swimming, gymnastics, and tennis. *Clin Sports Med* 2:247–270, 1983.
53. Stocker D, Pink M, Jobe FW: Comparison of shoulder injury in collegiate and masters level swimmers. *Clin J Sports Med* 5:4–8, 1995.
54. Ryu RK, McCormick J, Jobe FW: An EMG analysis of shoulder function in tennis players. *Am J Sports Med* 16:481–485, 1988.
55. Mero A, Kemi PV, Korjus T: Body segment contributions to javelin throwing during final thrust phases. *J Appl Biomech* 10:166–177, 1994.
56. Behm D: A kinesiological analysis of the tennis serve. *NSCA J* 19:4–14, 1988.
57. Gowan ID, Jobe FW, Tibone JE: A comparative EMG analysis of the shoulder during pitching. *Am J Sports Med* 15:586–590, 1987.
58. Leadbetter WB: An introduction to sports induced inflammation, in Leadbetter WB, Buckwalter JA, Gordon SL (eds): *Sports Induced Inflammation*. Park Ridge, Ill, American Academy of Orthopedic Surgeons, 1990, pp 3–23.
59. Kibler WB: Pathophysiology of overload injuries around the elbow. *Clin Sports Med*, 14:447–458, 1995.
60. Iannoti JP: Lesions of the rotator cuff: Pathology and pathogenesis, in Matsen FA, Fu FH, Hawkins RJ (eds): *The Shoulder: A Balance of Mobility and Stability*. Rosemont, Ill, American Academy of Orthopedic Surgeons, 1994, pp 239–253.
61. Kibler WB: Concepts in exercise rehabilitation, in Leadbetter WB, Buckwalter JA, Gordon SL (eds): *Sports Induced Inflammation*. Park Ridge, Ill, American Academy of Orthopedic Surgeons, 1990, pp 759–769.
62. Leadbetter WB: Cell matrix response in tendon injury. *Clin Sports Med* 11:533–577, 1992.
63. Kibler WB, Herring SA: Formulating an exercise program, in Griffin L (ed): *Rehabilitation of the Injured Knee*. St Louis, Mosby, 1994, pp 81–85.
64. Snyder SJ, Karzl W, DelPizzo W: S.L.A.P. lesions of the shoulder. *Arthroscopy* 6:274–279, 1990.
65. Jobe FW, Kvitine RS, Giangarra CE: Shoulder pain in the throwing athlete: The relationship of anterior instability and rotator cuff impingement. *Orthop Rev* 18:963–975, 1989.
66. Altchek DE, Warren RF, Skyhar MJ: T-plasty modification of the Bankhart procedure for multidirectional instability of the anterior and inferior types. *J Bone Joint Surg Am* 73:105–112, 1991.
67. Glousman R, Jobe FW, Tibone JE: Dynamic EMG analysis of the throwing shoulder with glenohumeral instability. *J Bone Joint Surg Am* 70:220–226, 1988.

68. Silliman FJ, Hawkins RJ: Current concepts and recent advances in the athlete's shoulder. *Clin Sports Med* 10:693–705, 1991.
69. Chandler TJ, Kibler WB, Uhl TL: Flexibility comparisons of junior elite tennis players to other athletes. *Am J Sports Med* 18:134–136, 1990.
70. Kibler WB, Chandler TJ, Uhl TL: A musculoskeletal approach to the preparticipation examination. Preventing injury and improving performance. *Am J Sports Med* 17:525–531, 1989.
71. Kibler WB, Chandler TJ: Musculoskeletal adaptations and injuries associated with intense participation in youth sports, in Cahill B (ed): *The Effect of Intense Training on Prepubescent Athletes*. Rosemont, Ill, American Academy of Orthopedic Surgeons, 1993, pp 203–216.
72. Lusardi DA, Wirth MA, Wurte D: Loss of external rotation following anterior capsulorraphy of the shoulder. *J Bone Joint Surg Am* 75:1185–1192, 1993.
73. Hawkins RH, Hawkins RJ: Glenohumeral osteoarthrosis. A complication of Putti-Platt repair. *J Bone Joint Surg Am* 22:1193–1197, 1990.
74. Payne RM, Voigth M: The role of the scapula. *J Orthop Sports Phys Ther* 18:386–391, 1993.
75. Warner JJP, Micheli LJ, Arslenian L: Scapulothoracic motion in normal shoulders and shoulders with glenohumeral instability and impingement syndrome. *Clin Orthop* 285:191–199, 1992.
76. Jobe FW, Moynes D: Delineation of diagnostic criteria and a rehabilitation program for rotator cuff injuries. *Am J Sports Med* 10:336–339, 1982.
77. Hinton RY: Isokinetic evaluation of shoulder rotational strength in high school baseball players. *Am J Sports Med* 16:274–279, 1988.
78. Warner JJP, Micheli LJ, Arslenian L: Patterns of flexibility, laxity and strength in normal shoulders and shoulders with instability and impingement. *Am J Sports Med* 18:366–375, 1990.
79. Ellenbecker TS: Rehabilitation of shoulder and elbow injuries in tennis players. *Clin Sports Med* 14:87–105, 1995.
80. Chandler TJ, Kibler WB, Stracener EC: Shoulder strength, power and endurance in college tennis players. *Am J Sports Med* 20:455–458, 1992.
81. Smith RH, Brunolti J: Shoulder kinesthesia after anterior glenohumeral joint dislocation. *Phys Ther* 69:106–112, 1989.
82. Irrgang JJ: Rehabilitation, in Fu FH, Stone DA (eds): *Sports Injuries—Mechanisms, Prevention, Treatment*. Baltimore, Williams & Wilkins, 1994, pp 81–95.
83. Barrack RL, Skinner HB, Brunet DW: Joint laxity and proprioception in the knee. *Phys Sports Med* 11:130–135, 1983.
84. Solomonow M, Baryatta R, Zholl BH: The synergistic action of the ACL and thigh muscles in maintaining joint stability. *Am J Sports Med* 15:207–213, 1987.
85. Kibler WB: Physical exam of the shoulder, in Pettrone F (ed): *The Shoulder in the Throwing Athlete*. New York, McGraw-Hill, 1995.
86. Andrews JR, Gillogly S: Physical exam of the shoulder in throwing athletes, in Zarins BA, Andrews JR, Carson WG (eds): *Injuries to the Throwing Arm*. Philadelphia, WB Saunders, 1985, pp 51–65.
87. American Shoulder and Elbow Surgeons Evaluation Form.
88. Kibler WB, Chandler TJ, Pace BK: Principles of rehabilitation after chronic tendon injuries. *Clin Sports Med* 11:661–673, 1992.
89. Kibler WB: Clinical implications of exercise: Injury and performance. *Instr Course Lect* 43:17–24, 1994.
90. Simkin PA: Anti-inflammatory medication in Matsen FA, Fu FH, Hawkins RJ (eds): *The Shoulder–A Balance of Mobility and Stability*. Rosemont, Ill, American Academy of Orthopedic Surgeons, 1994, pp 415–422.

91. Petri M, Dobrow R, Neiman R: Randomized, double blind, placebo controlled study of the treatment of the painful shoulder. *Arthritis Rheum* 30:1040–1045, 1987.
92. Gann N: Ultrasound: Current concepts. *Clin Management* 11:64–69, 1991.
93. Chan AK, Sigelman RA, Guy AW: Calculations of therapeutic heat generated by ultrasound in fat-muscle-bone layers. *IEEE Trans Biomed Eng* 21:280–284, 1973.
94. Micklovitz SL: *Thermal Agents in Rehabilitation.* Philadelphia, FA Davis, 1986.
95. Abramson DI, Burnett C, Bell Y: Changes in blood flow, oxygen uptake, and tissue temperature produced by therapeutic physical agents: I—effects of ultrasound. *Am J Phys Med* 39:51–62, 1960.
96. Gersten JW: Effects of ultrasound on tendon extensibility. *Am J Phys Med* 34:362–369, 1955.
97. Lehmann JF, Delateur BJ: Diathermy and superficial heat, laser and cold therapy, in Kottke PM, Ellwood F (eds): *Krusen's Handbook of Physical Medicine and Rehabilitation.* Philadelphia, WB Saunders, 1988.
98. Goodard DH, Revell PA, Cason J: Ultrasound has no anti-inflammatory effects. *Ann Rheum Dis* 42:582–584, 1983.
99. Dyson M: Mechanisms involved in therapeutic ultrasound. *Arch Phy Med Rehabil* 46:49–70, 1965.
100. McDiarmid J, Burns PN: Clinical applications of therapeutic ultrasound. *Physiotherapy* 73:155–162, 1987.
101. Patrick MK: Applications of therapeutic pulsed ultrasound. *Physiotherapy* 64:103–104, 1978.
102. Gieck JH, Saliba E: Therapeutic ultrasound: Influence on inflammation and healing, in Leadbetter WB, Buckwalter JA, Gordon SL (eds): *Sports Induced Inflammation* Park Ridge, Ill, American Academy of Orthopedic Surgeons, 1990, pp 479–492.
103. Griffin JE, Echternach JL, Price RE: Patients treated with ultrasonic driven hydrocortisone and with ultrasound alone. *Phys Ther* 47:594–601, 1967.
104. Davick JP, Martin RK, Albright JP: Distribution and deposition of tritiated cortisol using phonophoresis. *Phys Ther* 68:1672–1675, 1988.
105. Pollock RG, Flatow EL: Efficacy of physical therapy for the shoulder, in Matsen FA, Fu FH, Hawkins RJ (eds): *The Shoulder—A Balance of Mobility and Stability.* Rosemont, Ill, American Academy of Orthopedic Surgeons, 1994, pp 401–414.
106. Mohr TM, Akers TK, Wessman HC: Effects of high voltage stimulation on blood flow in the rat hind limb. *Phys Ther* 67:526–533, 1987.
107. Reed BV: Effect of high voltage pulsed electrical stimulation on microvascular permeability to plasma proteins: A possible mechanism in minimizing edema. *Phys Ther* 68:491–495, 1988.
108. Brukner P, Khan K: Principles of physiotherapy, in Brukner P, Khan K (eds): *Clinical Sports Medicine.* New York, McGraw-Hill, 1993, pp 103–129.
109. Arnheim DD: *Modern Principles of Athletic Training.* St Louis, Mosby, 1985.
110. Rippe B, Grega GJ: Effects of isoprenaline and cooling on histamine induced changes of capillary permeability in rat hindquarter vascular bed. *Acta Physiol Scand* 103:252–262, 1978.
111. Safran MR, Garrett WE, Seaber AV: The role of warm-up in muscle injury prevention. *Am J Sports Med* 16:123–129, 1988.
112. Kottke FJ, Pauley DL, Ptak RA: The rationale for prolonged stretching for correction of shortening of connective tissue. *Arch Phys Med Rehabil* 47:345–352, 1966.
113. Maitland GD: Treatment of the glenohumeral joint by passive movement. *Physiotherapy* 69:3–7, 1983.

114. Stone MH: *Weight Training: A Scientific Approach.* Minneapolis, Bellweather Press, 1987.
115. Kabat H: Proprioceptive facilitation in therapeutic exercise, in *Therapeutic Exercises.* Baltimore Waverly, 1965, pp 327–343.
116. Townsend H, Jobe FW, Pink M: EMG analysis of the glenohumeral muscles during a baseball rehabilitation program. *Am J Sports Med* 19:264–272, 1991.
117. Lephart SM, Kocher MS: The role of exercise in the prevention of shoulder disorders, In Matsen FA, Fu FH, Hawkins RJ (eds): *The Shoulder—A Balance of Mobility and Stability.* Rosemont, Ill, American Academy of Orthopedic Surgeons, 1994, pp 497–519.
118. Steindler A: *Kinesiology of the Human Body Under Normal and Pathological Conditions.* Springfield, Ill, Charles C Thomas, 1973.
119. Gray G: Rehabilitation of running injuries—biomechanical and proprioceptive considerations, in *Topics in Acute Care and Trauma Rehabilitation.* Rockville, Md, Aspen, 1986.
120. DeCarlo MS, Shelbourne DK, McCarroll JR: Traditional versus accelerated rehabilitation following ACL reconstruction: One year follow-up. *J Orthop Sports Phys Ther* 15:309–316, 1992.
121. Fu FH, Woo SLY, Irrgang JJ: Current concepts of rehabilitation following ACL reconstruction. *J Orthop Sports Phys Ther* 15:270–278, 1992.
122. Wilk KE, Andrews JR: Current concepts in the treatment of ACL disruption. *J Orthop Sports Phys Ther* 15:279–293, 1992.
123. Davies GJ, Dickoff-Hoffman S: Neuromuscular testing and rehabilitation of the shoulder complex. *J Orthop Sports Phys Ther* 18:449–458, 1993.
124. Kibler WB, Chandler TJ, Reuter BR: Advances in conditioning, in Griffin L (ed): *Orthopedic Knowledge Update—Sports Medicine.* Rosemont, Ill, American Academy of Orthopedic Surgeons, 1994, pp 65–72.
125. Asmussen E, Bonde-Peterson F: Storage of elastic energy in skeletal muscle in man. *Acta Physiol* 91:385–392, 1974.
126. Wilk KE, Voight ML, Keirns MA: Stretch-shortening exercises for the upper extremity: Theory and clinical application. *J Orthop Sports Phys Ther* 17:225–239, 1993.
127. Kibler WB, Pace BK: Functional rehabilitation of rotator cuff injuries. Video available through the American Academy of Orthopedic Surgeons, Rosemont, Ill.
128. Chandler TJ, Kibler WB: Muscle training in injury prevention, in Renstrom PFH (eds): *Sports Injuries—Basic Principles of Prevention and Care.* Oxford, Blackwell, 1993, pp 252–261.
129. Kibler WB, Chandler TJ: Sport specific conditioning. *Am J Sports Med* 22:424–432, 1994.
130. Johnson RJ: Outcomes research in the AOSSM. *Am J Sports Med* 22:734–738, 1994.

Appendix A

POSTOPERATIVE LABRAL REPAIR REHABILITATION PROTOCOL

I. Acute phase
  A. Goals
    1. Re-establish nonpainful range of motion
    2. Retard muscle atrophy of the entire upper extremity
    3. Neuromuscular control of the scapula in the neutral glenohumeral position
    4. Reduce pain and inflammation
    5. Maintain other components of the kinetic chain
  B. Range of motion
    1. Dependent
      a. Mobilization of the glenohumeral, clavicular, and scapulothoracic joints
      b. Manual capsular stretching and cross-friction massage
    2. Independent
      a. Codman's and/or pendulum exercises
      b. Ropes and pulleys
      c. T-bar
    3. Back
      a. Flexion/extension
      b. Rotation
  C. Muscle atrophy/neuromuscular control
    1. Local
      a. Isometrics
      b. Scapular control
      c. Closed-chain activities
    2. Distant
      a. Open chain—nonpathologic areas (elbow, back)
        (1) Concentrics
        (2) Eccentrics
    3. Aerobic/anerobic activities for the rest of kinetic chain
  D. Pain and inflammation
    1. Nonsteroidal anti-inflammatory drugs for 48–96 hr
    2. Modalities for 2–3 wk
    3. Joint mobilization
    4. Joint protection—sling, gradual progression out of the sling
  E. Criteria for advancement
    1. No swelling
    2. Level II pain
    3. Manual muscle testing strength 75% of the strength in other muscles
    4. Scapular control in the neutral position
    5. Back flexibility at 75%
    6. Kinetic chain function

II. Recovery phase
  A. Goals
    1. Regain and improve upper extremity muscle strength
    2. Improve upper extremity neuromuscular control
    3. Normalize shoulder arthrokinematics in single planes of motion
    4. Improve active/passive range-of-motion flexibility
    5. Normal back and hip flexibility, normal kinetic chain
  B. Strengthening
    1. Dependent
      a. Scapular proprioceptive neuromuscular facilitation
      b. Glenohumeral proprioceptive neuromuscular facilitation
    2. Independent single-plane motions
      a. Concentric and eccentric isotonics
      b. Isokinetics
      c. Tubing
      d. Rotator cuff isolation exercises (Jobe)
      e. Hip rotation
      f. Back flexion/extension
  C. Neuromuscular control
    1. Proprioceptive neuromuscular facilitation
    2. Closed chain—emphasis on force couples
      a. Scapular retractors/protractors
      b. Glenohumeral elevators/depressors
      c. Glenohumeral internal/external rotators
      d. Back/trunk rotation—"Swiss ball"
  D. Arthrokinematics
    1. Joint mobilization
    2. Kinetic chain movement patterns—rotation, stretch-shortening
  E. Criteria for advancement
    1. Full nonpainful scapulothoracic motion
    2. Almost full nonpainful glenohumeral motion
    3. Normal scapular stabilizer strength (lateral slide asymmetry less than 0.5 cm)
    4. Normal back motion
    5. Rotator cuff strength 75% of normal
    6. Normal throwing motion in the rest of the kinetic chain

III. Functional phase
  A. Goals
    1. Increase power and endurance in the upper extremity
    2. Increase normal multiple-plane neuromuscular control (eliminate subclinical adaptations)
    3. Sports-specific activity
  B. Power and endurance
    1. Multiple-plane motions—tubing, light weights
    2. Plyometrics
      a. Wall push-ups
      b. Ball throws
      c. Tubing or other elastic resistance
      d. Medicine ball

        3. Advanced closed-chain exercises
        4. Advanced open-chain exercises
        5. Conditioning based on principles of periodization
    C. Sports-specific functional progression
        1. Long toss–short toss
        2. Serving
        3. Other
IV. Criteria for return to play
    A. Normal arthrokinematics in multiple planes
    B. Isokinetic strength 90% of normal
    C. Completed progressions
    D. Negative clinical examination

Appendix B

POSTOPERATIVE SHOULDER INSTABILITY REHABILITATION PROTOCOL

I. Acute phase
  A. Goals
    1. Re-establish nonpainful range of motion
    2. Retard muscle atrophy of the entire upper extremity
    3. Neuromuscular control of the scapula in a neutral glenohumeral position
    4. Reduce pain and inflammation
    5. Maintain other components of the kinetic chain
  B. Range of motion
    1. Dependent
      a. Scapular, neck, and clavicle mobilization
      b. Elbow mobilization
    2. Independent
      a. Codman's and pendulum exercises
  C. Muscle atrophy/neuromuscular control
    1. Local
      a. Isometrics
      b. Scapular pinches and shrugs
      c. Closed chain, abduction less than 45 degrees
    2. Distant
      a. Open-chain exercises for the kinetic chain
      b. Aerobics for legs
      c. Anaerobics as tolerated
  D. Pain and inflammation
    1. Cryocuff postoperatively and after therapy
    2. Modalities for 2–3 wk
    3. Joint protection—sling or arm at less than 60-degree abduction/40-degree external rotation
  E. Criteria for advancement
    1. Tissue healing
    2. No swelling
    3. Level II pain
    4. Scapular control in the neutral position
    5. Back and leg flexibility
    6. Kinetic chain function

II. Recovery phase
  A. Goals
    1. Regain and improve upper extremity muscle strength
    2. Improve upper extremity neuromuscular control
    3. Normalize shoulder arthrokinematics in single planes of motion
    4. Improve active/passive range-of-motion flexibility
    5. Normal back and hip flexibility, normal kinetic chain

- B. Range of motion
    1. Wand-assistive abduction, external/internal rotation
    2. Active range-of-motion flexion/extension progressing to abduction/external rotation
- C. Strengthening
    1. Proprioceptive neuromuscular facilitation
        - a. Scapulothoracic
        - b. Glenohumeral
    2. Independent single-plane motions
        - a. 45 degrees' abduction
        - b. 60 degrees' abduction
        - c. 90 degrees' abduction
        - d. Isotonics
        - e. Tubing
- D. Neuromuscular control
    1. Closed chain—force couples
        - a. Scapular retractors/protractors
        - b. Glenohumeral elevators/depressors
        - c. Glenohumeral internal/external rotators
    2. Back flexion/extension
- E. Arthrokinematics
    1. Joint mobilization and cross-fiber friction massage
    2. Capsular stretching
    3. Kinetic chain movement patterns
        - a. Back and leg
        - b. Scapula
        - c. Shoulder and elbow
- F. Criteria for advancement
    1. Full scapulothoracic motion and stability
    2. Glenohumeral range of motion of 90 degrees in abduction, 60–80 degrees in external rotation
    3. Scapular slide, 0.5 cm

III. Functional phase

- A. Same as for labral repair, rotator cuff tendinitis, or scapular instability

Appendix C

SHOULDER AND FUNCTIONAL SCAPULAR STABILITY REHABILITATION PROTOCOL*

I. Phase of rehabilitation
  A. Acute
    1. Goals
      a. Re-establish nonpainful range of motion
      b. Retard muscle atrophy of the entire upper extremity complex
      c. Neuromuscular control of the scapula in neutral glenohumeral positions
      d. Decrease pain and inflammation
    2. Progression
      a. Range of Motion
        (1) Dependent
          (a) Grade I and II mobilization of the glenohumeral, sternoclavicular, acromioclavicular, and scapulothoracic joints
          (b) Manual capsular stretching and cross-friction massage
        (2) Independent
          (a) Codman's and/or pendulum exercises
          (b) Ropes and pullies
          (c) T-bar exercises
          (d) Active and passive flexibility exercises
      b. Muscle atrophy/neuromuscular control
        (1) Types
          (a) Isometrics
          (b) Scapular proprioceptive neuromuscular facilitation
          (c) Closed-chain activities (weight shift)
          (d) Open-chain activities and isotonics (nonpathologic area)
            1 Concentrics
            2 Eccentrics
      c. Pain and inflammation
        (1) Modalities
        (2) Joint mobilization
    3. Criteria for progression from acute to recovery
      a. Full passive range of motion
      b. Minimal pain and tenderness
      c. Manual muscle testing strength in the nonpathological area 4/5 and scapular control (no scapular slide) in the neutral glenohumeral posture

*The purpose of this protocol is to describe the basis for rehabilitation of the scapular and shoulder dysfunction that occurs in upper extremity athletic injuries. This program is based on scientific principles of anatomy, physiology, biomechanics, and kinesiology.

B. Recovery
  1. Goals
    a. Regain and improve upper extremity muscular strength
    b. Improve neuromuscular control of the entire upper extremity complex
    c. Normalize arthrokinematics of the shoulder in single planes of motion
  2. Progressions
    a. Strengthening
      (1) Dependent
        (a) Proprioceptive neuromuscular facilitation of the scapula and the glenohumeral areas
      (2) Independent
        (a) Exercise in single planes of motion
          1 Isotonics—concentric, eccentric
          2 Isokinetics
          3 Tubing exercises
          4 Jobe exercises
        (b) Neuromuscular control
          1 Proprioceptive neuromuscular facilitation
        (c) Arthrokinematics
          1 Joint mobilization
          2 Recognize the importance of movement patterns of the other joints that make up the shoulder complex
      (3) Criteria for progression from recovery to functional
        (a) Full nonpainful active and passive range of motion
        (b) No pain or tenderness
        (c) Strength 75% of the other side
        (d) Negative lateral or anterior slide

C. Functional
  1. Goals
    a. Increase power and endurance of the upper extremity complex
    b. Increase neuromuscular control in multiple planes of motion
    c. Prepare for return to the sport-specific activity
  2. Progression in the functional phase
    a. Power and endurance
      (1) Exercise in multiple planes of motion with concentration on power and endurance
      (2) Begin plyometrics
        (a) Wall push-ups to ball push-ups
        (b) Tubing exercises
        (c) Medicine ball
      (3) Return to periodization training program
    b. Neuromuscular control
    c. Sports-specific activity
  3. Criteria for progression from the functional phase to return to play
    a. Normal arthrokinematics in multiple-plane activities
    b. Isokinetic test 90% of the other side
    c. Satisfactory clinical examination by a physician

D. Return to play
   1. Goals
      a. Sport-specific training to full return of athletic activity
   2. Progression in return to play
      a. Functional sport-specific progression

II. Exercises for scapular dysfunction†
   A. Scapular depression
      1. Side lying
         a. Proprioceptive neuromuscular facilitation patterns: performed in the glenohumeral neutral position. Progress by varying the degrees of flexion and abduction at the glenohumeral joint
         b. Arm over the ball. Progress by moving anywhere from 0 to 90 degrees of shoulder flexion
      2. Sitting/standing
         a. Isometrics: push the elbow down into a chair
         b. Isotonics
            (1) Weights in hand
            (2) Wall slides: scapula against the wall with the arms in a 90/90 position
            (3) Arms forward-flexed and depression of the scapula so that the arm is being lifted away from the wall
            (4) Using tubing with a pull-back and the elbow at 90 degrees of flexion and progress to performing the exercise with the elbows straight
      3. Prone
         a. Begin in a glenohumeral neutral position, progress to arms in a 90/90 position, and then further increase the difficulty by adding weights to the hand
         b. Arms forward-flexed so that they are beside the head and lift the arms. The difficulty of this can be increased by trying various degrees of glenohumeral rotation
         c. Hand in the small of the back and lift the elbows away from the body. The difficulty of this can be increased by adding a weight on the elbow or performing this in varying degrees of rotation
   B. Scapular retraction
      1. Side lying
         a. Proprioceptive neuromuscular facilitation patterns to begin in the glenohumeral neutral position and progress to varying degrees of shoulder flexion and abduction
         b. Arm over the ball and moving through various degrees from 0 to 90 degrees of shoulder flexion
      2. Sitting/standing
         a. Isometrics. The difficulty can be varied from glenohumeral neutral to 90 degrees of abduction/external rotation

---

†These are some guidelines for rehabilitation of scapular and shoulder dysfunction. We must keep in mind that we are rehabilitating a whole athlete and while progressing through this program must also concentrate on strength and conditioning of the unaffected parts and energy systems in concert with this program.

b. Isotonics
   (1) One can use free weights in a glenohumeral neutral position to 90 degrees of abduction
   (2) Use tubing with the same variations for an increased degree of difficulty
3. Prone
   a. Perform glenohumeral neutral retraction and progress to a 90/90 position with weights in hand
   b. Perform retraction with a longer level arm (the elbow is straight) and increase difficulty by adding weight in hands
   c. Scapular retraction with 90 degrees of elbow flexion, weight in hands to increase difficulty

C. Scapular protraction
1. Side lying
   a. Proprioceptive neuromuscular facilitation patterns in a glenohumeral neutral position to progress to various degrees of shoulder flexion and abduction
   b. Arm over the ball and increase the difficulty by progressing from 0 to 90 degrees of shoulder flexion
2. Sitting/standing
   a. Isometric wall push-ups
   b. Isotonics with tubing or with weights. Varying the degrees of glenohumeral abduction to flexion from 0 to 90 degrees will increase the difficulty of these exercises
3. Supine
   a. Bench protraction with progressive resistance

D. Scapular elevation
1. Side lying
   a. Proprioceptive neuromuscular facilitation patterns in a glenohumeral neutral position to progress to various degrees of flexion/abduction.
   b. Arm over the ball, moving it to progress from 0 to 90 degrees of shoulder flexion
2. Sitting/standing
   a. Isometrics
   b. Isotonics with weights or tubing to perform an upright row or shrugs.
3. Supine
   a. Elevate by using weights/tubing in a glenohumeral neutral position
4. Prone utilizing tubing and/or weights
   a. Glenohumeral neutral
   b. Various degrees of abduction and flexion
   c. Various degrees of external rotation

Index

F

G

H

R

S

T

U

V

W

Z